Date Due

Women, Motherhood and Living with HIV/AIDS

Pranee Liamputtong

Editor

Women, Motherhood and Living with HIV/AIDS

A Cross-Cultural Perspective

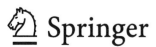 Springer

Editor
Pranee Liamputtong
School of Public Health
La Trobe University
Bundoora, VIC, Australia

ISBN 978-94-007-5886-5   ISBN 978-94-007-5887-2 (eBook)
DOI 10.1007/978-94-007-5887-2
Springer Dordrecht Heidelberg New York London

Library of Congress Control Number: 2013934115

Printed on acid-free paper

Springer is part of Springer Science+Business Media (www.springer.com)

To my parents: Saeng and Yindee Liamputtong
and
To my children: Zoe Sanipreeya and Emma Inturatana Rice

Preface

The HIV/AIDS epidemic has entered its fourth decade and continues to be a major public health problem worldwide. Ever since the diagnosis of the first case of AIDS in the early 1980s, the epidemic has risen rapidly, and although earlier on it has affected people ranging from injecting drug users and sex workers to heterosexual men, it has now affected a large number of women around the globe. Of the 34 million people worldwide who are living with HIV/AIDS in 2010, half were women. In recent times, we have witnessed more attention being given to the lived experiences of HIV-positive women, many of whom are also mothers of young children.

Up until now, many articles have been written to portray women who are mothers and living with HIV/AIDS in different parts of the world. But, to my knowledge, there has not been any recent book which attempts to put together results from empirical research relating to women, motherhood and living with HIV/AIDS. This book is formed with the intention to fill this gap. The focus of this text is on issues relevant to women, motherhood and living with HIV/AIDS which have occurred to individual women in different parts of the globe. The book comprises chapters written by researchers who carry out their research in different parts of the world. Each chapter contains empirical information which is based on real-life situations. This can be used as evidence for health-care providers to implement socially and culturally appropriate services to assist women who are living with HIV/AIDS in many societies. This body of work is significant as it has huge implications for policy makers and practitioners in the areas of HIV/AIDS. The book also contributes to the global debate regarding women, motherhood and HIV/AIDS.

From a cross-cultural perspective, *Women, Motherhood and Living with HIV/AIDS: A Cross-Cultural Perspective* will be of value to health-care providers who are interested in working with women who are mothers and living with HIV/AIDS. In particular, it will assist health workers in community health centers and hospitals in understanding issues related to womanhood, motherhood and HIV/AIDS and hence provide culturally sensitive health care to women from different social and cultural backgrounds who are mothers and living with HIV/AIDS. The volume will also attract many lay readers and professional groups in organizations which are interested in a cross-cultural perspective of women who are mothers and living with

HIV/AIDS. The book provides a valuable reference for students and lecturers in courses like women's studies, anthropology, sociology, social work, nursing, public health and medicine.

In constructing a book like this, it is impossible to include all groups and from all parts of the world. As readers will see, the volume has missed the inclusion of many groups of women living with HIV/AIDS who deserve to be known and understood. However, I have attempted to include as many groups of women as possible. What is included in this volume will, no doubt, provide crucial information which would not be easily accessible elsewhere.

Like any other publication, this book could not have been possible without assistance from others. First, I wish to express my gratitude to Esther Otten of Springer, who believed in the value of this book and contracted me to edit it. My thanks also go to Rosemary Oakes and Lee Koh who edited some chapters for me. But most importantly, I wish to express my sincere thanks to all the contributors in the volume who helped to make this book possible. Most of you worked so hard to meet my timetable and to endure my endless e-mails getting chapters from you. I hope that this journey has been a positive one for all of you.

This book is dedicated to my parents who brought their children up amidst poverty in Thailand. They believed that only education would improve the lives of their children and hence worked hard to send us to school. I have made my career thus far because of their beliefs and the opportunity that they both have provided for me. I thank them profoundly. I also dedicate this book to my two daughters who have been part of my life and for understanding the ongoing busy life of their mother.

Melbourne   Pranee Liamputtong

About the Editor

Pranee Liamputtong holds a personal chair in public health at the School of Public Health, La Trobe University, Melbourne, Australia. Pranee has previously taught in the School of Sociology and Anthropology and worked as a public health research fellow at the Centre for the Study of Mothers' and Children's Health, La Trobe University. Pranee has a particular interest in issues related to cultural and social influences on childbearing, childrearing and women's reproductive and sexual health. She has published several books and a large number of papers in these areas.

Her books in the health area include: *Maternity and reproductive health in Asian societies* (with Lenore Manderson, Harwood Academic Press, 1996); *Hmong women and reproduction* (Bergin & Garvey, 2000); *Coming of age in South and Southeast Asia: Youth, courtship and sexuality* (with Lenore Manderson, Curzon Press, 2002); *Health, social change and communities* (with Heather Gardner, Oxford University Press, 2003); *The journey of becoming a mother amongst women in northern Thailand* (Lexington Books, 2007); *Reproduction, childbearing and motherhood: A cross-cultural perspective* (Nova Science, 2007); *Childrearing and infant care: A cross-cultural perspective* (Nova Science, 2007); and *Community, health and population* (with Sansnee Jirojwong, Oxford University Press, 2008). Her most recent books include *Infant feeding practices: A cross-cultural perspective* (Springer, 2010); *Motherhood and postnatal depression: Narratives of women and their partners*, for Springer (with Carolyn Westall, Springer, 2011); and *Health, illness and well-being: Perspectives and social determinants* (with Rebecca Fanany and Glenda Verrinder, Oxford University Press, 2012).

Pranee has also published several method books. Her first method book is titled *Qualitative research methods: A health focus* (with Douglas Ezzy, Oxford University Press, 1999, reprinted in 2000, 2001, 2002, 2003, 2004), and the second edition of this book is titled *Qualitative research methods* (2005). This book is now in its fourth edition, and she is the sole author of this edition (Liamputtong 2013). Other method books include: *Health research in cyberspace: Methodological, practical and personal issues* (Nova Science, 2006); *Researching the vulnerable: A guide to sensitive research methods* (Sage, 2007); *Undertaking sensitive research: Managing boundaries, emotions and risk* (with Virginia Dickson-Swift and Erica James,

Cambridge University Press, 2008); and *Knowing differently: Arts-based and collaborative research methods* (with Jean Rumbold, Nova Science, 2008). She has published two books on the use of qualitative methodology in cross-cultural settings: *Doing cross-cultural research: Methodological and practical issues* (Springer, 2008) and *Performing qualitative cross-cultural research* (Cambridge University Press, 2010). Her most recent method books include *Focus group methodology: Principles and practice* (Sage, 2011) and *Research methods in health: Foundations for evidence-based practice*, 2nd edition (Oxford University Press, 2013).

Contents

About the Contributors

Tran Xuan Bach is an Alberta Innovates - Health Solutions postdoctoral fellow in the School of Public Health at the University of Alberta. He is also a lecturer in health economics at Hanoi Medical University. He has been working with the national HIV/AIDS program in Vietnam, focusing on the economic aspect of HIV/AIDS policies. He completed a PhD in health services and policy at the University of Alberta and was awarded the Charles WB Gravett Memorial Scholarship for superior academic achievement in health-care planning and evaluation. His doctoral work aimed to examine the role of methadone maintenance in HIV/AIDS care and treatment and cost-effectiveness of scaling up methadone and antiretroviral treatment in Vietnam's injection-driven HIV epidemics.

Donna B. Barnes is a medical sociologist with a research focus on social issues for women with HIV and AIDS. For the past 20 years as principal investigator supported by federal funding, she has conducted research on issues of motherhood, reproductive decision-making, disclosure of HIV status, stigma and access to health care. Currently, she is completing the results of a 10-year follow-up study on women with HIV and AIDS from Oakland, California and Rochester, New York, USA. In September 2009, Donna retired from 16 years of teaching women's studies with an emphasis on motherhood and women's health at California State University, East Bay in Hayward, California.

Jolly Beyeza-Kashesya received her medical degree (MBChB) from Makerere University in 1991 and a master's in obstetrics and gynecology from China Medical University (Peoples' Republic of China) in 1996. She has received additional training in HIV/AIDS research and management though the Makerere University-Karolinska Institutet Stockholm joint collaboration at doctorate level. Jolly has extensive experience in maternal and newborn health management both at clinical and programmatic level. As a clinician and teacher, Jolly has supervised several masters' students and doctors involved in patient care including those patients on PMTCT programs. She is currently holding the position of senior consultant obstetrician and gynecologist at the Mulago National and Teaching Hospital.

Lauren K. Birks is a postdoctoral fellow in the Faculty of Nursing at the University of Alberta, examining perinatal food choices in immigrant women. She completed her PhD in the population and public health at the University of Calgary, Canada, in 2012. Her research focused on knowledge mobilization, gender and mother-to-child HIV transmission among Maasai women in rural Northwestern Tanzania using Participatory Action Research. She worked actively in the field since 2008. Lauren's interest in international health and HIV has been long standing. She conducted her masters in health administration at the University of British Columbia, Vancouver, with research in Uganda focusing on immunization of orphaned children in rural areas. She hopes to build actively on the foundations of her doctoral degree by pursuing postdoctoral research that focuses on health promotion and social change that will lead to improved health for women and children.

Ineke Buskens is an international gender, research and facilitation consultant living in the Western Cape, South Africa. Having been one of the pioneers of women's studies in the 1970s in Europe, she currently leads the GRACE (Gender Research into Information Communication Technology for Empowerment) Network involving 25 research teams in 17 countries in Africa and the Middle East (grace-network. net). In her research, she focuses on emancipatory approaches that are aligned with a sustainable, just and loving world; in her research training on bringing out the genius in every participant; and in her facilitation work on gender awareness and authentic collaboration.

Pleumjit Chotiga is a lecturer at Boromarajonani College of Nursing, Chiang Mai in Thailand. She received her PhD in Nursing at the School of Nursing and Midwifery, University of East Anglia, UK, and conducted research exploring Burmese migrant women's experiences and decision-making with HIV testing and treatment in Northern Thailand.

Alex Coutinho is the executive director of the Infectious Diseases Institute at Makerere University in Kampala and also serves as chair of the board of the International Partnership for Microbicides. He has worked with the HIV epidemic since 1982 and his main focus is scaling up HIV prevention care and treatment programs in Africa.

Kenda Crozier is an experienced midwife who has an interest in aspects of women's health, particularly in relation to the antenatal period including mental health in pregnancy. She is a senior lecturer at University of East Anglia.

Susan L. Davies is associate professor of health behavior at the University of Alabama at Birmingham (UAB) School of Public Health and a scientist in the UAB Center for AIDS Research and the Center for the Study of Community Health. She has studied HIV and its prevention from many perspectives, including reducing sexual risk behaviors among 14–18-year-old African American adolescent girls, reducing secondary transmission of HIV among women living with HIV, identifying community barriers to HIV prevention among disenfranchised African American young adult males and increasing family functioning of mothers and families affected by HIV. For over 10 years, she has worked collaboratively with the community in designing, implementing and evaluating theory-based interventions for a broad array of special populations and in training health educators, peer educators and community volunteers.

Alice Desclaux is MD and directrice de recherches in medical anthropology in Institut de Recherche pour le Developpement (IRD, TRANSVIHMI). A former professor in Université Paul Cézanne d'Aix-Marseille, she as done extensive fieldwork on social transformations related to HIV, mainly in West Africa regarding women and children in the health system. She is currently working on the anthropology of long-term treatment among HIV-positive persons in Dakar (Sénégal).

Paula di Corrado is a psychologist and has been working at the Argentinean National Reference Center for AIDS (CNRS), School of Medicine, University of Buenos Aires, for 5 years now. She is a PhD student at the Psychology School (UBA). Paula was awarded a grant by Fogarty AIDS International Training and Research Program from 2008 to 2009 which allowed her to do research on women living with HIV and the accurate diagnosis of their newborns. She is currently an assistant researcher of a WHO-supported project jointly developed by CNRS, CEDES (Center for the Study of State and Society, Buenos Aires, Argentina), CENEP (Population Studies Center, Buenos Aires, Argentina) and the Gino Germani Institute (UBA): "Evidence as a basis for interventions aimed at promoting access to the prevention of unwanted pregnancies, HIV-infection/reinfection and mother-to-child transmission."

Silvia Beatriz Fernández is a sociologist at the School of Social Sciences, University of Buenos Aires as well as a researcher at the Ángel Roffo Institute (University of Buenos Aires). She has participated in research projects in the fields of sociology of health and public health, with a particular focus on sexual and reproductive health and cancer. She also holds a position of professor in public and private health institutions in Argentina and in universities in Argentina in the fields of qualitative and quantitative methodologies. She has published articles in specialized Argentine and foreign journals and has evaluated articles for Argentine journals.

Mónica Laura Gogna is a sociologist and obtained her PhD in social sciences (University of Buenos Aires, 2008). She is now a senior researcher at the Center for the Study of the State and Society (CEDES) and member of the National Research Council (CONICET) of Argentina. She holds a position of professor in postgraduate programs (gender studies, public health, family law) in public and private universities in Argentina. She is also a trainer in workshops on health research methodology and gender and rights perspectives conducted in Chile, Perú, Colombia, Cuba, El Salvador and Paraguay. She has authored numerous publications on sexual and reproductive health and rights issues (Spanish and English).

Niphattra Haritavorn is a lecturer in the Faculty of Public Health, Thammasat University, Thailand. She completed her PhD in anthropology at Macquarie University, Australia. Her research is related to intravenous drug users and their identity. In the last few years, she has been involved in numerous research projects concerning gender, HIV/AIDS and drug users.

Jennifer M. Hatfield is the associate dean of global/international health in the Faculty of Medicine at the University of Calgary. She is also an associate professor in the Department of Community Health Sciences and director of health and society major and global health in the O'Brien Centre for Bachelor of Health Sciences program, also at the University of Calgary. A former psychology clinician, Dr. Hatfield is leading many innovative research projects around the world on behalf of Canada and the University of Calgary. In 2008, she was named one of the 100 most powerful women in Canada by the Women's Executive Network, a list published annually in the Globe and Mail. As a Senior Mentor for the United Nations Institute for Training and Research, she participated in post-conflict reconstruction leadership development projects for civil service and NGO professionals in Afghanistan. As cochair of the Canadian Global Health Coalition Task Group on Global Health Research Partnerships, Dr. Hatfield is responsible for leading an international team working to promote and improve partnerships between researchers in Canada and lower-income countries.

Alan Jaffe has made his contributions to the South African health-care services as a medical officer, project manager and health researcher from 1981 until his death on 7 February 2009 in Durban, South Africa. One of the pioneers in the field of HIV/AIDS in South Africa, Alan has contributed to the development of innovative and community-oriented HIV policies, management protocols, educational materials, media, drama and training programs. Many of his initiatives won awards and were adopted nationally. Alan's last involvement before his death was with the Infant Feeding Research Project where he was key to the writing of research articles, the training of researchers and the development of the project's woman-centered counseling and counseling training program. He also managed the project's database.

Jessica Jerome is an assistant professor at St. John's College in Santa Fe, New Mexico. Her research uses ethnographic methods to investigate questions of citizenship, urban poverty and medical care in Northeastern Brazil. Most recently, she has focused on women's experiences with Brazil's universal health-care program.

Niyada Kiatying-Angsulee is the director of the Social Research Institute, Chulalongkorn University, Thailand. She is also an assistant professor at the Social Pharmacy Research Unit, Faculty of Pharmaceutical Sciences, Chulalongkorn University. Her interests include drug system monitoring and development, women's health, drug use among lay people and injecting drug users, HIV/AIDS, clinical trials and patients' rights, as well as access to ARVs.

Ray Lazarus is a clinical psychologist, with interests in the psychosocial aspects of HIV/AIDS, particularly with regard to children. She has worked in public health and NGO settings and has been involved in research, training and policy and materials development.

Josephine Mazonde was born in Botswana in a village called Gabane and came to Canada in 2003 to continue on her education journey where she got her master's of science in health research. Josephine took interest in social issues such as HIV/AIDS, development and poverty, domestic violence and women empowerment. She started a group of children and youth to teach them basic information on HIV/AIDS in 1999 in Kanye Village. Josephine participated in several HIV/AIDS committees in Botswana, Australia and Canada and participated in research. She was one of the founding team that started HIV/AIDS management in Botswana in 2000 when the country started treatment for people living with HIV and AIDS. She became a member of the American Association of Nurses in AIDS Care from 2000 to 2004, volunteered with Canadian HIV/AIDS Trials Network (Advisory Committee) from 2006 to 2010, and is currently a member of Canadian Association of Nurses in AIDS Care. She has worked in several levels of care across all age groups and populations.

Karalyn McDonald is a research fellow at Mother and Child Health Research and the Australian Research Centre in Sex, Health and Society at La Trobe University. She received a NHMRC CARG PhD scholarship and completed a PhD entitled "What about motherhood?": Women's journeys through HIV and AIDS. Karalyn's current research interests include women's sexual and reproductive health and the experience of living long term and aging with HIV.

Florence Maureen Mirembe is an associate professor at Makerere University. She has done extensive research and published work focusing on maternal mortality and morbidity, cervical cancer, adolescent health, STDs and HIV/AIDS and women's rights. Florence was instrumental in the introduction of the PMTCT program in Uganda, and she was PI for the first microbicide study in Uganda that has been a huge learning experience in the dynamics of HIV in the communities. She has delivered several key note addresses in the area of safe motherhood, reproductive health and HIV/AIDS at local and international scientific meetings. Florence has received several academic awards, including a Meritorious Award – Save the Mother Building in recognition to contribution in saving mothers and their children and another for her exemplary work with women and children (2007). Her current research is in the area of human papillomavirus diagnosis and control as well as family planning among women living with HIV/AIDS.

Philippe Msellati is an MD and had his PhD in epidemiology. He worked at the French Institut de Recherche pour le Développement, from 1992, as a directeur de recherches. He is now based in Yaoundé, Cameroon, in the Centre de Recherche et de Coordination du site ANRS Cameroun. He has been working mainly on AIDS in Africa (Rwanda, Côte d'Ivoire, Burkina Faso and recently Cameroon) from 1989, essentially on mother-to-child transmission of HIV, prevention of it, HIV infection in women and children, access to HAART in Africa and care management of HIV-infected children in Africa (including coinfections such as tuberculosis and hepatitis B).

Damalie Nakanjako is a physician and lecturer at Makerere University, College of Health Sciences, Department of Medicine, Infectious Diseases Division, Mulago Hospital. Damalie is involved in clinical and implementation research in the field of HIV/AIDS diagnosis and treatment in sub-Saharan Africa. Damalie has been involved in a series of studies that have transformed HIV care and treatment in resource-limited settings in the areas of HIV testing as well as prevention and treatment of opportunistic infections. She has presented her work at various international HIV/AIDS meetings in Africa, Europe and America. She has published papers in areas of HIV/AIDS and behavior, HIV testing and access to HIV treatment, scaling up HIV treatment among mother after PMTCT and outcomes of antiretroviral therapy among people living with HIV/AIDS in Africa. She has a passion to achieve universal access to HIV/AIDS care for all in need as well as improve the treatment outcomes among women and girls living with HIV/AIDS.

María Julieta Obiols is a psychologist and has been working at the Argentinean National Reference Center for AIDS (CNRS), School of Medicine, University of Buenos Aires, for 2 years now performing counseling and interviewing women with HIV infection. She is also a teaching assistant of Mental Health and Public Health (Prof. Alicia Stolkiner's Chair) at the School of Psychology, University of Buenos Aires. She is currently collaborating with several projects related to public health systems in Argentina, including the WHO-supported project conducted by CNRS, CEDES, CENEP and the GGI, under the coordination of Mónica Gogna.

Pauline Oosterhoff is an international public health practitioner, political scientist and medical anthropologist. Since 2003 she has been based in Vietnam. Her key areas of interest are: critical analysis of social determinants of health, HIV/AIDS, gender inequity, human rights, environmental health issues and ethnic minorities. Her regional focus is Asia.

Michael Pfeil is a senior lecturer at the University of East Anglia and a clinical academic research fellow of the NHS East of England. His research interests focus on the ways in which patients, families and professionals experience living with health challenges and undergo health-care interventions. He employs primarily qualitative methodologies, either on their own or in order to complement and enhance randomized trials.

Yadira Roggeveen is a medical doctor, originally from the Netherlands, where she finished the Dutch "Tropenopleiding," a training that specializes on working in remote hospitals. From 2008–2010 she worked as a medical doctor in Ngorongoro Conservation Area, Tanzania, serving the mainly Maasai community. She started and chaired the Safe Motherhood Project of the hospital to improve maternal health-care services and strengthen relationships between the hospital and the community. Aside her work – as a general clinician with special interest for maternal and child health – she worked with Lauren Birks as a coresearcher. She has experienced participatory research as being directly beneficial to the hospital, as the research immediately led to increased insight in and connection with the community. She now combines writing her PhD thesis with being a registrar in Obstetrics and Gynecology.

Ratchneewan Ross is an associate professor and director of international activities at the Kent State University College of Nursing in the United States, where, since 2002, she has taught parent-newborn nursing, research methodology and statistics to nursing students from the bachelor to doctorate levels. In addition to being a teacher and research methodologist, she has been principal investigator for various international research projects focusing on psychological distress among vulnerable populations such as pregnant and postpartum women with HIV. In her early career as midwife and nurse, she cared extensively for pregnant and postpartum women and their newborns and families, including those with HIV.

Jamie L. Stiller is project manager at the University of North Carolina at Chapel Hill Gillings School of Global Public Health. She has experience in behavioral health research related to HIV/AIDS in various populations and federally funded multisite program implementation and evaluation. She works collaboratively with federal clients, key stakeholders and program administrators within public health, medical and academic professions.

Helen Struthers is a director of Anova Health Institute based in Johannesburg and an honorary research associate in the Department of Medicine at the University of Cape Town. She has masters degrees in science and business administration and has been involved in HIV-related research for the past 10 years.

Herpreet Kaur Thind is PhD candidate at the University of Alabama at Birmingham (UAB) School of Public Health. As a physician in India, she has closely interacted with HIV-positive patients receiving care at government clinics and hospitals. She is familiar with the social and economic barriers that affect not only treatment seeking but overall quality of life of HIV-positive patients. She has also studied the attitudes and practises of health-care providers in relation to HIV. She has completed professional development training on HIV/AIDS administered by the Wockhardt-Harvard Medical International HIV/AIDS Education and Research Foundation.

Wilfreda (Billie) Thurston has a BA in psychology, a masters and a doctorate in health research and social epidemiology. She worked in family and children's services and addictions and was director of a shelter for women escaping abusive relationships. She is a professor in the Department of Community Health Sciences, Faculty of Medicine and in the Department of Ecosystems and Public Health in the Faculty of Veterinary Medicine. She is past director of the University of Calgary Institute for Gender Research and past director of the Office of Gender and Equity, Faculty of Medicine, at the University of Calgary. Her program of research and training includes development and evaluation of population health promotion programs that address social inequities. Particular foci include the interplay of gender, culture and socioeconomics as determinants of health; prevention of gender-based interpersonal violence (IPV) against women through the health sector; and public participation as a key tenet of population health. Projects include a national study of farm family health, a longitudinal study of the health of women who have experienced interpersonal violence, a participatory project for prevention of diabetes in

Aboriginal female youth, preventing Aboriginal homelessness and development of a primary health-care research network to promote urban Aboriginal health. She supervises several students doing research in social justice subjects.

Jenny Trinitapoli is an assistant professor of sociology, demography and religious studies and an associate of the Population Research Institute at Penn State University. Most of her research takes place at the intersection between the sociology of religion and social demography. She is the principal investigator of Tsogolo la Thanzi, a study of reproduction and AIDS in Malawi.

Avy Violari currently heads the pediatric division of the Perinatal HIV Research Unit of the University of the Witwatersrand, based at the Chris Hani Baragwanath Hospital. She has been involved in many clinical trials in pediatric and PMTCT research, and her research interest focuses on developing new strategies for the treatment of HIV in infants.

Sara Yeatman is a social demographer in the Department of Health and Behavioral Sciences at the University of Colorado Denver. Sara has been working in Malawi since 2005 and is currently collecting longitudinal data from 2,500 young men and women in the southern Malawian town of Balaka. Her research focuses on the inter-relationships between fertility, reproductive health and HIV.

Chapter 1
Women, Motherhood, and Living with HIV/AIDS: An Introduction

Pranee Liamputtong

1 Introduction

Globally, we have witnessed a dramatic increase in the rates of women living with HIV/AIDS, and many of these women are also mothers with young infants (Wilson 2007; Desclaux et al. 2009). At the end of 2010, among 34 million people worldwide who are living with HIV/AIDS, half are women and two million are children (UNAIDS 2008; The Joint United Nations Programme on HIV/AIDS (UNAIDS) AIDS epidemic update 2009; Desclaux et al. 2009; Héjoaka 2009; WHO/UNAIDS/UNICEF 2011). Among young women in developing countries in particular, the rates of infection are increasing rapidly. Women suffer more from the adverse impact of HIV and AIDS than their male counterparts (Fleischman 2003; National AIDS Control Organization (NACO) 2006; Thomas et al. 2009: Wilcher and Cates 2010; Magadi 2011a; see also Chaps. 16 and 18 in this volume). Today, in sub-Saharan Africa, the region most heavily affected by HIV, for example, women account for half of all the people living with HIV and approximately 60% of infection (UNAIDS 2008; Magadi 2011a). Overwhelmingly, the HIV/AIDS pandemic has disproportionately affected women of reproductive age (Cooper et al. 2007; UNAIDS 2010). In sub-Saharan Africa, 75% of infections occurred among young women aged 15–24 (UNAIDS 2008; Wilcher and Cates 2010).

It is suggested that the number of individuals living with HIV/AIDS will continue to grow in sub-Saharan Africa (UNAIDS 2010; Magadi 2011b). In Malawi, a nation of 12 million, there are about 900,000 people living with HIV/AIDS. According to Kasenga et al. (2010), in Malawi in 2003, 520,000 women of childbearing age were estimated to be infected with HIV. Among pregnant women who attend antenatal care in Malawi, it is estimated that HIV prevalence ranges from 16 to 36%. Similarly,

P. Liamputtong (✉)
School of Public Health, La Trobe University, Kingsbury Drive,
Bundoora, VIC 3086, Australia
e-mail: pranee@latrobe.edu.au

P. Liamputtong (ed.), *Women, Motherhood and Living with HIV/AIDS:*
A Cross-Cultural Perspective, DOI 10.1007/978-94-007-5887-2_1,
© Springer Science+Business Media Dordrecht 2013

in Uganda, at the end of 2007, one million people were living with HIV, and across the age range from birth to age 45–49 years, women were infected more than men (60% for women and 40% for men) (Nassalia et al. 2009). In Brazil too, among the 13,933 new AIDS patients in the first 6 months of 2004, 5,567 (40%) were women, and most of these women (81.1%) aged between 20 and 49 years (Nóbrega et al. 2007). According to Murray et al. (2011), since 1998, there has been an increase in the number of AIDS cases among young women in Brazil. In Haiti, the male to female proportion is about 1:1.14, and young women of childbearing age are most at risk of contracting HIV and subsequently transmit the disease to their infants (Deschampsa et al. 2009). See Chaps. 2, 3, 5, 6, 10, 11, 16, 17, and 19 in this volume.

In Asia, 29% of HIV-positive adults are women, and this percentage is increasing (Desclaux et al. 2009). For example, it has been estimated that by the end of 2009, there were about 740,000 people living with HIV in China (Li et al. 2011), and as in other parts of Asia, almost half would be women. Research in India has shown an increase in HIV among monogamous married women (Pallikadavath and Stones 2003; Chatterjee and Hosain 2006). In recent years, the percentage of HIV cases attributed to mother-to-child transmission (MTCT) has increased significantly (Gupta et al. 2007; Thomas et al. 2009). See also Chaps. 9, 12, 14, and 15 on HIV/AIDS in Asia.

Existing statistics suggest that women bear the brunt of HIV/AIDS pandemic as well as men. However, it has also been noted, not only that most women living with HIV/AIDS are of reproductive age, these women are more likely to live in poverty (*see most chapters in this volume*). Often too, many of them are associated with substance use activities; they may be using drugs themselves or have a partner who is also a drug user (Zierler et al. 1996; Latham et al. 2001). As such, as Latham et al. (2001: 348) put it, "already, these women are likely to be stigmatized due to race, poverty, and/or association with drug use. Women who are involved in drug use may be particularly isolated from caring relationships and be consumed by shame and disconnectedness. A diagnosis of HIV infection can intensify this stigma and lead to rejection by family and friends." See Chap. 9 in this volume.

2 Being a Woman/Mother and Living with HIV/AIDS

When a woman is being labeled as having HIV, she is treated with suspicion, her morality is questioned, and, often, blame is placed on her (Cullinane 2007; Liamputtong et al. 2009; Thomas et al. 2009). Japanese women living with HIV/AIDS, for example, "are blamed for eschewing marriage and motherhood in favor of material pursuits" (Cullinane 2007: 255). Because of their HIV status, many women experience violence from their partners or significant others (WHO 2000; Jewkes et al. 2003; Türmen 2003; Kaye 2004; Strebel et al. 2006; see also Chap. 13 in this volume). Previous research has also suggested that due to perceived gender differences, delay in diagnosis, inferior access to healthcare services, internalized stigma, and poor utilization of health services can occur to women living with HIV/AIDS (Kremer and Sonnenberg-Schwan 2003; Rosenfield and Yanda 2002; Thomas et al. 2005; Turan et al. 2008). This makes it extremely difficult for women to take care of their own health needs (Thomas et al. 2009). Women who are living with HIV/AIDS and who are mothers carry a triple burden of being HIV infected; they are mothers of children who may or may not be positive themselves and often are also caregivers to their HIV-positive partners (Thomas 2006; Héjoaka 2009; Thomas et al. 2009). Héjoaka (2009: 869) puts it clearly: "HIV/AIDS also strikes women by significantly increasing the burden of care they shoulder." See Chaps. 7, 8, 9, 15, and 18 in this volume.

Stigma can have particularly painful consequences for women and mothers living with HIV (Simbayi et al. 2007; Wilson 2007; Davies et al. 2009; Liamputtong 2013; Wyrod 2013). For example, if their HIV status becomes known in the community, their children may be stigmatized and their family members may see them as "unfit" mothers (Davies et al. 2009: 553). Hence, these mothers may decide not to disclose their HIV status to anyone including their children for fear of experiencing negative consequences such as physical feelings of shame, social ostracism, violence, or expulsion from home (Black and Miles 2002; Ciambrone 2002; Maman et al. 2002; Sandelowski and Barroso 2003; Héjoaka 2009; Qiao et al. 2011; Greeff 2013; Chaps. 5, 8, and 18 in this volume). Women may even isolate themselves from their social networks in order to hide their illness so that their families can be protected from the stigma associated with it (Sowell et al. 1997; Latham et al. 2001). According to Herek and Capitanio (1993), HIV/AIDS is "an epidemic of stigma" which can change the relationships that the women have with others. Latham et al. (2001: 348) content, "stigma can emanate from family, friends, lovers, employers, and health care professionals, altering the stigmatized individual's ability to obtain needed emotional and tangible support, as well as undermining their ability to receive quality health care and maintain a sense of well-being" (see also Liamputtong 2013; Chaps. 15 and 18 in this volume). Not surprisingly, we witness many mothers living with HIV/AIDS "live in social isolation to avoid stigmatization" and frequently experiencing "anxiety and depression in confronting their seropositive status" (Davies et al. 2009: 552; see also Li et al. 2011; chapter in Parts I and II in this volume).

Often too, mothers living with HIV/AIDS do not have sufficient social support from their social networks (Davies et al. 2009). Social support is referred to here as "a process in which resources are provided or exchanged between at least two individuals with a purpose to enhance the well-being of the recipient" (Zhao et al. 2011: 671; see also Rosenfeld 1997: 5). Generally, it acts as a "buffer" to diminish distress and strengthen resilience for individuals who experience stressful life events (Richmond et al. 2007; Zhao et al. 2011). It is grounded in the individual's "social network or the web of relationships of which the person is a part" (Bogossian 2007: 170). Social support includes emotional, tangible, and informational support (Bogossian 2007; Mbekenga et al. 2011). It also includes formal support provided by health professionals and informal support that an individual receives from her social networks such as family and other significant members. Social networks, both formal and informal, are one essential component of the social capital concept (Ferlander 2007; Mbekenga et al. 2011). According to Nyqvist (2009), social capital permits an individual to have access to resources including support which might otherwise not be attainable.

According to Davies et al. (2009: 553), for people living with HIV/AIDS (and other highly stigmatized condition, "a supportive group environment" can have a tremendous positive impact on their mental and physical health (see also Davison et al. 2000). It has been illustrated that HIV-positive individuals with extensive social support have less depression, feeling of hopelessness, and physical symptoms than those who lack or have lower levels of support (Serovich et al. 2001; Mizuno et al. 2003; Lindau et al. 2006). It is likely that people who have social support will disclose their illness status as well as actively seek ways of dealing with the illness instead of avoiding it (Kalichman et al. 2003; Lindau et al. 2006; Liamputtong et al. 2009; see also Chaps. 1, 15, and 18 in this volume).

Additionally, social support can impact on willpower for survival as well as access to, acceptance of, and adherence to therapy among individuals living with HIV/AIDS (Cohen 2001; Crosby et al. 2001; Gielen et al. 2001; Cox 2002; Burgoyne 2004; Lindau et al. 2006). In the United States, for example, shame and stigma associated with HIV/AIDS, especially for pregnant women, have produced and continued to cause "a formidable societal barrier to care" (Lindau et al. 2006: 67; see also Black and Miles 2002; Parker and Aggleton 2003; Chaps. 7 and 18 in this volume). However, these effects have been particularly moderated by social support (Catz et al. 2002; Ciambrone 2002; Kalichman et al. 2003). Social support is also linked with better health and quality of life in people living with HIV (Cox 2002; Gielen et al. 2001; Burgoyne 2004; Gregson 2004).

The availability of "culturally appropriate HIV-related resources" is a crucial factor which has positive impact on the health of women living with HIV/AIDS (Davies et al. 2009: 559; see also Blankenship et al. 2000; Plowden et al. 2005). Davies et al. (2009: 559) suggest that "psycho-educational support groups" such as the "Making Our Mothers Stronger (MOMS)" program can be a useful means for providing emotional support and required information to mothers who, because of their HIV status, lacked or resisted social interactions (see also Chaps. 18 in this volume).

3   HIV-Positive Women, Reproduction, and Motherhood

Motherhood for the HIV-positive women was a source of strength and esteem, an anchor in a turbulent life, and a refuge from and buffer against physical and social adversity. (Sandelowski and Barroso 2003: 477)

Significant progress has been made in HIV antiretroviral treatment (ARV) in recent years. This has improved the quality of life of many HIV-positive women. For example, it has become possible to reduce vertical transmission of HIV through use of antiretroviral therapy for the mother and her newborn infant, in combination with elective caesarean section, control of comorbidities, and suppression of breast-feeding (see Chaps. 10, 11, and 19 in this volume). These advances have allowed HIV-positive women to change their expectations about having children (Rossi et al. 2005; Cooper et al. 2007; Hebling and Hardy 2007; Nóbrega et al. 2007; Kanniappana et al. 2008; Agadjanian and Hayford 2009; Nduna and Farlane 2009; Cliffe et al.

2011). Although women have their rights to children, in the case of HIV-positive women, having a child is not a simple matter. Not only do they have to follow specific biomedical recommendations, they also have to deal with the psychological, social, and cultural issues associated with the disease, and death (Hebling and Hardy 2007: 1095). Too often, as Sandelowski and Barroso (2003: 475) put, "motherhood aggravated the symptoms of the infection and intensified the stigmatization associated with it because HIV-infected mothers were seen to place "innocent" children at risk." See chapters in Part I and Chaps. 7 and 8 in this volume.

Many HIV-positive women of childbearing age express their desire and commitment to have children (Wesley et al. 2000; Sandelowski and Barroso 2003; Nakayiwa et al. 2006; Craft et al. 2007; Barnes and Murphy 2009; Nattabi et al. 2009; Awiti Ujiji et al. 2010; Finocchario-Kessler et al. 2010; Kisakye et al. 2010; Wilcher and Cates 2010; see also chapters in Part II in this volume). In their study, Hebling and Hardy (2007: 1098) suggest that for most participants, motherhood was the reason for them to live and to look after themselves. Similar to many women in general, motherhood is essential for HIV-positive women. It is seen as an integral constituent of their femininity. For many HIV-positive women, despite living with a serious illness, becoming a mother permits them to "come back to life." Motherhood enables the women to "reclaim their social identity", which was put into question by the infection. On becoming a mother, they can continue saying, "I am a woman just like any other." In a way, motherhood "symbolizes life and represents a challenge to staying alive." Similarly, in Barnes and Murphy's study (2009: 489) with HIV-positive women in the USA, they found that "birthing a child and mothering was an opportunity for experiencing every day the shifting in attitude from dying to making progress toward living with HIV" (see also Chap. 7 in this volume).

Additionally, having a child is treated as a means for many women to manage the hostile social impacts of living with HIV and associated anxieties about their future (Kisakye et al. 2010). Sandelowski and Barroso (2003: 477) contend that the discourse of motherhood is used by many HIV-positive mothers "to negotiate their identities—to draw attention away from their "deviant" conditions and toward themselves as mothers." However, these women often have to work very hard to "pass" as mothers (Grue and Laerum 2002: 678).

Some women discover that they are HIV-positive during their pregnancies (see Chaps. 3, 4, 15, 16, 17, and 18 in this volume). Others seek to become pregnant after being diagnosed with the illness (Paiva et al. 2007; Awiti Ujiji et al. 2010). In a research conducted by Awiti Ujiji et al. (2010: 8) in an urban slum setting in Kenya, their findings reveal that the women sought to become pregnant by "activating motherhood"; that is, they actively planned and strategized to get pregnant and have children. This is because becoming a mother offered them "identity and recognition in the community, and thus happiness and fulfillment as women." Due to the increased availability of antiretroviral therapy, these women had an opportunity to "restore their status through motherhood." Other studies have also illustrated this (see Panozzo et al. 2003; Blair et al. 2004).

In many societies, childlessness is seen as undesirable, and it has huge social repercussions on the life of childless women (Inhorn 1996, 2003; Matsubayashi et al.

2001; Doyal and Anderson 2005; Johnson-Hanks 2006; Donkor and Sandall 2007; Rashid 2007; Hollos and Larsen 2008; Liamputtong 2009; see also Chap. 16 in this volume). For many women living with HIV/AIDS, they have to live not only with fear of death but also with grief because they realize that they may "die without having children" (Smith and Mbakwem 2007; Kisakye et al. 2010). As in many other societies, in African cultures, women are usually blamed for childlessness (Gerrits 1997; Johnson-Hanks 2006; Chapman 2007; Donkor and Sandall 2007; Dyer 2007; Hollos, and Larsen 2008; Larsen et al. 2010). In the Ugandan context, where child-bearing plays a crucial role in the social identity of a woman, for example, a woman's failure to bear children could also lead to stigmatization and discrimination (Donkor and Sandall 2007; Kisakye et al. 2010; See Chaps. 5 and 6 in this volume). As such, motherhood has a huge meaning to women living with HIV/AIDS. However, with the scale-up of antiretroviral therapy in many parts of the world, women living with HIV are offered a chance to have children with a decreased risk of mother-to-child transmission (Agadjanian and Hayford 2009; Awiti Ujiji et al. 2010).

4   HIV Mothers and Infant Feeding Practises

Every day globally, more than 1,500 unborn or newborn babies are infected with HIV. Most of these babies will die before they reach their fifth birthday (Kasenga et al. 2010). And not surprisingly, these children are born in poor nations, particularly in sub-Saharan Africa (Deschampsa et al. 2009; UNICEF/UNAIDS/WHO/UNFPA 2010; Desclaux and Alfieri 2011; Doherty 2011). Approximately, 40% of HIV-positive children are infected through breastfeeding. This makes breastfeeding the most widespread means of MTCT (mother-to-child transmission) of HIV (Maru et al. 2009: 1114; see also Kourtis et al. 2006; Kasenga et al. 2010; Doherty 2011). For HIV-positive mothers who practise prolonged breastfeeding, the risk of MTCT HIV span from 25 to 48% (De Cock et al. 2000; Nassalia et al. 2009).

As part of prevention of mother-to-child HIV transmission (PMTCT) strategies, there are two options that HIV-positive women are asked to select about the feeding of their infant. These are exclusive breastfeeding with early weaning or replacement feeding (with breast-milk substitutes) (WHO/UNICEF/UNFPA/UNAIDS 2007a, b; Desclaux and Alfieri 2009). The options may be feasible for women who can afford to do so, but for many HIV-positive mothers residing in resource-poor nations, who also practise prolonged breastfeeding due to economic, social, and cultural grounds, asking them to adopt exclusive replacement feeding with their infants can be problematic and a challenge indeed (Kamau-Mbuthia et al. 2008; Deschampsa et al. 2009; see Chaps. 10, 11, and 16 in this volume).

Very often too, women living with HIV/AIDS are advised not to breastfeed their infants. Most of these mothers are from poor backgrounds, and their poverty has a great impact on their feeding practises (Liamputtong 2011; see also Chap. 4 in this volume). In poor nations, where sanitary conditions are not good, this can be much more difficult as unsuitable handling of infant formula may result in dehydration and diarrhea, which are major causes of infant mortality (UNICEF 2007; Maru et al. 2009; Desclaux and Alfieri 2009). Maru et al. (2009: 1114) content that in settings where there is poor access to clean water and sanitation, such as those in sub-Saharan Africa, HIV-positive mothers are confronted with "the choice of breastfeeding, which confers an increased risk of HIV, or formula feeding, which increases the risk of malnutrition, respiratory tract infections, and diarrheal diseases."

The transmission of HIV through breast milk has created a dilemma for HIV-positive mothers. Often, the benefits of breastfeeding as well as the risks of not breastfeeding must be considered against the risk of HIV transmission through breastfeeding (Desclaux and Alfieri 2011; Doherty 2011). Public or child health specialists and healthcare workers in many resource-poor settings are challenged by the infant feeding dilemma posed by HIV. Whereas previously breastfeeding, especially exclusive breastfeeding, was a key child-survival strategy, the finding that HIV is present in breast milk has led to the reassessment of the benefits of breastfeeding, and avoiding prolonged breastfeeding is now recommended to eliminate the transmission of HIV through breast milk (Desclaux and Alfieri 2011; Doherty 2011). How do these mothers deal with these issues? What can the government and local authorities do to assist these women? Some of these discussions will be included in several chapters in this volume. See Chaps. 10, 11, and 19 in this volume.

Nevertheless, what is clear is that women should receive sufficient guidance and counseling regarding the benefits and risks of infant feeding options so that women could make an "informed choice" (Desclaux and Alfieri 2009). They must be given particular guidance in choosing the option which is appropriate for their living situation, and they should be supported in the choice that they have made (WHO/UNICEF/UNFPA/UNAIDS 2007b; Desclaux and Alfieri 2009; Doherty 2011). However, counseling regarding infant feeding in the context of HIV provided by healthcare providers is often problematic. Presently, counseling is provided to HIV-positive mothers in very different ways (Desclaux and Alfieri 2009). For example, Piwoz et al. (2006) reveal in their study that there were marked differences between the attitudes and practices of the health workers and the recommendations from the World Health Organization (WHO). Accordingly, "health workers with counselling experience believed that HIV-infected mothers should breastfeed exclusively, rather than infant formula feed, citing poverty as the primary reason. Because of high levels of malnutrition, all the workers had concerns about early cessation of breastfeeding" (Piwoz et al. 2006: 1). Clearly, the attitudes of health workers were influenced by social contexts of the mothers, and this was reflected in the way they provided counseling to HIV-positive mothers (see more discussions in Chap. 19).

5   Gender Lens Perspective

Chapters in this volume provide theoretical understanding about the perceptions and experiences of women. As such, I contend that the experiences of women should be seen through the gender lens perspective (see Gysae and Øverland 2002;

Türmen 2003; Strebel et al. 2006). Sociologically, gender is understood as a social construct, referring to the distinguishing characteristics of being female or male (Lorber 1994). Gender can be seen as the full range of personality traits, attitudes, feelings, values, behaviors, and activities that "society ascribes to the two sexes on a differential basis" (Keleher and MacDougall 2009: 56; Türmen 2003). In its broadest sense, according to Türmen (2003: 411), gender is concerned with "what is meant to be male or female, and how that defines a person's opportunities, roles, responsibilities, and relationships." It is different from sex, which is a "biological construct premised upon biological characteristics enabling sexual reproduction" (Krieger 2003: 653).

Gender does not operate in isolation. It often intersects with other social determinants including ethnicity and social class (Risman 2004; Hankivsky et al. 2009; Hunt and Annandale 2012; Liamputtong et al. 2012). Here, ethnicity is referred to as "a shared cultural background"; it is a characteristic of a group within a society (Julian 2009: 177). Ethnicity includes other dimensions than biological determinants (which is referred to as race). Gender is also interconnected with social class which refers to the position of a person in "a system of structured inequality" which is grounded in the unequal distribution of income, wealth, status, and power (Germov 2009: 86). As readers will see in this volume, the intersection of gender, ethnicity, and social class has recreated health inequalities among many women in many corners of the world (Lorber 1994, 1997; Broom 2009), and for women who are mothers and living with HIV/AIDS, this inequality is even more evident (*see chapters in this volume*).

Although gender is frequently conceptualized as "a characteristic of an individual" as presented above, Wyrod (2013) contends that it should be perceived more as "a type of social structure." Risman (2011: 19), for example, argues that we need to understand gender as having a structure:

> Just as every society has a political structure (e.g., democracy, monarchy) and an economic structure (e.g., capitalist, socialist), so, too, every society has a gender structure (from patriarchal to at least hypothetically egalitarian).

According to Risman (2004), there are three dimensions or levels of the social structure of gender: individual, interactional, and institutional. On the individual, or intrapersonal, dimension, gender functions through gender identity development occurring through the socialization process of an individual's life (Wyrod 2013). The senses of "gendered selves" (Risman 2004: 433) dictate how an individual thinks of him/herself as gendered and has particular expectations of him/herself as a gendered individual (Butler 1990; Risman 2011; Wyrod 2013). It is at this level that cultural orders which produce gender inequalities are personally learned. It is also at this level that norms governing gender identity become a norm to individuals within the society (Epstein 2007; Wyrod 2013).

On the interactional dimension, gender shapes how individuals interact with each other in their everyday life by structuring certain social orders about expectations and proper behavior for gendered members of a given society. As such, women and men, regardless of their identical ethnic and class positions, have different cultural expectations. It is at this level that social interactions create gender hierarchies and inequalities (Risman 2004; Wyrod 2013). At the institutional level, gender hierarchies are reinforced through organizational practises, allocation of essential resources and material goods, and legal regulations which prejudice men over women (Risman 2004: 437, 2011: 20; see also Giddens 1984; Lorber 1994, 1997; Wyrod 2013).

As readers will see throughout this volume, often it is gender hierarchies and inequalities that have caused HIV/AIDS to women in many parts of the globe (see also Ackermann and De Klerk 2002; Jewkes et al. 2003; Türmen 2003; Dunkle et al. 2004; Upchurch and Kusunoki 2004; Magadi 2011a). It is also because of these hierarchies and inequalities that women suffer more from the epidemic. All too often, they are blamed for having the illness, and sensitive healthcare are denied to them. But some positive attempts have also emerged to make the lives of these HIV-positive women better. These will be discussed in the chapters in this volume.

6 About the Book

The book is divided into three parts. Chapter 1, written by Pranee Liamputtong, sets the scene of this book. It provides a background understanding about women living with HIV/AIDS. It discusses salient issues concerning women who are mothers and the essence of having children as well as infant feeding practices. A gender lens perspective is also introduced as all chapters in the volume are argued to be situated within this approach. The chapter also introduces the book, and it outlines details of all chapters which are included in the volume.

Part I contains chapters concerning women, reproduction, and HIV/AIDS. Chapter 2 is about family planning by HIV-positive mothers in a South African urban setting and is written by Ray Lazarus, Helen Struthers, and Avy Violari. The authors suggest that prevention of unintended pregnancy among HIV-positive women is a critical intervention to reduce maternal mortality and prevent HIV infection of infants. In their qualitative study carried out in Soweto, South Africa, HIV-positive mothers of HIV-negative or HIV-positive infants were interviewed shortly after the birth of their babies in order to explore their perceptions, understandings, and experiences on a range of issues. The interviews were subjected to thematic analysis to identify themes significant to the women themselves, as well as those relevant to healthcare provision. Their chapter focuses on findings regarding fertility desires, intentions, and practise. Some implications for healthcare provision are also highlighted in this chapter.

Pregnancy and motherhood in the narratives of women with HIV infection from the metropolitan area of Buenos Aires (Argentina) are presented in Chap. 3 by Mónica Gogna, Silvia Fernández, Paula di Corrado, and María Julieta Obiols. This chapter discusses qualitative data from a broader research project supported by WHO that aims at identifying the obstacles to the provision of more integral healthcare to women living with HIV in the metropolitan area of Buenos Aires. The first phase of the study explored women's experiences, needs, and expectations regarding pregnancy, vertical transmission prevention, condom use, and reproductive intentions through a survey applied to women attending CNRS (National Reference Center for AIDS) for their viral load or CD4 tests or for their babies' diagnosis ($N = 169$). Based on the results of a 2009 survey, the authors interviewed a dozen of women taking their babies for lab tests. Interview guidelines focused on time and circumstances when they were notified about their HIV infection; experience in relation to diagnosis, reconstruction of the steps taken since then, and perception of difficulties and facilitators in the care provided by the health services; partner's role; pregnancy experience; and reproductive intentions. Their findings indicate that getting an HIV-positive result, particularly during pregnancy, is a very difficult situation that awakes strong and contradictory feelings (fear, shame, anger, sorrow). Nevertheless, the fact that an offspring, whether wanted or unexpected, is associated with life counterbalances in some way the feelings elicited by the diagnosis. After the "initial shock," HIV infection becomes part of the women's lives and does not have a unique impact on their sexual and reproductive behavior. Interviewees complied with treatment to prevent vertical transmission as part of their responsibilities to their offspring but tended to postpone their own care. The priority given to children, whether it is that women delay treatment or follow treatment "because of them," confirms the centrality motherhood has in these women's lives. Coping with the infection and other adverse situations seemed to have empowered women regarding their contraceptive and reproductive needs and wishes.

Pleumjit Chotiga, Kenda Crozier, and Michael Pfeil write about the experience of Burmese migrant women in northern Thailand in making decisions in pregnancy about HIV testing and treatment in Chap. 4. The chapter presents a number of case studies which will be discussed to illustrate the decision-making processes for migrant women when considering HIV testing and treatment in pregnancy. The case studies are drawn from research which was conducted among 38 Burmese migrant pregnant women and 26 healthcare workers in the Thai-Burmese border provinces in the northern part of Thailand during 2008 and 2009. With its high rate of HIV infections and high numbers of Burmese migrants, this area was selected in order to access the desired group of participants. The complex issues that surround decisions to accept or refuse HIV testing and treatment are presented from the point of view of women and also healthcare workers who are engaged in caring for them in the antenatal period. In this chapter, they also make suggestions for improved communication and information sharing to enable the women to be actively involved in decisions at this time.

In Chap. 5, Lauren K. Birks, Yadira Roggeveen, and Jennifer M. Hatfield present motherhood, infertility, and HIV from the perspective of the Maasai of northern Tanzania. They point out that in a culture emphasizing procreation and sexual relations as an integral part of everyday life and success in society, the Maasai of northern Tanzania face a difficult task when confronting HIV/AIDS. Reproduction and motherhood are inextricably linked to prosperity and success for the Maasai. In fact, Maasai women are expected to produce children to fulfill life's purpose, and women without children are most certainly pitied. Therefore, an absence of children gives said women license to engage in sexual practises that may be considered as high risk in order to cure her affliction of infertility. HIV/AIDS becomes of particular concern with infertility is a factor for Maasai women because such women are more likely to engage in unprotected sexual intercourse with greater numbers of male partners in an attempt to conceive, thereby increasing the likelihood of exposure to HIV and other diseases. This chapter will explore the unique cultural and sexual practices of the Maasai that seek to mitigate infertility and achieve motherhood, while also examining how such practices contribute to risk of exposure to HIV/ AIDS. The research discussed in this chapter was collected over the course of 2 years, between 2008 and 2010 in the Maasai community of the Ngorongoro Conservation Area (NCA) in northern Tanzania. To gather data in a culturally sensitive manner and emphasize a participatory approach, Participatory Action Research (PAR) methodology was employed in their research.

Sara Yeatman and Jenny Trinitapoli introduce their chapter on HIV-positive childbearing in rural Malawi in Chap. 6. They suggest that a number of studies have demonstrated that HIV-positive women across sub-Saharan Africa are less likely than uninfected women to want more children; however, every relevant study has also found that at least a sizeable minority continue to desire a/another child in spite of their infection. In this chapter, they shed light on evolving social norms around HIV-positive childbearing and the heterogeneity of reproductive goals held by HIV-positive women in a town in southern Malawi. They argue that although HIV has had a dramatic impact on the community, it has not altered the fundamental motivations for childbearing: achieving full adulthood, maintaining the moral order, and cementing a relationship. Compared to these intrinsic values of childbearing, HIV is a relatively minor factor and is unlikely to alter a woman's desire for children until the others have been satisfied. At this point in the epidemic, a broader social consensus about HIV-positive childbearing is emerging, and there is some fuzzy minimal threshold of children that women—even HIV-positive women—are expected and encouraged to achieve.

Part II is concerned with motherhood, infant feeding, and HIV/AIDS. Donna Barnes, in Chap. 7, presents motherhood experiences for women living longer than expected with HIV/AIDS. She contends that for women living longer than expected with HIV/AIDS, the opportunity to see their "babies grow up" becomes possible with access to improved medical care. Motherhood offers women with HIV/AIDS a reason for living and a valued position. Fifty-nine women living with HIV, from Oakland, California ($n = 30$) and Rochester, New York ($n = 29$), participated in an initial study on reproductive decisions (1995–2001). In the follow-up study (2005–2009), 51 women were living. Donna completed face-to-face interviews with women ($n = 36$) for a follow-up rate of 70.6%. Grounded theory qualitative methods of collaborative coding, memo writing, diagramming, and participant verification of analysis were used. The sample ($n = 36$) was predominantly women of color, with a mean age of 42.6 years. Half of the participants reported an annual household income of less than $15 K. The majority had a current HIV status as asymptomatic. Most participants were single, and more than half had children living with them. Participants were living with HIV for an average of 14.8 years. How women with increased longevity with HIV managed their lost mothering opportunities, as they defined loss, was interrelated with their attitudes about how mothers should care for their children and how participants' related HIV stigmatization may affect their children. Mothering and reconciliation of past reproductive choices were influenced by the contexts of their social worlds and the historical contexts of the AIDS epidemic changing from a death sentence to a chronic disease. Multiple marginalization of social conditions emanate from gender, race, ethnicity and class, family relations, child custody issues, acute and chronic episodes and stage of illness, and, for some, substance use and incarceration. Donna developed the concept of *lost mothering,* interpreting the interacting elements in situations. She suggests that the findings of her study have implications for developing innovative programs on mothering skills and assistance in reuniting families.

Chapter 8 discusses issues relevant to HIV-positive mothers, disclosure and stigma, and is written by Karalyn McDonald. Karalyn contends that HIV-positive mothers face the complex and challenging decision about whether to disclose their HIV status to their children. Not only do HIV-positive mothers worry about the potential emotional burden this disclosure may impose on their children, but there is also the risk of unwanted disclosure by children and the possibility of ensuing stigma. When thinking about the disclosure of one's HIV status to another, stigma is implicit. In-depth interviews were conducted in 2001 with 34 HIV-positive women in Australia who were diagnosed during their childbearing years, 28 of whom were mothers. In this chapter, she explores HIV-positive women's accounts of disclosure and how women construct both public and private accounts of living with HIV as a way of deriving meaning from their diagnosis as well as a way of managing disclosure and its potential ramifications. Karalyn also examines the role of stigma in the decisions made about disclosure to children as well as family, friends, and broader social networks.

Niphattra Haritavorn writes about tactics of mothers with HIV and drug uses in dealing with life in Chap. 9. In this chapter, Niphattra argues that throughout their lives, women injecting drug users in Thailand have been subjected to stigmatization, a socially informed, painful experience that has become part of their disposition. Stigma, in fact, dominates their everyday lives. She suggests that Thai women injecting drugs are in effect "doubly stigmatized": As drug users, they fail to fit the Thai "good" women/mothers image, that is, to meet their socially expected or stereotypical gender roles. Constant exposure to stigma sees their clear sense of self dissipate and replaced by the relational self, in the process rendering their gender and identity hazy and complex. Being a mother requires bridging the public and private lives of women injecting drugs, who find themselves faced with coping with the dual roles of motherhood and drug users. This chapter is based upon her ethnographic data and on in-depth interviews conducted with 25 Thai women living with HIV and injecting drugs, most of whom were informed of their HIV status when tested for pregnancy. Pregnancies among female drug users are invariably unplanned: The women do not consider the absence of menstruation as indicative of pregnancy because taking drugs may cause irregular menstrual periods; thus, they wait until more overt physical signs appear. Drug-using pregnant women are reluctant to share information concerning their drug use with doctors because of the guilt they (are often made to) feel regarding fetal well-being. This chapter explores female drug users as mothers and looks at the specific ways in which they deal with their lives in a habitus that constitutes conditions for social suffering. The tactics they use could be informed by the particular form of drug culture they pursue and how it is integrated with their gendered habitus.

In Chap. 10, Alice Desclaux presents Senegalese women living with HIV in relation to the 2009 WHO recommendations for PMTCT, particularly meanings for resistance regarding infant feeding among these women. The 2009 WHO recommendations for the prevention of HIV transmission through breastfeeding advise the use of pharmaceutical prophylaxis with a single infant feeding mode selected at the regional or national level, that is, exclusive breastfeeding for West African countries. HIV-positive women should be "educated" to increase the efficacy of this new strategy. These recommendations engendered unexpected resistance in Senegal from HIV-positive women who protested publicly. This collective protest was quite new in a setting where PLHIV-organization members are considered social counselors rather than activists and women are seen as natural caregivers and good patients rather than community health experts. Based on a study held with an association of HIV-positive women and within the public health system, this chapter is based on the analysis of international policies regarding HIV transmission through breastfeeding and women's roles in prevention before 2009, the local determinants for adoption of the new strategy, and women's perceptions of HIV risk and protest. Contrary to international policies and stakeholders who believe that the implementation of a pharmaceutical strategy for prevention is a step toward eradication of mother-to-child HIV transmission, women think that the efficacy of this strategy is not sufficient to protect their infants. The women call for their participation in making decisions on public health strategies that concern them as mothers and as associative caregivers and counselors. Their protest is also a quest to be acknowledged for their autonomy and expertise.

Improving access to PMTCT programs in Africa is discussed in Chap. 11 by Philippe Msellati. For more than 10 years, pediatric AIDS has been virtually eradicated from North developed countries. In Africa, despite technical means and apparent political will, the percentage of pregnant women involved in PMTCT interventions is not increasing as fast as public health authorities would expect. There have been real progress during the last years, but these changes are still limited to southern and east Africa. Eradication of pediatric AIDS in Africa in 2015, as UNAIDS has targeted, seems a difficult objective to reach. This chapter is based on the combination of a literature review, an analysis of databases and empirical evidence collected during 15 years of PMTCT implementation, childcare research, and treatment programs in West Africa. Philippe contends that one way to progress is to analyze why in some countries PMTCT programs do not work properly and how in some others it works well. It seems important to analyze the process of PMTCT programs at several levels (site, regional, and national), step-by-step through literature, databases, and qualitative studies. It should be the better way to understand the successes and failures of the programs and how to "scale up" PMTCT programs, where there are gaps or obstacles and how to try to go through these obstacles. It includes analyses of the health system, of health workers expectations and limitations, of mothers' expectations, and of relationships between mothers and the care system.

Perinatal intervention itself changes with new recommendations by the World Health Organization (WHO). Women can, however, give up or vanish at any time during the whole process. With new recommendations by WHO on breastfeeding and antiretroviral drugs, we can expect a dramatic decrease of postnatal transmission of HIV, but new problems arise, such as difficulties in getting infant formula when HIV-infected mothers make that choice. This additional step gives many problems as women and exposed children have to be followed longer, and the final diagnosis cannot be given before the end of breastfeeding.

In Part III, issues relevant to women, mothers, and care are included. Ratchneewan Ross presents psychological distress among HIV-positive pregnant and postpartum women in Thailand in Chap. 12. In this chapter, she points out that the HIV infection rates among women have been reported at 1–3% in different parts of Thailand. Most HIV transmission has been found to be heterosexual through husband/partner's promiscuity in Thailand. However, when infected with the virus, Thai women can feel stigmatized and depressed. This chapter will include topics concerning HIV-positive pregnant and postpartum Thai women in relation to their lived experiences, psychological disturbances (depressive symptoms), physical symptoms, a Buddhist way to cope with HIV infection, and recommendations for healthcare professionals.

In Chap. 13, entitled "HIV is my 'Best' Problem: Living with Racism, HIV and Interpersonal Violence," Josephine Mazonde and Wilfreda Thurston tell the story of an HIV-positive Aboriginal woman. They contend that gender-based violence is a problem for women around the world. Although HIV/AIDS and interpersonal violence (IPV) have been studied extensively as separate entities, the connection between the two has received less attention than should be warranted. They argue that studying HIV/AIDS and IPV as intersecting issues is essential in understanding women's experiences of either or both, and the results have implications for health policy. Through telling her story of living with HIV and IPV, an Aboriginal woman reveals a life where gender-based violence took place in the context of a history of colonialism and marginalization of her people. HIV was a much easier issue to discuss than the violence she had experienced in her life. Using a socio-ecological framework to interpret her story revealed that relationships with her children were just one casualty of intersecting oppressions. Services tended to treat either HIV or IPV but failed to see her as a whole person. The experience of surviving HIV/AIDS and IPV on a day-to-day basis negatively impacted her life and created a cycle of abuse, including self-abuse, which was difficult to escape. The results demonstrate the intertwined relationships of HIV/AIDS and IPV, and factors at the personal, interpersonal, community, and environmental levels that impact this relationship. The value of culturally safe approaches to care for HIV/AIDS is also highlighted in this chapter.

In Chap. 14, Pauline Oosterhoff and Tran Xuan Bach write about the effects of collective action on the confidence of individual HIV-positive mothers in Vietnam.

They suggest that women's social roles and identities as mothers can be prescriptive and constricting. Young Vietnamese women face intense pressure to marry and have (male) children, putting them at risk of contracting HIV. However, being a mother also provides women with some status and power within the family. Although most HIV-positive women were infected by their husbands, they are not passive victims but take action to improve their lot. This chapter examines changes in the circumstances and priorities of 419 HIV-positive mothers in five support groups (the "Sunflowers") across four provinces in northern Vietnam, starting with the first group's inception in 2004, before the arrival of large-scale antiretroviral therapy (ART) programs, followed by the formation of four new groups in 2005. In this context, access to medical resources was both a stimulus for and a result of grassroots group mobilization. On first joining a group, most women reported feelings of worthlessness, isolation, lack of confidence, and social stigma within their families. Over time, and following participation in the mothers' groups, both women's perceptions of stigmatization and their reported needs changed. Members accessed essential social, health, and economic services including ART, PMTCT, loans, and social and legal support through the referral network of the support groups. Most women also reported being able to participate in family meals and send their children to school. Their health concerns rapidly decreased, and they came to focus on economic problems. However, successes in mobilizing access to essential services, support, and resources had little impact on the prevailing problem of individual women's perceptions of their personal ability to make strategic decisions; group members still reported a lack of confidence and low self-esteem.

In Chap. 15, Pranee Liamputtong and colleagues write about the living positively discourse among Thai women living with HIV/AIDS. In this chapter, they contend that living with an incurable illness such as HIV/AIDS is a stressful experience. However, many HIV-positive individuals are able to maintain their emotional well-being. This begs the question of what strategies these individuals employ to allow them to do so. This chapter examines how Thai women living with HIV/AIDS dealt with the illness. The women adopted several strategies to deal with their HIV status including taking care of own self, accepting one's own faith, disclosing their HIV status to family, and joining AIDS support groups. These strategies can be situated within the "living positively" discourse which helps to create a sense of optimism to combat the HIV epidemic among the women. Additionally, the acceptance of their HIV status plays an essential role in the meaning making process because it assists the women to sustain the equilibrium of their emotional well-being.

Damalie Nakanjako, Florence Mirembe, Jolly Beyeza, and Alex Coutinh, in Chap. 16, write about cross-cultural barriers in scaling up HIV/AIDS care among women in sub-Saharan Africa. The HIV/AIDS epidemic wears a female face, as evidenced by the disproportionately high women's vulnerability to HIV infection particularly in the sub-Saharan Africa (SSA) region. Women and girls continue to be affected disproportionately by HIV infection than men and boys, and they account for approximately 60% of the estimated HIV infections worldwide. Women in the developing world confront serious sociocultural, economic, and gender disadvantages that influence the dynamics of the HIV/AIDS among females. It is critical, therefore, to have strategies to expand the culturally appropriate care for women. In this chapter, they review the cross-cultural norms and practises around motherhood, pregnancy, childbirth, newborn care, adolescence, breastfeeding, and family planning and how these have affected the uptake and scale-up of HIV/AIDS prevention, treatment, and care programs. They discuss sociocultural beliefs and practises about motherhood in Africa, which are pertinent to the scale-up of HIV prevention and treatment interventions among women. These include knowledge of HIV sero-status, disclosure of HIV sero-status, HIV sero-discordance, PMTCT, family planning in the context of HIV/AIDS, and the need to foster a new sociocultural perspective in the context of HIV/AIDS epidemic that has been around for over three decades. They also highlight some strategies to make the current prevention and treatment interventions adaptable to the various regions affected by the cross-cultural HIV/AIDS epidemic.

Women's access, uptake, and adherence to comprehensive HIV/AIDS prevention and treatment/care programs including PMTCT and HAART are hampered by numerous sociocultural constraints including the socioeconomic power-gender inequalities, male dominance of women's decision-making processes, and continuous thrive of women to conform to societal expectations and prestige surrounding motherhood. Therefore, in order to reach all the women in need of HIV/AIDS care, and change the tide of the HIV/AIDS epidemic, the prevention and treatment interventions need to be tailored to the sociocultural perspectives, norms, and practices of the communities affected by the epidemic.

Chapter 17 is about mothers with HIV within the perspective of a human rights approach to HIV/AIDS care in northeastern Brazil and is written by Jessica Jerome. In this chapter, Jessica asks: How do Brazilian healthcare policies, designed to support human rights, affect mothers with HIV? Drawing on semi-structured in-depth interviews with a group of urban poor mothers in northeastern Brazil, this chapter examines the broader social and political contexts within which these women live their lives with HIV. The chapter looks specifically at women's attitudes toward HIV diagnosis, their motivations for accepting HIV treatment and care, and their experiences with medical caregivers. It argues that strong social and institutional networks as well as a Universal HIV treatment program provide northeastern Brazilian mothers with forms of support that may be absent in other countries. It further suggests that particular forms of healthcare, such as the human rights-based approach Brazil has taken to HIV/AIDS, may improve patient-provider relationships.

Susan Davies, Herpreet Thind, and Jamie Stiller, in Chap. 18, write about the use of intervention mapping to develop a culturally tailored parenting intervention for mothers living with HIV in the southern USA, which they refer to as The MOMS (Making Our Mothers Stronger) Project. They suggest that The Southeastern region of the United States has had the highest increase of new HIV/AIDS cases among all regions in the country and now has the highest incidence of HIV-positive women. The MOMS Project was a randomized, controlled behavioral trial that aimed to improve functioning of families affected by HIV by reducing childbearing stressors among HIV-positive mothers. Participants were randomly assigned to 1 of 2 intervention conditions: a Social Cognitive Theory (SCT)-based intervention (focused on reducing parenting stress) or an attention control intervention (focused on reducing health-related stress). The parenting intervention focused on building 4 key skills: *communicating clearly* and *effectively* with their children; using *positive* and *negative consequences* with their children to effectively change child's behavior; enjoying their children more by finding ways to *build quality time together* into their normal routine; and *taking care of themselves* so they can best care for their children. Post-intervention, there was significant decline in parenting-related stress in both the intervention conditions. Implications and future directions based on study findings are discussed in their chapter.

Ineke Buskens and Alan Jaffe present their chapter on coping with patriarchy in an era of HIV/AIDS and female sexism in infant feeding counseling in southern Africa in the last chapter (Chap. 19). In an 11-site ethnographic field work study into mothers' experiences with primary healthcare infant feeding counseling in the context of HIV/AIDS, conducted in southern Africa from 2003 until 2005, the relationship between the infant feeding counselors and the mothers was found to be wrought with interpersonal problems, so much so that the initial intent of contributing to the fight against pediatric AIDS through the design of a woman-centered infant feeding counseling format was deemed to be ineffectual. Further analysis of this relationship and of the relationship between the mothers and other health workers in the clinics necessitated the introduction of the concept of female sexism, as developed by Phyllis Chesler in her seminal work *Woman's Inhumanity towards Woman*, to make sense of what was going on.

Female sexism is linked to a country's general sexism rate, and southern Africa can be characterized as very sexist. Female sexism reveals itself as women judging, shaming, and shunning other women because they are women. This is particularly so for women who break the accepted patterns of what a "good woman" should be and do as HIV-positive women are being framed despite ample evidence to the contrary. Eighty percent of African women are faithful to their husbands and contract the disease within their marriage. Married women are also at higher risk of contracting the disease than unmarried women. Being a good woman in the traditional sense can be considered a life-threatening attitude in the context of HIV/AIDS. The judgment that is part of the syndrome of female sexism allows the judging woman to maintain a distance from the woman she judges and attribute her unfortunate situation to personal characteristics and not to a systemic social context that would also implicate her. Just like their clients, the female counselors would not be able to control their sexual and reproductive health because they would not be in a position to negotiate safe sex or sexual fidelity with their partners. Judging their clients as personally and morally lacking would give the health workers a way of denying that what happened with their clients could also happen to them. The authors argue that the concept of female sexism allowed them to understand the negative attitude of the health workers as a strategy for these women to cope with feeling helpless and overburdened regarding the task at hand and being confronted with their own anxiety in the interface with their clients without being able to process what they were experiencing. It was obvious that this coping strategy, dysfunctional as it was, actually created additional stress to the health workers. The systemic gender perspective that the researchers developed offers the health services a perspective on a problem that needs systemic understanding in order to design interventions that would support the health workers to find positive coping strategies, without condoning abusive health worker behavior.

References

Ackermann L, De Klerk GW (2002) Social factors that make South African women vulnerable to HIV infection. Health Care Woman Int 23(2):163–172

Agadjanian V, Hayford SR (2009) PMTCT, HAART, and childbearing in Mozambique: an institutional perspective. AIDS Behav 13:S103–S112

Awiti Ujiji A, Ilako F, Indalo D, Rubenson B (2010) I will not let my HIV status stand in the way. Decisions on motherhood among women on ART in a slum in Kenya- a qualitative study. BMC Women's Health 10, 13. Retrieved 20 May 2010 from: http://www.biomedcentral.com/1472-6874/10/13

Barnes DB, Murphy S (2009) Reproductive decisions for women With HIV: motherhood's role in envisioning a future. Qual Health Res 19(4):481–491

Black BP, Miles MS (2002) Calculating the risks and benefits of disclosure in African American women who have HIV. J Obstet Gynecol Neonatal Nurs 31(6):688–697

Blair JM, Hanson DL, Jones JL, Dworkin MS (2004) Trends in pregnancy rates among women with human immunodeficiency virus. Obstet Gynecol 103(4):663–668

Blankenship KM, Bray SJ, Merson MH (2000) Structural interventions in public health. AIDS 14(1):S11–S21

Bogossian FE (2007) Social support: proposing a conceptual model for application to midwifery practice. Women Birth 20:169–171

Broom D (2009) Gender and health. In: Germov J (ed) Second opinion: an introduction to health sociology, 4th edn. Oxford University Press, Melbourne, pp 130–155

Burgoyne R (2004) Social support and quality of life over time among adults living with HIV in the HAART era. Soc Sci Med 58(7):1353–1366

Butler J (1990) Gender trouble: feminism and the subversion of identity. Routledge, New York

Catz SL, Gore-Felton C, McClure JB (2002) Psychological distress among minority and low-income women living with HIV. Behav Med 28(2):53–60

Chapman RR (2007) Chikotsa – secrets, silence, and hiding: social risk and reproductive vulnerability in central Mozambique. Med Anthropol Q 20(4):487–515

Chatterjee N, Hosain GM (2006) Perceptions of risk and behavior change for prevention of HIV among married women in Mumbai, India. J Health Popul Nutr 24(1):81–88

Ciambrone D (2002) Informal networks among women with HIV/AIDS: present support and future prospects. Qual Health Res 12(7):876–896

Cliffe S, Townsend CL, Cortina-Borja M, Newell M-L (2011) Fertility intentions of HIV-infected women in the United Kingdom. AIDS Care 23(9):1093–1101

Cohen MH (2001) Women and HIV: creating an ambiance of caring. J Am Med Womens Assoc 56(1):9–10

Cooper D, Harries J, Myer L, Orner P, Bracken H, Zweigenthal V (2007) "Life is still going on": reproductive intentions among HIV-positive women and men in South Africa. Soc Sci Med 65:274–283

Cox LE (2002) Social support, medication compliance and HIV/AIDS. Soc Work Health Care 35(1–2):425–460

Craft SM, Delaney RO, Bautista DT, Serovich JM (2007) Pregnancy decisions among women with HIV. AIDS Behav 11:927–935

Crosby RA, DiClemente RJ, Wingood GM, Cobb BK, Harrington K, Davies SL, Hook EW III, Oh MK (2001) HIV/STD-protective benefits of living with mothers in perceived supportive families: a study of high risk African American female teens. Prev Med 33(3):175–178

Cullinane J (2007) The domestication of AIDS: stigma, gender, and the body politic in Japan. Med Anthropol 26(3):255–292

Davies SL, Horton TV, Williams AG, Martin MY, Stewart LE (2009) MOMS: formative evaluation and subsequent intervention for mothers living with HIV. AIDS Care 21(5):552–560

Davison KP, Pennebaker JW, Dickerson SS (2000) Who talks? The social psychology of illness support groups. Am Psychol 55(2):205–217

De Cock KM, Fowler MG, Mercier E, de Vincenzi I, Saba J, Hoff E et al (2000) Prevention of mother-to-child HIV transmission in resource-poor countries: translating research into policy and practice. JAMA 283(9):1175–1182

Deschampsa M-M, Dévieuxb JG, Théodorea H, Saint-Jeanc G, Antillusa L, Cadota L et al (2009) A feeding education program to prevent mother-to-child transmission of HIV in Haiti. AIDS Care 21(3):349–354

Desclaux A, Alfieri C (2009) Counseling and choosing between infant-feeding options: overall limits and local interpretations by health care providers and women living with HIV in resource-poor countries (Burkina Faso, Cambodia, Cameroon). Soc Sci Med 69:821–829

Desclaux A, Alfieri C (2011) Facing competing cultures of breastfeeding: the experience of HIV-positive women in Burkina Faso. In: Liamputtong P (ed) Infant feeding practices: a cross-cultural perspective. Springer, New York, pp 195–200

Desclaux A, Msellati P, Walentowitz S (2009) Women, mothers and HIV care in resource-poor settings. Soc Sci Med 69:803–806

Doherty T (2011) Infant feeding in the era of HIV: challenges and opportunities. In: Liamputtong P (ed) Infant feeding practices: a cross-cultural perspective. Springer, New York, pp 175–193

Donkor ES, Sandall J (2007) The impact of perceived stigma and mediating social factors on infertility-related stress among women seeking infertility treatment in Southern Ghana. Soc Sci Med 65:1683–1694

Doyal L, Anderson A (2005) My fear is to fall in love again. How HIV-positive African women survive in London. Soc Sci Med 60:1729–1738

Dunkle KL, Jewkes RK, Brown HC, Gray GE, McIntryre JA, Harlow SD (2004) Gender-based violence, relationship power, and risk of HIV infection in women attending antenatal clinics in South Africa. Lancet 363(9419):1415–1421

Dyer SJ (2007) The value of children in African countries: insights from studies on infertility. J Psychosom Obstet Gynaecol 28(2):69–77

Epstein CF (2007) Great divides: the cultural, cognitive, and social bases of the global subordination of women. Am Sociol Rev 72(1):1–22

Ferlander S (2007) The importance of different forms of social capital for health. Acta Sociol 50(2):115–128

Finocchario-Kessler S, Sweat MD, Dariotis JK, Trent ME, Kerrigan DL, Keller JM, Anderson JR (2010) Understanding high fertility desires and intentions among a sample of urban women living with HIV in the United States. AIDS Behav 14(5):1106–1114

Fleischman J (2003) Fatal vulnerabilities: reducing the acute risk of HIV/AIDS among women and girls. CSIS, Washington, DC. Retrieved 13 May 2008 from: http://www.csis.org/media/csis/pubs/020103_fatal_vulnerabilities.pdf

Germov J (2009) The class origins of health inequality. In: Germov J (ed) Second opinion: an introduction to health sociology, 4th edn. Oxford University Press, Melbourne, pp 85–110

Gerrits T (1997) Social and cultural aspects of infertility in Mozambique. Patient Educ Couns 31(1):39–48

Giddens A (1984) The constitution of society: outline of the theory of structuration. University of California Press, Berkeley

Gielen AC, McDonnell KA, Wu AW, O'Campo P, Faden R (2001) Quality of life among women living with HIV: the importance violence, social support, and self care behaviors. Soc Sci Med 52(2):315–322

Greeff M (2013) Chapter 6: Disclosure and stigma: a cultural perspective. In: Liamputtong P (ed) Stigma, discrimination and HIV/AIDS: a cross-cultural perspective. Springer, Dordrecht

Gregson S (2004) Community group participation: can it help young women to avoid HIV? An exploratory study of social capital and school education in rural Zimbabwe. Soc Sci Med 58(11):2119–2132

Grue L, Laerum KT (2002) "Doing motherhood": some experiences of mothers with physical disabilities. Disabil Soc 17:671–683

Gupta A, Gupte N, Sastry J, Bharucha KE, Bhosale R, Kulkarni P et al (2007) Mother-to-child transmission of HIV among women who chose not to exclusively breastfeed their infants in Pune, India. Int J Med Res 126(2):131–134

Gysae M, Øverland L (2002) Monitoring HIV/AIDS: reporting through gender lens. Retrieved 11 Oct 2011 from: http://www.womensmediawatch.org.za/publication/monitoringHIVaids.pdf

Hankivsky O, Cormier R, deMerich D (2009) Intersectionality: moving women's health research and policy forward. Women's Health Research Network, Vancouver

Héjoaka F (2009) Care and secrecy: being a mother of children living with HIV in Burkina Faso. Soc Sci Med 69:869–876

Hebling EM, Hardy E (2007) Feelings related to motherhood among women living with HIV in Brazil: a qualitative study. AIDS Care 19(9):1095–1100

Herek GM, Capitanio JP (1993) Public reactions to AIDS in the United States: a second decade of stigma. Am J Public Health 83:574–577

Hollos M, Larsen U (2008) Motherhood in sub-Saharan Africa: the social consequences of infertility in an urban population in northern Tanzania. Cult Health Sex 10(2):159–173

Hunt K, Annandale E (2012) General introduction. In: Hunt K, Annandale E (eds) Gender and health: Major themes in health and social welfare. Routledge: London 1:1–11

Inhorn MC (1996) Infertility and patriarchy: the cultural politics of gender and family life in Egypt. University of Pennsylvania Press, Philadelphia

Inhorn MC (2003) 'The worms are weak': male infertility and patriarchal paradoxes in Egypt. Men Masculinities 5(3):236–256

Jewkes R, Levin J, Penn-Kekana L (2003) Gender inequalities, intimate partner violence and HIV preventive practices: findings of a South African cross-sectional study. Soc Sci Med 56:125–134

Johnson-Hanks J (2006) Uncertain honor: modern motherhood in an African crisis. University of Chicago Press, Chicago

Julian R (2009) Ethnicity, health, and multiculturalism. In: Germov J (ed) Second opinion: an introduction to health sociology, 4th edn. Oxford University Press, Melbourne, pp 175–196

Kalichman SC, DiMarco M, Austin J, Luke W, DiFonzo K (2003) Stress, social support and HIV-status disclosure to family and friends among HIV-positive men and women. J Behav Med 26(4):315–332

Kamau-Mbuthia E, Elmadfa I, Mwonya R (2008) The impact of maternal HIV status on infant feeding patterns in Nakuru, Kenya. J Hum Lact 24:34–41

Kanniappana S, Jeyapaula MJ, Kalyanwala S (2008) Desire for motherhood: exploring HIV-positive women's desires, intentions and decision-making in attaining motherhood. AIDS Care 20(6):625–630

Kasenga F, Hurtig A-K, Emmelin M (2010) HIV-positive women's experiences of a PMTCT programme in rural Malawi. Midwifery 26:27–37

Kaye D (2004) Gender inequality and domestic violence: implications for human immunodeficiency virus (HIV) prevention. Afr Health Sci 4(1):67–70

Keleher H, MacDougall C (2009) Understanding health. In: Keleher H, MacDougall C (eds) Understanding health: a determinants approach, 2nd edn. Oxford University Press, Melbourne, pp 3–16

Kisakye P, Owot Akena W, Kabonge Kaye D (2010) Pregnancy decisions among HIV-positive pregnant women in Mulago Hospital, Uganda. Cult Health Sex 12(4):445–454

Kourtis AP, Lee FK, Abrams EJ, Jamieson DJ, Bulterys M (2006) Mother-to-child transmission of HIV-1: timing and implications for prevention. Lancet Infect Dis 6(11):726–732

Kremer H, Sonnenberg-Schwan U (2003) Women living with HIV does sex and gender matter? A current literature review. Eur J Med Res 8(1):8–16

Krieger N (2003) Genders, sexes and health: what are the connections—and why does it matter? Int J Epidemiol 32:652–657

Larsen U, Hollos M, Obono O, Whitehouse B (2010) Suffering infertility: the impact of infertility on women's life experiences in two Nigerian communities. J Biosoc Sci 42(6):787–814

Latham BC, Sowell RL, Phillips KD, Murdaugh C (2001) Family functioning and motivation for Childbearing among HIV-infected women at increased risk for pregnancy. J Fam Nurs 7(4): 345–370

Li L, Ji G, Liang L-J, Ding Y, Tian J, Xiao Y (2011) A multilevel intervention for HIV-affected families in China: Together for Empowerment Activities (TEA). Soc Sci Med 73(8): 1214–1221

Liamputtong P (2009) Treating the afflicted body: perceptions of infertility and ethnomedicine among fertile Hmong women in Australia. In: Culley L, Hudson N, van Rooij F (eds) Marginalized reproduction: ethnicity, infertility and reproductive technologies. Earthscan Publisher, Oxford, pp 151–164

Liamputtong P (2011) Infant feeding beliefs and practices across cultures: an introduction. In: Liamputtong P (ed) Infant feeding practices: a cross-cultural perspective. Springer, New York, pp 1–20

Liamputtong P (ed) (2013) Stigma, discrimination and HIV/AIDS: a cross-cultural perspective. Springer, Dordrecht

Liamputtong P, Haritavorn N, Kiatying-Angsulee N (2009) HIV and AIDS, stigma and AIDS support groups: perspectives from women living with HIV and AIDS in central Thailand. Soc Sci Med 69(6):862–868

Liamputtong P, Fanany R, Verrinder G (2012) Health, illness and well-being: an introduction. In: Liamputtong P, Fanany R, Verrinder G (eds) Health, illness and well-being: perspectives and social determinants. Oxford University Press, Melbourne, pp 1–17

Lindau ST, Jerome J, Miller K, Monk E, Garcia P, Cohen M (2006) Mothers on the margins: implications for eradicating perinatal HIV. Soc Sci Med 62:59–69

Lorber J (1994) Paradoxes of gender. Yale University Press, New Haven

Lorber J (1997) Gender and the social construction of illness. Sage, Thousand Oaks

Magadi MA (2011a) Understanding the gender disparity in HIV infection across countries in sub-Saharan Africa: evidence from the Demographic and Health Surveys. Sociol Health Illn 33(4):522–539

Magadi MA (2011b) Household and community HIV/AIDS status and child malnutrition in sub-Saharan Africa: evidence from the demographic and health surveys. Soc Sci Med 73(3):436–446

Maman S, Mbwambo JK, Hogan NM, Kilonzo GP, Campbell JC, Weiss E et al (2002) HIV-positive women report more life time partner violence: findings from a voluntary welfare. Am J Public Health 92(8):1331–1337

Maru S, Datong P, Selleng D, Mang E, Inyang B, Ajene A et al (2009) Social determinants of mixed feeding behavior among HIV-infected mothers in Jos, Nigeria. AIDS Care 21(9): 1114–1123

Matsubayashi H, Hosaka T, Izumi S, Suzuki T, Makino T (2001) Emotional distress of infertile women in Japan. Hum Reprod 16(5):966–969

Mbekenga CK, Christensson K, Lugina H, Olsson P (2011) Joy, struggle and support: postpartum experiences of first-time mothers in a Tanzanian suburb. Women Birth 24:24–31

Mizuno Y, Purcell DW, Dawson-Rose C, Parsons JT (2003) Correlates of depressive symptoms among HIV-positive injection drug users: the role of social support. AIDS Care 15(5): 689–698

Murray LR, Garcia J, Muñoz-Laboy M, Parker RG (2011) Strange bedfellows: the Catholic Church and Brazilian National AIDS Program in the response to HIV/AIDS in Brazil. Soc Sci Med 72(6):945–952

Nakayiwa S, Abang B, Packel L, Lifshay J, Purcell DW, King E et al (2006) Desire for children and pregnancy risk behavior among HIV-infected men and women in Uganda. AIDS Behav 10:95–104

Nassalia M, Nakanjakob D, Kyabayinzec D, Beyezaa J, Okotha A, Mutyaba T (2009) Access to HIV/AIDS care for mothers and children in sub-Saharan Africa: adherence to the postnatal PMTCT program. AIDS Care 21(9):1124–1131

National AIDS Control Organization (NACO) (2006) HIV/AIDS epidemiological surveillance & estimation report for the year 2005. Government of India: Ministry of Health & Family

Nattabi B, Li J, Thompson SC, Garimoi Orach C, Earnest J (2009) A systematic review of factors influencing fertility desires and intentions among people living with HIV/AIDS: implications for policy and service delivery. AIDS Behav 13(5):949–968

Nduna M, Farlane L (2009) Women living with HIV in South Africa and their concerns about fertility. AIDS Behav 13:S62–S65

Nóbrega AA, Oliveira FAS, Galvão MTG, Mota RS, Barbosa RM, Dourado I et al (2007) Desire for a child among women living with HIV/AIDS in Northeast Brazil. AIDS Patient Care STDS 21(4):261–267

Nyqvist F (2009) Social capital and health: variations, associations and challenges. Abo Academi University, Vasa

Paiva V, Santos N, Franca-Junior I, Filipe E, Ayres JR, Segurado A (2007) Desire to have children: gender and reproductive rights of men and women living with HIV: a challenge to health care in Brazil. AIDS Patient Care STDS 21(4):268–277

Pallikadavath S, Stones RW (2003) Disseminating knowledge about AIDS through Indian family planning programme: prospects and limitations. AIDS (London, England) 17, 2008–2009

Panozzo L, Battegay M, Friedl A, Vernazza PL (2003) Swiss Cohort Study: high risk behaviour and fertility desires among heterosexual HIV-positive patients with a serodiscordant partner–two challenging issues. Swiss Med Wkly 133(7–8):124–127

Parker R, Aggleton P (2003) HIV and AIDS-related stigma and discrimination: a conceptual framework and implications for action. Soc Sci Med 57:13–24

Piwoz EG, Ferguson YO, Bentley ME, Corneli AL, Moses A, Nkhoma J, Tohill BC, Mtimuni B, Ahmed Y, Jamieson DJ, van der Horst C, Kazembe P, the UNC Project BAN Study Team (2006) Differences between international recommendations on breastfeeding in the presence of HIV and the attitudes and counselling messages of health workers in Lilongwe, Malawi. Int Breastfeed J 1:2. Retrieved 17 May 2010 from: http://www.internationalbreastfeedingjournal.com/content/1/1/2

Plowden KO, Fletcher A, Miller JL (2005) Factors influencing HIV-risk behaviors among HIV-positive urban African Americans. J Assoc Nurses AIDS Care 16(1):21–28

Qiao S, Li X, Stanton B (2011) Disclosure of parental HIV infection to children: a systematic review of global literature. AIDS Behav. doi:10.1007/s10461-011-0069-x

Rashid SF (2007) *Kal dristi*, stolen babies and 'blocked uteruses': poverty and infertility anxieties among married adolescent women living in a slum in Dhaka, Bangladesh. Anthropol Med 14(2):153–166

Richmond CAM, Ross NA, Egeland GM (2007) Social support and thriving health: a new approach to understanding the health of indigenous Canadians. Am J Public Health 97(9):1827–1833

Risman BJ (2004) Gender as a social structure: theory wrestling with activism. Gend Soc 18(4):429–450

Risman BJ (2011) Gender as structure or trump card? J Family Theory Rev 3:18–22

Rosenfeld E (1997) Social support and health status: a literature review. South Australian Community Health Research Unit, Adelaide

Rosenfield A, Yanda K (2002) AIDS treatment and maternal mortality in resource-poor countries. J Am Med Womens Assoc 57(3):167–168

Rossi AS, Fonsequi-Carvasan GA, Makuch MY, Amaral E, Bahamondes L (2005) Factors associated with reproductive options in HIV infected women. Contraception 71(1):45–50

Sandelowski M, Barroso J (2003) Motherhood in the context of maternal HIV infection. Res Nurs Health 26:470–482

Serovich JM, Kimberly JA, Mosack KE, Lewis TL (2001) The role of family and friend social support in reducing emotional distress among HIV positive women. AIDS Care 13(3): 335–341

Simbayi LC, Kalichman S, Strebel A, Cloete A, Henda N, Mqeketo A (2007) Internalized stigma, discrimination, and depression among men and women living with HIV/AIDS in Cape Town, South Africa. Soc Sci Med 64(9):1823–1831

Smith DJ, Mbakwem BC (2007) Life projects and therapeutic itineraries: marriage, fertility, and antiretroviral therapy in Nigeria. AIDS 21(5):37–41

Sowell RL, Seals BF, Moneyham L, Demi A, Cohen L, Brake S (1997) Quality of life in HIV-infected women in the southeastern United States. AIDS Care 9:501–512

Strebel A, Crawford M, Shefer T, Cloete A, Henda N, Kaufman M et al (2006) Social constructions of gender roles, gender-based violence and HIV/AIDS in two communities in the Western Cape, South Africa. J Soc Aspects HIV/AIDS 3(3):516–528

The Joint United Nations Programme on HIV/AIDS (2009) AIDS epidemic update, December 2009. The Joint United Nations Programme on HIV/AIDS, Geneva. Retrieved 25 Mar 2010 from: http://data.unaids.org/pub/Report/2009/JC1700_Epi_Update_2009_en.pdf

Thomas F (2006) Stigma, fatigue and social breakdown: exploring the impacts of HIV/AIDS on patient and carer well-being in the Caprivi Region, Namibia. Soc Sci Med 63(12):3174–3187

Thomas BE, Rehman F, Suryanarayanan D, Josephine K, Dilip M, Dorairaj VS et al (2005) How stigmatizing is stigma in the life of people living with HIV: a study on HIV-positive individuals from Chennai, South India. AIDS Care 17(7):795–801

Thomas B, Nyamathi A, Swaminathan S (2009) Impact of HIV/AIDS on mothers in Southern India: a qualitative study. AIDS Behav 13:989–996

Türmen T (2003) Gender and HIV/AIDS. Int J Gynecol Obstet 82:411–418

Turan JM, Miller S, Bukusi EA, Sande J, Cohen CR (2008) HIV/AIDS and maternity care in Kenya: how fears of stigma and discrimination affect uptake and provision of labor and delivery services. AIDS Care 20(8):938–945

UNAIDS (2008) Report on the global HIV/AIDS epidemic 2008. UNAIDS, Geneva

UNAIDS (2010) UNAIDS report on the global AIDS epidemic. UNAIDS, Geneva

UNICEF (2007) The state of the world's children 2008. Child survival. UNICEF, New York. Retrieved 23 Oct 2011 from: http://www.unicef.org/publications/index_42623.html

UNICEF/UNAIDS/WHO/UNFPA (2010) Children and AIDS: fifth stocktaking report. UNICEF/UNAIDS/WHO/UNFPA, New York. Retrieved 18 Oct 2011 from: http://www.childinfo.org/files/ChildrenAndAIDS_Fifth_Stocktaking_Report_2010_EN.pdf

Upchurch DM, Kusunoki Y (2004) Associations between forced sex, sexual and protective practices, and sexually transmitted diseases among a national sample of adolescent girls. Womens Health Issues 14(3):75–84

Wesley Y, Smeltzer SC, Redeker NS, Walker S, Palumbo P, Whipple B (2000) Reproductive decision making in mothers with HIV-1. Health Care Women Int 21:291–304

WHO/UNAIDS/UNICEF (2011) Global HIV response: progress report 2011. WHO/UNAIDS/UNICEF, Geneva. Retrieved 30 Aug 2012 from: http://www.who.int/hiv/pub/progress_report2011/hiv_full_report_2011.pdf

WHO/UNICEF/UNFPA/UNAIDS (2007a) HIV and infant feeding. New evidence and programmatic experience. Report of a technical consultation. World Health Organization, Geneva

WHO/UNICEF/UNFPA/UNAIDS (2007b) HIV and infant feeding. Update. World Health Organization, Geneva. Retrieved 28 Nov 2008 from: http://whqlibdoc.who.int/publications/2007/9789241595964_eng.pdf

Wilcher R, Cates W Jr (2010) Reaching the underserved: family planning for women with HIV. Stud Fam Plann 41(2):125–128

Wilson S (2007) 'When you have children, you're obliged to live': motherhood, chronic illness and biographical disruption. Sociol Health Illn 29(4):610–626

World Health Organization (2000) Violence against women and HIV/AIDS. World Health Organization, Geneva

Wyrod R (2013) Chapter 5: Gender and AIDS stigma. In: Liamputtong P (ed) Stigma, discrimination and HIV/AIDS: a cross-cultural perspective. Springer, Dordrecht

Zhao G, Li X, Fang X, Zhao J, Hong Y, Lin X, Stanton B (2011) Functions and sources of perceived social support among children affected by HIV/AIDS in China. AIDS Care 23(6): 671–679

Zierler S, Whitbeck B, Mayer K (1996) Sexual violence among women living with or at risk for HIV infection. Am J Prev Med 12:304–310

Part I
Women, Reproduction and HIV/AIDS

Chapter 2
Growing Confidence? Family Planning by HIV-Positive Mothers in a South African Urban Setting

Ray Lazarus, Helen Struthers, and Avy Violari

1 Introduction

In sub-Saharan Africa, more than half of the 22.5 million people living with HIV/AIDS (PLWHA) are women (UNAIDS 2010). HIV poses additional risks during pregnancy: a report on maternal mortality in South Africa for the period 2005–2007 identified HIV/AIDS as the largest cause of maternal mortality (NCCEMD 2008). Worldwide, in 2011 despite a drop of 24% since 2009, 330,000 children were newly infected with HIV, the majority through mother-to-child transmission (MTCT) (UNAIDS 2012). Although this was a significant decrease from previous years, much remains to be done to achieve the goal of virtual elimination of MTCT by 2015 (UNICEF/UNAIDS/WHO/UNPF 2010). Preventing unintended pregnancies amongst women living with HIV is a critical strategy both to reduce mortality related to pregnancy and to prevent mother-to-child transmission (PMTCT) (NDOH/SANAC 2010; WHO 2010).

However, despite wide support for family planning[1] and for strengthening linkages between HIV/AIDS services and sexual and reproductive health (SRH)

---

[1] The term, family planning, is used rather than the alternative, reproductive choices, since the former is the term in general use in many guidelines and, in South Africa, amongst women themselves and healthcare workers.

R. Lazarus (✉)
Perinatal HIV Research Unit, University of the Witwatersrand,
Chris Hani Baragwanath Hospital, 20 22nd Street, Menlo Park, Pretoria 0081, South Africa
e-mail: ianray@telkomsa.net

H. Struthers
Anova Health Institute, Postnet Suite 242, Private Bag X30500,
Houghton, Johannesburg 2041, South Africa
e-mail: struthers@anovahealth.co.za

A. Violari
Paediatric Division, Perinatal HIV Research Unit, University of the Witwatersrand,
Chris Hani Baragwanath Hospital, P.O. Box 114, Diepkloof Soweto 1864, South Africa
e-mail: violari@mweb.co.za

P. Liamputtong (ed.), *Women, Motherhood and Living with HIV/AIDS:*
A Cross-Cultural Perspective, DOI 10.1007/978-94-007-5887-2_2,
© Springer Science+Business Media Dordrecht 2013

services[2] (FHI 2010a, b), operationalization remains disappointing (Wilcher and Cates 2010). Moreover, there is little in the way of specific guidance on how to engage with PLWHA on family planning, increasing the likelihood that health workers' own values and attitudes will affect how guidelines are implemented (London et al. 2008). South African guidelines (NDOH/SANAC 2010), for example, provide detailed protocols on counseling and testing, antiretroviral prophylaxis and promotion of safe feeding practises, but refer to family planning only under the general rubric of "counseling on safer sex, family planning and contraception". Such a directive fails to address the complicated set of issues that counseling on family planning needs to deal with, including information on risks of pregnancy for HIV-positive women and transmission to infants, contraceptive options (including termination of pregnancy, where appropriate), attitudes and possible involvement of male partners or other family members, gender norms and, not least, rights to autonomous decision-making (Gruskin et al. 2007). With regard to the latter, it is important to distinguish between desires to have (or not have) children (fertility desires), intentions or decisions to pursue or to avoid pregnancy, and actual practise, expressed in pregnancy rates (Ndlovu 2009).

The focus of this chapter is to explore issues related to family planning for HIV-positive women. The chapter starts with a brief literature review, focusing primarily on studies in sub-Saharan Africa. We then report on a qualitative study carried out in Soweto, South Africa, focusing on findings relevant to the fertility desires and family planning intentions and practise of a group of HIV-positive mothers of young HIV-negative or HIV-positive babies. We conclude by discussing the findings and drawing out some implications for healthcare guidelines and practise.

2 Literature Review

Demographic, cultural, psychosocial and socio-economic factors all play a role in the desire and final decision to have children (Nóbrega et al. 2007; Nattabi et al. 2009). Some of the significant interlinked factors impacting on the childbearing decision-making process for PLWHA – both as motivators to fall pregnant and as pressures not to fall pregnant – are age and gender, already having children, family and partner attitudes towards childbearing, health concerns, understanding of and access to PMTCT and highly active antiretroviral therapy (HAART), duration of HAART, disclosure (or not) of HIV status, stigma-related concerns and health worker attitudes and practises.

---

[2] Although the focus in this chapter is on prevention of unintended pregnancy, linkages/integration of HIV/AIDS and SRH services are also intended to offer more effective services to support maternal health during pregnancy and delivery and offer PLWHA who wish to have children appropriate counselling related to child spacing and ways to limit risks of transmission to partners during conception and from mother to child.

2.1 HIV Status and Fertility Desires

Studies in sub-Saharan Africa have shown that being HIV-positive does not eliminate women's desire to have children (Gray et al. 1998; Boerma and Urassa 2000; Hunter et al. 2003). However, fertility desires are generally relatively low and considerably lower than in the case of HIV-negative women (Rutenberg and Baek 2005; Nakayiwa et al. 2006; Elul et al. 2009). Importantly, studies undertaken after the introduction of broader access to HAART have shown that desire for children may increase amongst women who have access to HAART (Maier et al. 2009; Ndlovu 2009), who express optimism about HAART (Kaida et al. 2009), who have improved health due to HAART (Panozzo et al. 2003) and with longer duration of HAART (Smith and Mbakwem 2007). Whether increase in desire leads to increases in pregnancy rates is not clear.

2.2 Age and Existing Children

A number of studies (Nakayiwa et al. 2006; Myer et al. 2007; Nóbrega et al. 2007; Cooper et al. 2009; Peltzer et al. 2009; Kakaire et al. 2010) have found a significant correlation between fertility desires and age, with younger women more likely to want children than older women. Possibly linked to this association, some studies suggest that already having (surviving) children may decrease the likelihood of strong fertility desires amongst PLWHA (Nakayiwa et al. 2006; Myer et al. 2007; Nóbrega et al. 2007). However, in contrast, Peltzer et al. (2009) found no association between the number of prior children and fertility desire in HIV-positive women.

2.3 Social Roles

Realizing parenthood is part of a broader set of social relations and pressures that impact on PLWHA's desires and intentions to bear children. The possibility of discussion or negotiation between partners (or indeed, others) on these matters is largely dependent on deep-seated "cultural scripts" that dictate the respective roles of women and men in sexual behavior and in decisions on limiting fertility (UNICEF/UNAIDS/WHO/UNPF 2010).

The desire for children amongst PLWHA – especially women – often reflects a central belief that to fulfil their role in society, women *must* have children (Nakayiwa et al. 2006; Cooper et al. 2007; Myer et al. 2007; Long 2009). Childbearing serves as a significant marker of various aspects of womanhood, providing proof of a relationship with a man and raising women's status in the family; however, because of the high value placed on children and a tendency to blame women for infertility, in many African societies, childlessness and infertility are highly stigmatizing and can result in negative social repercussions such as loss of social status, blame and rejection for women (Long 2009; Ujiji et al. 2010; see also Chaps. 1, 5 and 6 in this volume).

For both men and women, the desire for children is linked to the idea of lineage and posterity (Beyeza-Kashesya et al. 2009). For men, fertility is also considered proof of virility – central to South African male social identity (Cooper et al. 2007). Some studies (Nakayiwa et al. 2006; Myer et al. 2007; Cooper et al. 2009) have found that HIV-positive men were more likely than HIV-positive women to want additional children, implying the possibility of pressure on female partners, even when contrary to the latter's wishes. Very high rates of sexual violence in South Africa, within and outside intimate relationships and legitimated by patriarchal attitudes (Gender Links/MRC 2010), may also contribute to unintended pregnancies.

There is some evidence of challenges to these entrenched attitudes, at least in the case of PLWHA. Most HIV-positive women participants in a study in Zimbabwe (Feldman and Maposhere 2003) thought that HIV-positive women should not have children, a belief they assumed was shared by relatives and community members. These findings require replication but may in any case reflect an aspect of HIV stigma rather than a more general change in underlying attitudes.

2.4 Stigma and Disclosure

Many HIV-positive women are at pains not to disclose their status to others, including their male partners, for fear of rejection, abandonment or violence (Greeff 2013; see also Chap. 15 in this volume). On the other hand, lack of disclosure potentially exposes them to pressure from their families and from their male partners regarding their fertility. To choose not to have (further) children on the grounds of their HIV status thus exposes HIV-positive women to a double stigma: that of not having children and (potentially) that associated with being known to be HIV-positive. Even when wanting to fall pregnant, they are caught in a dilemma that discussing their fertility intentions and HIV status with their partners could expose them to rejection (Ujiji et al. 2010). On the other hand, nondisclosure increases the risk of pregnancy even when this is not desired.

2.5 Knowledge

A critical factor affecting the childbearing desires and intentions of PLWHA is the extent of their knowledge about transmission, the effectiveness of PMTCT measures and effects of pregnancy on their own health. Laher et al. (2009) have argued that much of the decision-making process around pregnancy intentions is based on exaggerated fears about the likelihood of MTCT and negative consequences of pregnancy on their own health and life expectancy (e.g. risk of re-infection with a different HIV strain during attempts to conceive, a decrease in CD4 count in pregnancy, illness during pregnancy and loss of blood at delivery). A number of studies (Feldman and Maposhere 2003; Rutenberg and Baek 2005; Cooper et al. 2007; Kanniappan et al. 2008) have confirmed that such fears are common. Thus, it is not surprising that knowledge of PMTCT strategies (Peltzer et al. 2009) and optimism about HAART (Kaida et al. 2009) have been found to increase the fertility desires of HIV-positive women.

2.6 Health Workers and Healthcare Practise

The focus of HIV prevention campaigns on avoiding unprotected sex and using condoms can imply that PLWHA should not have (further) children. Many HIV-positive women have internalized this message and find it reinforced by health workers, whose attitudes and beliefs – often judgmental and moralistic – can powerfully influence decision-making with regard to fertility (Tavrow 2010). Negative attitudes towards termination as an option to deal with unintended pregnancy remain common amongst health workers (Harries et al. 2009).

Health workers may act as gatekeepers of knowledge, sometimes providing incorrect or outdated information (Tavrow 2010) or information filtered through their own attitudes towards sexual activity or pregnancy in PLWHA (Harries et al. 2007). Rather than providing a balanced appraisal of risks and preventive measures, the negative aspects of pregnancy tend to be stressed (Oladapo et al. 2005; Laher et al. 2009). Even when not overtly prescriptive, counseling tends to emphasise biomedical consideration (Harries et al. 2007) rather than the myriad other factors influencing fertility desires and intentions – let alone practise, which is often strongly influenced by male partners.

In routine clinical care, counseling around issues of fertility and contraception generally takes place around the time of the birth of a child and/or HAART initiation (Myer et al. 2007; Nduna and Farlane 2009). Yet, since fertility desires may change over time (and specifically over time on HAART), a more responsive form of engagement is necessary in long-term care, adapting counseling and contraceptive advice to the changing needs of clients (Myer et al. 2007; Laher et al. 2009).

What we have discussed above sketches only some of the competing influences on the fertility desires, intentions and practises of HIV-positive women, together creating a nexus of personal, social, economic and cultural factors that constrain their ability to make decisions on their own terms and to follow through with decisions once made.

3 The Study

This chapter draws on findings from a qualitative study that explored the understandings, attitudes and concerns of HIV-positive women in the context of learning their baby's HIV status in the first few weeks of life. Certain findings have been reported in two earlier papers (Lazarus et al. 2009, 2010). Here, we provide a more in-depth account of reported fertility desires, intentions and practises of mothers of

HIV-negative or HIV-positive babies and attempt to situate what they had to say in the context of social norms and pressures influencing them.

3.1 Study Context[3]

Fieldwork took place at an HIV research and treatment site in Soweto, a township of Johannesburg. At the time of this study, the site provided polymerase chain reaction (PCR) testing for HIV for 60% of HIV-exposed babies in Soweto and follow-up healthcare for the majority of those testing HIV-positive. Fieldwork was carried out over a 10-week period in November 2006–January 2007.

Soweto, a township with a population of around two million, is located about 15 km from the Johannesburg city centre. Unemployment rates were (and remain) high. Most residents use the public health system (Gray et al. 2006). There is widespread awareness of HIV and AIDS. Nevertheless, seroprevalence rates in pregnant women are high (just under 30%) (NDOH 2010). However, uptake of HIV testing and the PMTCT regimen by pregnant women during antenatal care is high, as is subsequent testing of their babies for HIV on a PCR test at 4–6 weeks. Perinatal transmission rates on the single-dose nevirapine (NVP) regimen at the time of this study were around 8.4% (Struthers et al. 2006).[4] Babies who test HIV-positive are eligible for enrolment in HAART programmes at government health services or donor-funded partner sites (Mphatswe et al. 2007; Violari et al. 2007).

3.2 Methods

3.2.1 Recruitment of Study Participants

A sample of convenience of HIV-positive mothers was recruited when they brought their babies for PCR testing. Mothers of HIV-negative babies were interviewed[5] on average 2 weeks after receiving the PCR test results; mothers of HIV-positive

---

[3] Ethical approval for the study was obtained from the Ethics Committee of the University of the Witwatersrand, Johannesburg, South Africa.

[4] In 2011, following a year of implementing the 2010 revised WHO PMTCT guidelines, national rates had fallen to 2.7% (Dinh et al. 2012); based on a previous study (Goga et al. 2012), rates in Soweto were likely to be similar or lower, though still a matter for concern.

[5] Written informed consent to participate in tape-recorded interviews was obtained before the interviews. Confidentiality was assured by recording all data under anonymous codes, removing any identifying information during interview transcription and destroying interview tape recordings on completion of the study.

babies were interviewed about 5 weeks after receiving their baby's results, hence when their babies were on average somewhat older than the HIV-positive babies (see below). The difference reflects primarily an ethical decision to defer interviews of mothers of HIV-positive babies in order to minimise possible stress on receiving the result. In addition, some mothers (more often of HIV-positive babies) were interviewed later due to scheduling of clinic visits or to the baby having been ill and/or needing hospitalization.

3.2.2 Data Collection and Analysis

A trained fieldworker conducted qualitative, in-depth interviews with participants in their preferred language, using an interview guide comprising open-ended questions on a range of issues (see Box 1).

A second fieldworker translated and transcribed the recordings into English. The transcriptions were then reviewed for accuracy by the fieldworker responsible for the interviews. Both fieldworkers assisted in clarifying uncertainties or ambiguities in meaning encountered during data analysis.

Thematic analysis was used to identify themes that appeared significant to participants, as well as those of interest from a healthcare perspective (Ritchie and Spencer 1994). Generally, there was no attempt to quantify the occurrence of themes. Rather, following a qualitative paradigm, the intention was to highlight not only themes that seemed characteristic across participants (indicated by shorthand references such as "most" or "often") but also less common themes, which may reflect ideas that are less often expressed, but are nevertheless potentially significant in a healthcare context.

Box 1 Questions from Interview Guide

- Was this baby planned? How did you feel when you found out you were pregnant?
- After getting the PCR result, what are your thoughts about the possibility of falling pregnant again?
- As far as you know, what are the risks for you of having a HIV-positive child if you were to fall pregnant again?
- Are you using any method of family planning at present? If yes, what and why? What do you plan to do about family planning in future?
- What are/would be the difficulties for you in sticking to the method you prefer? (Do other people cause difficulties?) What would make it easier for you to stick to the method?

Because of significant commonality across participants in the findings reported here, themes are not differentiated by status of the baby, except where there appear to be clear differences. Selected quotations have been used to illustrate the themes described in the report.

3.2.3 Participant Profile

Two groups of women – 20 mothers of HIV-negative babies and 18 mothers of HIV-positive babies – participated in the study. Mothers of HIV-negative and HIV-positive babies were similar in age (average 29 and 27 years, respectively), education (all with at least some high school education), employment status (the majority unemployed) and household composition (living with an average of 3.5 other people, generally not including a male partner). These profiles are fairly typical of young women living in Soweto (Gray et al. 2006).

For both groups, the median number of children was two. For two mothers of HIV-negative babies and six mothers of HIV-positive babies, this was their first baby. Interview data suggested that most (but not all) mothers in both groups had no other HIV-infected children.

A minority of the women were on HAART – five mothers of HIV-negative babies and just one mother of an HIV-positive baby – and most described their health as good, apart from minor complaints. All except three women had taken PMTCT prophylaxis, as had their babies.

Median age of the babies at the time of the interview was 5.7 weeks (range = 4.9–13.7 weeks) for HIV-negative and 10.6 weeks (6.7–16.0 weeks) for HIV-positive babies. Just more than two-thirds of the HIV-positive babies were on HAART. A third of HIV-positive babies had been ill or hospitalised at least once, while this applied to only two (10%) of the HIV-negative babies.

Most women (18 mothers of HIV-negative babies and 17 mothers of HIV-positive babies) had disclosed their HIV status to at least one other person, generally a female member of her extended family. Slightly more than half of the women had disclosed their status to a male partner; those who had not done so were generally no longer involved with the partner.

4   Findings

4.1   Prior Intentions and Reactions to Finding Themselves Pregnant

Most women from both groups said their current baby was not planned. Some women who had been using some form of contraception said their contraception had failed; those who were not assumed that they were protected for a time after stopping contraception, or because they did not like the side effects of contraception, or they were intending to use contraception but had not yet gotten round to doing so:

> I had been using contraceptives, but I had previously gone for three years without using them ... so before realizing that I was pregnant, I was telling myself that I was going to use contraceptives again, because I wasn't prepared to have another baby. [Lerato (12)[6]]

Some women had fallen pregnant while knowing they were HIV-positive, sometimes due to contraceptive failure or their partners' unwillingness to use condoms and their own fear of rejection if they were to insist. Some accounts suggested that where earlier children had tested negative, this might have reduced the felt pressure to use contraception and do so consistently.

For some women, their feelings about finding out that they were pregnant were coloured by their learning at more or less the same time that they themselves were HIV-positive: pregnancy and HIV were thus intimately connected. A few who had wanted to have a baby were nevertheless happy to find themselves pregnant:

> I was beginning to think that I was now unable to bear children, because we had been trying for a long time to conceive – even my boyfriend thought that he was infertile. [Tumi (5)]

In contrast, most said that the pregnancy was problematic in some way, although some said they found a way to come to terms with the fact:

> What came into my mind is that God wanted to give me this baby because he came when I was using protection and I [had] miscarried twice, so God wanted me to have a baby, with or without HIV. [Nomonde (8)]

Overall, ambivalent acceptance of the pregnancy was perhaps the most common response – but not solely because of the implications of their HIV-positive status for the baby. Concerns expressed included being too young, not married, fearing the reaction of their parents, being financially stressed, already having the responsibility of another young child and the possible effect of pregnancy on their own health. Additionally, there were the dilemmas and tragedy that HIV can bring to the relationship with a sexual partner:

> It's the first time ever that I have met someone who loves me and treats me the way he does ... [but] when I had this baby I found out that I am HIV-positive, so I was very disappointed... because I loved and trusted his father so much, but he infected me. [Eva (9)]

Close to a third of the women – more of them with HIV-positive babies – reported considering termination of pregnancy but were dissuaded by their own moral beliefs,

---

[6] Not her real name – pseudonyms are used throughout to protect the identity of participants. Number in brackets – participant number (numbers less than 30, mothers of HIV-negative babies; numbers 30 and above, mothers of HIV-positive babies).

to a lesser extent by male partners or relatives, or because of the timing of discovering they were pregnant:

> I would have terminated it, but I found out late, and my partner knew [about the pregnancy] … so it was difficult for me to terminate it, but if he hadn't known, I would have done it because my CD4 was low and the baby can't fight for himself. [Lindiwe (44)]

Two mothers, whose babies tested positive, now regretted that they had not terminated the pregnancy. One mother said:

> I thought of aborting, but something came to my mind that … there is a possibility that she might be negative, so now when I learned that she was positive, I realized that aborting would have been the right choice. [Tshidi (35)]

However, whether other women might have shared this view is not known.

4.2   Falling Pregnant Again

Mothers of HIV-negative babies generally said they would not want to have another baby, with only one expressing some ambivalence. Although the majority of mothers of HIV-positive babies also said they did not plan to have more children, a number did allow the possibility of further pregnancy. Some spoke about pregnancy as a vague possibility sometime in the future, rather than as a definite intention, or expressed ambivalence. Others placed conditions on their having another baby ('I want to have another baby, but after 5 years' [Lindiwe (44)], 'if I get married' [Susan (37)]).

Reasons for not having more children varied, but were similar in both groups. Some referred simply to their own status as self-evidently sufficient reason for not having any more children: "Why would one want to bring a child into this world knowing full well that you are positive?" [Thandi (14)]. For some, a decision already taken and implemented to be sterilised or use other contraception effectively closed discussion on the issue of future pregnancy.

Concern about the possibility of having an(other) HIV-positive child was mentioned but as one amongst many other reasons given. Only one woman explicitly mentioned that taking prophylaxis does not guarantee PMTCT. For some mothers of HIV-positive babies, particularly those whose babies had in the first few weeks of their lives already been seriously ill, there were painful disincentives:

> I don't want her [another baby] to go through the suffering that my baby is going through … coming to the clinic this much, having your blood drawn through your neck and eventually having to live on treatment is too much for a baby. [Mahlodi (47)]

Many women said they were satisfied with the number of children they already had, taking into account their wish and capacity to provide good care for them. It seemed likely that this position was reinforced by the fact of their own and, in the case of HIV-positive babies, their baby's status. As regards capacity to care for their children, some referred to their own constrained material and financial circumstances, factors that may have assumed extra significance because of their HIV-positive status.

The need to be vigilant in protecting their own health was also highlighted. Some understood that being HIV-positive meant their health was compromised: "How can I have another baby when I am sick? … even though I am not yet showing [signs], I am sick" [Karabo (2)]. One woman gave a clear account of the risk of re-infection that would flow from having unprotected sex in order to have another baby. Many were aware that their HIV status meant that there were risks to their health additional to those ordinarily applying in the case of pregnancy and childbirth. These views might reflect or be reinforced by views circulating in the community:

> I sometimes hear people saying that some people die immediately after giving birth [and] that if an HIV-positive person has more than two children, she gets sick…. [Tumi (5)]

4.3 Contraception

Responses regarding the use of contraception may have reflected attitudes and practices relating to the resumption of sexual intercourse relatively soon after delivery when the interviews took place. A few women talked about abstaining from sexual intercourse, either because they had recently given birth or because they were not currently in a relationship with a man, or, in one case (a mother of an HIV-positive baby), because her partner was refusing to use condoms. However, most women indicated that they were using or intending to use some form of contraception (see also Chap. 3). Some women were undecided about whether or what contraceptive to use, either because of lack of knowledge or based on past negative experience with one or more forms of contraceptive. Amongst those not currently using contraception, responses implied some lack of urgency to arrange contraception, possibly because they were not currently in a sexual relationship or were not yet ready or under pressure to resume sexual intercourse. However, the history of contraceptive use by some of the women suggested that delay might carry risks of unintended pregnancy.

Health-related concerns (including the possibility of infecting partners or being reinfected – see further below) were a major motivator. For some women, the possibility of unplanned pregnancy as a result of the ever-present threat of rape in South Africa was a factor:

> I am going to use prevention because there are so many rapists and maybe I can be a victim, so to prevent conception, I will have to use contraception. [Nontobeko (32)]

The most frequently mentioned forms of contraception were sterilization, injectable contraceptives and condoms. Contraceptive pills were generally not favored because of the risk of forgetting to take them regularly.

A number of women had already been sterilized (sometimes in consultation with their male partners), while others were considering sterilization. At least one woman was not sure what sterilization entailed – it is possible that others were in a similar position. Some women saw sterilization as an effective form of contraception, while others doubted its reliability and permanence:

> I spoke to other people [patients] at the clinic – some said it is possible to fall pregnant if you have sterilized and others said it's a lie, so I don't know who to believe, because some from that group I spoke to, they said they have sterilized and they fell pregnant. [Tsietsi (39)]

The "injection" was a commonly chosen form of contraception. Many women had used it previously, and it was seen as convenient and reliable. Some women, however, referred to unpleasant side effects such as dizziness or weight gain, which prevented them from using it.

There was frequent reference to using condoms. Some women who had not yet started or resumed using injectable or other contraceptive measure were using or intending to use condoms meanwhile. Those not currently having sexual relationships also anticipated using condoms should they become sexually active in future. A few women were using condoms as their primary form of contraception, but more often – reflecting strong compliance with a central healthcare message – it was to prevent re-infection (or infection of a partner) or as backup to another primary contraceptive method. The risk of condoms bursting during intercourse was mentioned by a number of women.

Only one woman spoke about the possibility of using a female condom, citing her ability to do so without her partner's knowledge as a strong advantage:

> If I could get female condoms, that would be fine … female condoms are more helpful, because once I used it and he didn't notice, because you put it in six hours before … when you are through with it, you throw it away. I don't think he knows anything about it – he did not feel it and I did not let him see me throwing it away. [Tshidi (35)]

The issue of limited availability is, however, implicit in her statement.

4.4   (En)countering Pressures

Decisions on further childbearing were not always free of pressure from others. As indicated in the profile of participants above, most of the women had disclosed their HIV status to at least one other person, and about half had done so to their male partners, thus mitigating a potential source of difficulty in regard to using contraception. However, male partners still played a role in making and potentially undermining decisions around having children:

> When we decided to fall pregnant [both being HIV-positive], my partner said his reason for wanting to have a baby was for him to leave a picture on earth when he dies … we agreed that we were not going to have another baby after this one … it's something I am sure of, but I'm not sure about my partner, though we had an agreement beforehand that the two we are having now is fine…. [Tumi (5)]

In a few cases, other family members (sometimes at some remove from the woman) played a role in supporting or obstructing decisions on further children. However, women generally represented themselves as relatively autonomous decision-makers:

> It is a problem [pressure to have more children], especially with my partner's family, but I would tell them that maybe God doesn't want me to have other children ... no-one will know about it [use of contraceptives]. [Tsietsi (39)]

Such resistance to family pressure (and, here, subversive use of religious belief) would perhaps not be found amongst other groups of women, particularly in rural areas.

Relatively few women in fact anticipated difficulties in sticking to their chosen form of contraception. With regard to contraception other than condoms, women tended to make decisions independently and without the knowledge of their male partners:

> He doesn't want to use a condom, so I told myself that I am going to use contraceptives [injection] and I won't tell him. [Lindiwe (44)]

However, the need to negotiate with male partners about the use of condoms was an issue, with protection of health (rather than contraception) generally presented as the primary motivation. Many of the women presented themselves as surprisingly assertive in these negotiations:

> I told the baby's father so that he should be aware that from that time, we will no longer have sexual intercourse without a condom. [Tshepiso (3)]

However, women often delayed or avoided talking to their partners about condom use:

> As time goes on, when I feel better, I will discuss it with my boyfriend, because I will have to use them ... but with him, I don't know – I will have to see what he has to say. [Eva (9)]

In some cases, partners reportedly agreed to use condoms relatively easily. In others – perhaps coincidentally, more so amongst the mothers of HIV-positive babies – there was resistance from partners. The result might be resigned acquiescence by the woman:

> I am not using protection [condoms] with my partner, because he doesn't want to use it – he said we can have many babies, he doesn't mind. [Mandisa (18)]

> You know men are men – sometimes he wants to do it flesh to flesh, but sometimes we stick to condoms. [Ellen (43)]

Alternatively, some women reported ongoing disagreement and contestation:

> I tell him that if I have sex without protection, I will be re-infected... [but] he says that there is no HIV and if there is, who came with it and why and we are all going to die, so there is no need for us to use plastic... when he comes by to spend a night, we usually fight about condoms. [Sthembile (33)]

The latter picture is one commonly assumed characteristic of condom negotiation in southern Africa, but, as indicated above, is clearly not the only pattern.

4.5   The Influence of Health Workers

In discussing their intentions in relation to family planning and contraception, women tended to refer to their own prior experiences and the opinions of other women, rather than to advice from health workers. It seemed that health workers encountered in antenatal and postnatal care were primarily focussed on PMTCT and limiting risks to women's health through pregnancy. Condom use was encouraged to prevent re-infection, transmission to sexual partners and conception, and women were given access to other forms of contraception. However, women did not appear to receive in-depth or ongoing counselling on the broader issues involved in family planning.

Of the women who considered termination of the recent pregnancy, only one mentioned discussing the possibility with health workers, as opposed to making a decision on their own or in consultation with their male partner or another relative. On the other hand, health workers played a critical and sometimes contradictory role in influencing intentions and access to sterilization:

> They [health workers] told me that I don't have a choice – I should do it [be sterilized] ...
> because I had already had three children. [Tintswalo (12)]

> They [health workers] told me that if I decide to have [more] children, they can't reverse it
> ... ... they even said what if I get somebody who wants to marry me and maybe that person
> wants to have children? [Nonhlanhla (11)]

Such contradictions, expressed by health workers from the same district health system, must impact on women's decision-making.

5   Discussion

Our findings in many respects concur with other studies mentioned earlier (e.g. Feldman and Maposhere 2003; Rutenberg and Baek 2005; Nakayiwa et al. 2006; Cooper et al. 2009; Elul et al. 2009; Laher et al. 2009), although there are also some unique features. Unintended pregnancy was common, emphasizing the importance of effective reproductive health services for HIV-positive women. Desire for further pregnancy was relatively low. Despite an average of only two children and less certainty amongst women for whom this was the first baby, most women were satisfied with their existing number of children. A link with the related factor of age was not explored in the interviews but may have played a role, given that the women were on average in their mid to late twenties. Health risks were a definite concern: possible infection of any future infants, effects on their own health (such as re-infection, increased maternal risk during pregnancy and childbirth) and possible infection of a sexual partner.

An additional factor affecting fertility desires and intentions which came strongly to the fore in this study was women's assessment of their capacity to provide for their children, not only because of possible effects of illness or death but more importantly taking into account their financial and material circumstances. This strong sense of responsibility to ensure the well-being of their existing children seemed likely to provide significant motivation against unintended pregnancy.

In this study, emotional factors clearly affected women's current views on further pregnancy. Bearing in mind the intimate connection between confirming the most recent pregnancy and learning their own HIV status, loss of trust in the partner who had infected them and their ambivalent acceptance of the most recent pregnancy, this should not be surprising, especially as the interviews took place not long after the birth of their babies. However, emotional factors seem to be under-acknowledged in the literature.

Although possibly an artefact of the small sample, the fact that some women who already had an HIV-positive baby were less certain than mothers of HIV-negative babies about future pregnancy seems contrary to what might be expected. Whether this reflected an element of denial of the reality of their situation was not clear. Knowledge of PMTCT and HAART did not, as found in other studies (Cooper et al. 2009; Kaida et al. 2009; Peltzer et al. 2009), appear to increase fertility desires. However, this might change with increasing time since the birth of the current baby and, as suggested by other studies (e.g. Cooper et al. 2009), as more of these women are on HAART.

Amongst this group of women, there was general acceptance of the need to use contraception. Against a background of high rates of rape, the danger of rape added a uniquely South African dimension. Similar to the findings of Feldman and Maposhere (2003) in Zimbabwe, women mentioned a range of contraceptive options and were generally able to give reasons for their choice. However, delay in starting intended contraceptive use was common, sometimes on the basis of not being currently involved in a sexual relationship but also due to confused understanding of the risks of pregnancy following delivery, or about the various contraceptive options, or concern about the side effects of some options. Having had previous children test HIV-negative may also have diluted the felt pressure to start contraception. As in other studies (e.g. Feldman and Maposhere 2003; Cooper et al. 2009), male partners and, sometimes, family members played a role in making and potentially undermining decisions on contraception. A lack of a sense of urgency in starting contraception clearly increases the risk of unintended pregnancy.

Termination of the most recent pregnancy had been considered by some women but appeared to have been an issue fraught with moral concerns and affected by the attitude of their male partner to the pregnancy. Sterilization was an option a number of women had taken up or were considering following the recent pregnancy. Some confusion and doubts about its effectiveness were expressed, suggesting lack of in-depth information. Contradictory approaches by health workers, as also described by Harries et al. (2007), could have increased doubts about this option.

Stigma and disclosure, or lack thereof, seemed to play a relatively limited role in the family planning intentions and decisions of these women. Most had disclosed to a small number of people, generally within a restricted circle of intimates, sometimes including their male partner. Despite generally accepting or supportive responses, women were, however, not free of fear of negative consequences, especially from male partners, and these fears sometimes affected how family planning intentions were (or were not) put into practise. However, women in this group, perhaps because they already had at least one child and had "survived" disclosure, did not seem to be significantly affected by the double stigma of infertility and HIV and related dilemmas referred to elsewhere (Long 2009; Ujiji et al. 2010).

As in other studies (Nakayiwa et al. 2006; Cooper et al. 2007; Myer et al. 2007; Long 2009), social role requirements affected women's fertility desires and intentions. These were reflected in the need to have children as part of a woman's self-identity and pressure from male partners (with respect to the sexual responsibilities expected of a wife or female partner, as well as lineage and posterity) and to lesser extent family members (with regard to childbearing). Community views on the health risks of childbirth for HIV-positive women may have indirectly reduced pressure on women but, as previously noted, may simultaneously serve a stigmatizing function.

Nevertheless, women in our study generally represented themselves as relatively autonomous in their fertility intentions and decisions. The pressures of family and community affected them, but could to some extent be discounted or subverted, perhaps reflecting a loosening of extended family ties and community cohesion in an urban setting. As regards male partners, many were supportive; where not, although some women were resigned to having to acquiesce if their male partners disagreed, others were prepared to resort to subterfuge or confrontation to achieve what they wanted. The question arises whether findings of greater confidence amongst many of these women and co-operation by their male partners reflect a trend, at least amongst younger urban women and their partners in South Africa.

The main point of contact of these women with the health services had been with antenatal and postnatal care, primarily for their babies. In this context, as shown elsewhere (Harries et al. 2007), health workers appeared to have focussed mainly on the biomedical rather than personal and social aspects of family planning and sometimes expressed contradictory views. Interestingly, the views of other lay people seemed to carry at least as much if not more weight than those of health workers. There was no indication of longer-term responsive family planning counseling to deal with the changing realities of women's lives.

6   Conclusion

In summary, our qualitative study found that HIV-positive mothers of young babies in an urban area in South Africa were aware of the need and ways to prevent unintended pregnancy. Their motivations reflect a complex of health, material and emotional concerns. Fertility desires were low, but might change over time. Although the views of male partners and family, as well as community perceptions, could affect women's practise, they generally appeared surprisingly confident of their capacity to carry out their intentions to limit further childbearing. The influence of health workers appeared relatively limited and primarily important for access to the various contraceptive options.

Improved linkages or integration between HIV and reproductive health services could assist women such as these to continue to avoid unintended pregnancy. Family planning counseling should, however, extend beyond biomedical factors to take account of emotional, material and social factors. As HAART becomes a reality for more and more HIV-positive women in low- and middle-income countries, in-depth and ongoing responsive family planning counseling will be crucial to assist them and their partners negotiate their fertility desires and intentions and avoid unintended pregnancy over the longer term.

Acknowledgments The work reported in this chapter was undertaken at the Perinatal HIV Research Unit, University of the Witwatersrand, Johannesburg, South Africa. The Unit is based at Chris Hani Baragwanath Hospital, Soweto. We would like to thank the women who participated in the study; fieldworkers Boitumelo Rakosa for conducting and, together with Thomas Mogale, transcribing interviews; and Janet Jobson for assisting with the literature review.

References

Beyeza-Kashesya J, Kaharuza F, Mirembe F, Neema S, Ekstrom AM, Kulane A (2009) The dilemma of safe sex and having children: challenges facing HIV sero-discordant couples in Uganda. Afr Health Sci 9(1):2–12

Boerma J, Urassa M (2000) Associations between female infertility, HIV and sexual behaviour in rural Tanzania. In: Boerma J, Mgalla Z (eds) Women and infertility in Sub-Saharan Africa: a multidisciplinary perspective. KIT Publishers, Amsterdam, pp 175–187

Cooper D, Harries J, Myer L, Orner P, Bracken H (2007) 'Life is still going on': reproductive intentions among HIV-positive women and men in South Africa. Soc Sci Med 65:274–283

Cooper D, Moodley J, Zweigenthal V, Bekker L, Shah I, Myer L (2009) Fertility intentions and reproductive health care needs of people living with HIV in Cape Town, South Africa: implications for Integrating reproductive health and HIV care services. AIDS Behav 13:S38–S46

Dinh TH, Goga A, Jackson D, Lombard C, Woldesenbet S, Puren A et al (2012) Impact of the South Africa's PMTCT programs on perinatal HIV transmission: results of the 1st year implementing the 2010 WHO recommended guidelines. Presentation. 4th international workshop on HIV paediatrics, Washington, DC

Elul B, Delvaux T, Munyana E, Lahuerta M, Horowitz D, Ndagije F et al (2009) Pregnancy desires, and contraceptive knowledge and use among prevention of mother-to-child transmission clients in Rwanda. AIDS 23(Suppl 1):S19–S26

Family Health International (FHI) (2010a) Family planning and HIV integration: approaching a tipping point. In: The case for integrating family planning and HIV/AIDS services: evidence, policy support and programmatic experience, Research Triangle Park, NC, USA

Family Health International (FHI) (2010b) Policy support for strengthening family planning and HIV/AIDS linkages. In: The case for integrating family planning and HIV/AIDS services: evidence, policy support and programmatic experience, Research Triangle Park, NC, USA

Feldman R, Maposhere C (2003) Safer sex and reproductive choice: findings from 'positive women: voices and choices' in Zimbabwe. Reprod Health Matter 11(22):162–173

Gender Links/Medical Research Council (MRC) (2010) The war @ home: preliminary findings of the Gauteng Gender Violence Prevalence Study. Retrieved 7 Dec 2010 from:http://www.genderlinks.org.za/article/gauteng-gender-violence-prevalence-study-2010-11-22

Goga AE, Dinh TH, Jackson DJ, for the SAPMTCTE Study Group (2012) Evaluation of the effectiveness of the national prevention of mother-to-child transmission (PMTCT) programme measured at six weeks postpartum in South Africa, 2010. South African Medical Research Council, National Department of Health of South Africa & PEPFAR/US Centers for Disease Control and Prevention, Pretoria, SA

Gray RH, Wawer MJ, Serwadda D, Sewankambo N, Li C, Wabwire-Mangen F et al (1998) Population-based study of fertility in women with HIV-1 infection in Uganda. Lancet 351:98–103

Gray GE, Van Niekerk R, Struthers H, Violari A, Martinson N, McIntyre J, Naidu V (2006) The effects of adult morbidity and mortality on household welfare and the wellbeing of children in Soweto. Vulnerable Child Youth Stud 1(1):17–30

Greeff M (2013) Chapter 5: Disclosure and stigma: a cultural perspective. In: Liamputtong P (ed) Stigma, discrimination and HIV/AIDS: a cross-cultural perspective. Springer, Dordrecht

Gruskin S, Ferguson L, O'Malley J (2007) Ensuring sexual and reproductive health for people living with HIV: an overview of key human rights, policy and health system issues. Reprod Health Matter 15(Suppl 29):4–26

Harries J, Cooper D, Myer L, Bracken H, Zweigenthal V, Orner P (2007) Policy maker and health care provider perspectives on reproductive decision-making amongst HIV-infected individuals in South Africa. BMC Publ Health 7:282–288

Harries J, Stinson K, Orner P (2009) Health care providers' attitudes towards termination of pregnancy: a qualitative study in South Africa. BMC Publ Health 9:296–307

Hunter SC, Isingo R, Boerma JT, Urassa M, Mwaluko GM, Zaba B (2003) The association between HIV and fertility in a cohort study in rural Tanzania. J Biosoc Sci 35:189–199

Kaida A, Lima VD, Andia I, Kabakyenga J, Mbabazi P, Emenyonu N et al (2009) The WHOMEN's Scale (Women's HAART Optimism Monitoring and EvaluatioN Scale v.1) and the association with fertility intentions and sexual behaviours among HIV-positive women in Uganda. AIDS Behav 13:S72–S81

Kakaire O, Osinde MO, Kaye DK (2010) Factors that predict fertility desires for people living with HIV infection at a support and treatment centre in Kabale, Uganda. Reprod Heal 7:27

Kanniappan S, Jeyapaul MJ, Kalyanwala S (2008) Desire for motherhood: exploring HIV-positive women's desires, intentions and decision-making in attaining motherhood. AIDS Care 20(6):625–630

Laher F, Todd CS, Stibich MA, Phofa R, Behane X, Mohapi L, Gray G (2009) A qualitative assessment of decisions affecting contraceptive utilization and fertility intentions among HIV-positive women in Soweto, South Africa. AIDS Behav 13:S47–S54

Lazarus R, Struthers H, Violari A (2009) Hopes, fears, knowledge and misunderstandings: responses of HIV-positive mothers to early knowledge of the status of their baby. AIDS Care 21(3):329–334

Lazarus R, Struthers H, Violari A (2010) Starting HIV-positive babies on antiretroviral treatment: perspectives of mothers in Soweto, South Africa. J Pediatr Health Care 24(3):176–183

London L, Orner PJ, Myer L (2008) 'Even if you're positive, you still have rights because you are a person': human rights and the reproductive choice of HIV-positive persons. Dev World Bioeth 8(1):11–22

Long C (2009) Contradicting maternity: HIV-positive motherhood in South Africa. Wits University Press, Johannesburg

Maier M, Andia I, Emenyonu N, Guzman D, Kaida A, Pepper L, Hogg R, Bangsberg D (2009) Antiretroviral therapy is associated with increased fertility desire, but not pregnancy or live birth, among HIV+women in an early HIV treatment program in rural Uganda. AIDS Behav 13:28–37

Mphatswe W, Blankenberg N, Tudor-Williams G, Prendergast A, Thobakgale C, Mkhwanazi N et al (2007) High frequency of rapid immunological progression in African infants infected in the era of perinatal HIV prophylaxis. AIDS 21:1253–1261

Myer L, Morroni C, Rebe K (2007) Prevalence and determinants of fertility intentions of HIV-infected women and men receiving antiretroviral therapy in South Africa. AIDS Patient Care STDS 21(4):278–285

Nakayiwa S, Abang B, Packel L, Lifshay J, Purcell DW, King R et al (2006) Desire for children and pregnancy risk behavior among HIV-infected men and women in Uganda. AIDS Behav 10:95–104

National Committee on Confidential Enquiries into Maternal Deaths (NCCEMD) (2008) Saving mothers 2005–2007: fourth report on confidential enquiries into maternal deaths in South Africa. NDOH, Pretoria. Retrieved 21 Dec 2010 from: http://www.doh.gov.za/docs/reports/2007/savingmothers.pdf

National Department of Health, South Africa (NDOH) (2010) National antenatal sentinel HIV and syphilis prevalence survey in South Africa, 2009. NDOH, Pretoria. Retrieved 23 Dec 2010 from: www.doh.gov.za/docs/index.html

National Department of Health, South Africa/South African National AIDS Council (NDOH/SANAC) (2010) Clinical guidelines: PMTCT (Prevention of mother-to-child transmission). NDOH, Pretoria

Nattabi B, Jianghong L, Thompson SC, Orach CG, Earnest J (2009) A systematic review of factors influencing fertility desires and intentions among people living with HIV/AIDS: implications for policy and service delivery. AIDS Behav 13:949–968

Ndlovu V (2009) Considering childbearing in the age of highly active antiretroviral therapy (HAART): views of HIV-positive couples. J Soc Aspects HIV/AIDS 6(2):58–68

Nduna M, Farlane L (2009) Women living with HIV in South Africa and their concerns about fertility. AIDS Behav 13:S62–S65

Nóbrega AA, Oliveira FA, Galvão MT, Mota RS, Barbosa RM, Dourado I et al (2007) Desire for a child among women living with HIV/AIDS in Northeast Brazil. AIDS Patient Care STDS 21(4):261–267

Oladapo OT, Daniel OJ, Odusoga OL, Ayoola-Sotubo O (2005) Fertility desires and intentions of HIV-positive patients at a suburban specialist center. J Natl Med Assoc 97(12):1672–1681

Panozzo L, Battegay M, Friedl A, Vernazza PL (2003) High risk behaviour and fertility desires among heterosexual HIV-positive patients with a serodiscordant partner—two challenging issues. Swiss Med Wkly 133:124–127

Peltzer K, Chao L-W, Dana P (2009) Family-planning among HIV-positive and negative prevention of mother to child transmission (PMTCT) clients in a resource poor setting in South Africa. AIDS Behav 13:973–979

Ritchie J, Spencer L (1994) Qualitative data analysis for applied policy research. In: Bryman A, Burgess RG (eds) Analysing qualitative data. Routledge, London, pp 173–194

Rutenberg N, Baek C (2005) Addressing the family-planning needs of HIV-positive PMTCT clients: baseline findings from an operations research study. Horizons Research Update, Washington, DC

Smith DJ, Mbakwem BC (2007) Life projects and therapeutic itineraries: marriage, fertility, and antiretroviral therapy in Nigeria. AIDS 21:S37–S41

Struthers H, Violari A, Myeni Z, McIntyre J (2006) PMTCT in Soweto: a large scale intervention. PEPFAR HIV/AIDS Implementers' Meeting, Durban, 12–15 June

Tavrow P (2010) Promote or discourage: how providers can influence service use. In: Maalarchar S (ed) Social determinants of sexual and reproductive health: informing future research and programme implementation. World Health Organisation, Geneva, pp 17–36

Ujiji OA, Ekstrom AM, Ilako F, Indalo D, Rubenson B (2010) 'I will not let my HIV status stand in the way.' Decisions on motherhood among women on ART in a slum in Kenya – a qualitative study. BMC Women's Health 10:13–22

UNAIDS (Joint United Nations Programme on HIV/AIDS) (2010) Global report: UNAIDS report on the global AIDS epidemic 2010. UNAIDS, Geneva

UNAIDS (2012) Global report: UNAIDS report on the global AIDS epidemic 2012, UNAIDS, Geneva

UNICEF/UNAIDS/WHO/UNPF (2010) Children and AIDS: 5th stocktaking report. UNICEF/UNAIDS/WHO/UNPF, Geneva

Violari A, Cotton M, Gibb D, Babiker A, Steyn J, Jean-Philippe P, et al (2007) Antiretroviral therapy initiated before 12 weeks of age reduces early mortality in young HIV-infected infant: Evidence from the children with HIV Early Antiretroviral Therapy (CHER) Study. In: Fourth IAS conference on HIV Pathogenesis and Treatment, Sydney, Australia

Wilcher R, Cates W (2010) Reaching the underserved: family planning for women with HIV. Stud Fam Plann 41:125–128

World Health Organisation (WHO) (2010) PMTCT strategic vision 2010–2015: preventing mother-to-child transmission of HIV to reach the UNGASS and Millennium Development Goals. World Health Organisation, Geneva

Chapter 3
Pregnancy and Motherhood in the Narratives of Women with HIV Infection Living in the Metropolitan Area of Buenos Aires, Argentina

Mónica Laura Gogna, Silvia Beatriz Fernández, Paula di Corrado, and María Julieta Obiols

1 Introduction

Argentina, a middle-income country located in the Southern Cone of Latin America, has had an HIV/AIDS epidemic for 25 years. As in most Latin American countries, the epidemic is currently of a "concentrated" type. It affects less than 1% of the population (specifically, 0.4% of people over 15 years old), but it goes up to 5% or more in certain subpopulations (5% in commercial sex workers, 12% among men who have sex with men, and 34% in transsexuals) (Ministerio de Salud 2010). In 2008, the annual rate of infection for HIV was 13 per 100,000 inhabitants for the whole country, but it was significantly higher in Buenos Aires city (23.2 per 100,000 inhabitants). Currently, it is estimated that 130,000 individuals live with HIV, out of

M.L. Gogna (✉)
Interdisciplinary Institute, Av. Las Heras 3231, 12 A, CP 1425,
Ciudad Autónoma de Buenos Aires, Argentina
e-mail: mgogna.conicet.IIEGE@gmail.com

S.B. Fernández
National University of Avellaneda (UNDAV),
Honorio Pueyrredón 765-P.B.C, CP 1405, Ciudad Autónoma de Buenos Aires, Argentina
e-mail: silviabff@yahoo.com.ar

P. di Corrado
Former staff at CNRS, Francia 2297, CP 1602, Florida – Buenos Aires, Argentina
e-mail: pauladicorrado@hotmail.com

M.J. Obiols
Psychology School, University of Buenos Aires and CONICET
(National Scientific and Technological Research Council),
Zapiola 1340 Departamento 7, CP 1426, Buenos Aires, Argentina
e-mail: julieta.obiols@gmail.com

P. Liamputtong (ed.), *Women, Motherhood and Living with HIV/AIDS:*
A Cross-Cultural Perspective, DOI 10.1007/978-94-007-5887-2_3,
© Springer Science+Business Media Dordrecht 2013

which only half of them know their condition. Most of the notified cases (69%) are assisted by the public health system[1] (Ministerio de Salud 2010).

The progression of the infection via heterosexual sex raised the relative weight and number of women with HIV, with new infections tending toward a smaller male-to-female ratio. In the 2007–2009 period, the male-to-female ratio of new HIV infections was 1.7 males per each woman diagnosed (Ministerio de Salud 2010).

Legislation grants universal access to treatment and highly active antiretroviral therapy (HAART) has been available, but not without difficulties, since 1997. During 2009, 29,886 persons received HAART from the public health sector (Ministerio de Salud 2010).

The country has also adopted protocols to prevent mother-to-child transmission (MTCT) which establish the legal obligation to systematically offer every pregnant woman to undergo voluntary counseling and HIV testing as part of prenatal care. Currently, the prevalence of HIV in pregnant women is 0.32% and up to 1% in some hospitals in the metropolitan area of Buenos Aires (Bianco and Mariño 2010).

The rate of global perinatal transmission in the deliveries of women with HIV performed in Buenos Aires city during the period 2003–2009 was 5.5%.[2] The time of diagnosis, in relation to the pregnancy, had a great impact in the transmission rate: 3.1% in women diagnosed during pregnancy, 22.6% in those diagnosed during labor work, and 35.1% in those diagnosed during puerperium. The mother's level of education was another factor associated to HIV vertical transmission (Coordinación Sida/GCBA 2010).

In Argentina, as elsewhere, the extended use of HAART substantially diminished the morbidity and mortality associated to HIV and transformed it into a chronic pathology. As social representations of AIDS as a synonymous of death gradually began to fade, the personal and family projects of people living with HIV started to emerge or gain visibility (Grimberg 2003; Gianni 2006; Segurado and Paiva 2007; Pecheny et al. 2008).

A quanti-qualitative national study conducted in 2006 showed that parenthood can be a deeply cherished wish for many people living with HIV (Gogna et al. 2009). Data from a probabilistic sample of PLWHA aged 18 or more attending health-care centers for follow-up or treatment showed that women without children are six times more likely than women with children to want to have children. In contrast, men without children are nearly two times more likely than men with children to want to have children. The comparison highlights the centrality of motherhood for women in our country. The study also revealed the unmet need of contraception in this population since half the pregnancies that occurred after HIV diagnosis had been unexpected (Pecheny et al. 2008).

---

[1] The Argentine health care system has three relatively independent subsystems: public, private, and social security. For more details, see Belmartino (2000).

[2] 39.6% of those deliveries corresponded to women resident in Buenos Aires City, 57.8% to residents from the metropolitan area of Buenos Aires, and 3.05% to residents from other jurisdictions.

Studies performed in Argentina and Brazil show that women who live with HIV do not talk with the health professionals that assist them about their desire to have children because they fear a negative reaction, nor do they ask about birth control methods because the condom is the only alternative promoted by infectious disease specialists, who usually act as family doctors for the people who live with HIV (Paiva et al. 2002; Oliveira and Junior 2003; Weller et al. 2004; Pecheny et al. 2008).

As Gruskin and colleagues (2007) maintain, the rights as well as the needs and aspirations related to sexual and reproductive health of PLWHA are not different from those that people who do not live with the virus have, although living with the infection causes specific needs and aspirations (see also Chap. 2 in this volume). Women with HIV are more exposed to certain issues (for instance, there is evidence of a greater relation between cervical cancer and HIV than in the general population; and risk of mother-child transmission if there is no access to prevention in time and manner; among others). Also, women with HIV may have different expectations and pressures when compared to other women as regards whether they should or should not have children, and both men and women often report feeling pressured (by family, society, health services, and so on) as to the fact that they should not be sexually active, even if they do not have symptoms (Gruskin et al. 2007).

In this chapter, we focus on pregnancy and motherhood in women who live with HIV, an issue that has only recently began to be analyzed in depth in our country (Biagini et al. 2008; García 2009). The findings are part of a larger study (see Sect. 3).

2 Theoretical Framework

According to Greco (2008: 33), the reproductive event falls within the "wide field of women's health, in which the social discourses regarding maternity, womanhood and the health-disease-medical care process coincide. These discourses, threaded by the crosscutting axis of gender, give the pregnant women's body a series of meanings which organize her experience and at the same time, transcend it, dehumanizing, tugging or silencing its singularity." In the social representation, Fernandez (1994) contends, motherhood is seen as the "paradigmatic" function of women and as that which gives them identity and meaning to their lives; see also Chap. 1 and other chapters in Part I in this volume.

Some authors (see López 2006; Zamberlin 2005; Biagini et al. 2008; Greco 2008) argue that women from disadvantaged social groups, with few or no options of participation in the public sphere, "choose" to follow the "road of motherhood" – culturally imposed from generation to generation – since it guarantees them a certain social recognition they would not achieve through other means.

However, as Greco herself (2008: 89) points out, the issue of pregnancy, whether planned or unplanned, inevitably leads to the complex issue of the desire to be a mother which cannot be analyzed solely from the sociocultural point of view, seeing it as a gender mandate. It is important to also consider the sociopsychological aspects involved in it. From this point of view, it is important to have in mind that desire is always built in virtue of, and at expense of, a part of unconscious knowledge, that is, to say, unavailable, which is what prevents these women from accounting for their attitudes and behaviors (especially those visualized as contradictory or "illogical").

The HIV infection and the possibility of avoiding its transmission from mother to child have made a matter which is already difficult to deal with and to understand, even more complex. Research carried out in different contexts indicates that a diagnosis of HIV infection during pregnancy is an experience that causes deep uncertainties and a specific psychological burden (Bennetts et al. 1999; Kwalombota 2002; Nelms 2005; Torres de Carvalho and Piccinini 2006; Gonçalvez and Piccinini 2007; Sanders 2008; García 2009). While some authors emphasize the psychic suffering which these women undergo (Kwalombota 2002), others stress the ways in which the HIV diagnosis increases the medicalization of pregnancy, labor, and puerperium. Thus, for example, Gonçalvez and Piccinini (2007) maintain that apart from the fear of transmitting the virus to the baby and of the usual anxiety pregnancy elicits, women must submit themselves to a highly medicalized process in which most of the decisions are out of their control, a situation which has an impact at a subjective level. García (2009: 257), in turn, points out that the body "becomes -both for the medical intervention and for women themselves- to some extent split, separated from their own histories and feelings. It becomes a means that, as mothers-to-be, they must make available for studies and therapeutic practises in order to protect the child they are expecting."

Regarding motherhood, a meta-analysis conducted by Sandelowski and Barroso (2003)[3] concluded that it entailed work directed toward the illness itself and the social consequences of having HIV infection in the service of two primary goals: (a) the protection of children from HIV infection and HIV-related stigma and (b) the preservation of a positive maternal identity. According to the authors, motherhood both intensified and mitigated the negative physical and social effects of HIV infection. HIV-positive mothers engaged in a distinctive kind of maternal practise to resist forces that disrupted their relationships with and ability to care for their children, as well as their identities as mothers.

Similarly, a qualitative study conducted by Hebling and Hardy (2007), aimed at describing the feelings of a dozen HIV-positive women regarding motherhood, indicated that it was seen as an essential attribute of women and a reason for living. The study also revealed that some women made provisions with their family for the care of their children and that thinking about the possibility of their children becoming orphans made women feel impotent and guilty. Such painful feelings were minimized through mechanisms of defense like compensation, denial, rationalization, and projection.

The contradictions associated to motherhood in women with HIV infection also arise in the study carried out by Long (2009) in South Africa. The psychologist concludes that HIV infection promotes social representations and more specifically

---

[3] It integrated findings from 56 reports of qualitative studies conducted with HIV-positive women.

prejudices and stigma which associate it with a negative situation while the pregnancy is meant as a positive event that contributes to the complete fulfillment of a woman. Other research carried out in Vietnam maintains that motherhood grants women a certain status, while being childless is stigmatized. At the same time HIV-positive mothers reported feeling like unfit parents, a reflection of negative broader social opinions on HIV and its association with "social evils" (Oosterhoff et al. 2008; see also Chap. 14 in this volume).

3 The Study

This chapter discusses findings produced within the framework of a collaborative study between CEDES and CENEP (Center for the Study of State and Society)[4] and CENEP (Center for Population Studies),[5] supported by WHO. The research has a double purpose: (a) to identify, from the woman's and health service providers' point of view, the obstacles to the provision of integral health care to women of reproductive age who live with HIV/Aids and (b) to promote greater interaction between the several health services which provide care to this population (infectology, obstetrics, gynecology, and family planning) in two selected hospitals in Buenos Aires city[6] and to document and monitor this experience.

The qualitative analysis presented here is based on 11 semi-structured interviews with women taking their babies to be tested for HIV to CNRS[7] during January of 2010. The interviews were performed by the authors and took place in a private room after the blood test to the baby for an accurate diagnosis was performed. As customary, an informed consent was applied. Upon finishing the interviews, counseling was provided to those women who required it, and informative material was provided to all of them. The interviews were recorded (with the women's prior authorization) and then they were transcribed and coded for their analysis.

The central themes of the interview guideline were the following: basic sociodemographic characteristics; time and circumstances when they were notified about their HIV infection; experience in relation to diagnosis, reconstruction of the steps taken since then, and perception of difficulties and facilitators in the care provided by the health services; partner's role; pregnancy experience; and reproductive intentions.

---

[4] CEDES – Centro de Estudios de Estado y Sociedad.

[5] CENEP – Centro de Estudios de Población.

[6] Hospitals were chosen by researchers and Coordinación Sida. Both provide health care to people living with HIV/AIDS. One of them is a general hospital, while the other specializes in infectious diseases.

[7] We thank Horacio Salomón M.D. (Director) and the staff at the Centro Nacional de Referencia de Sida (National Aids Reference Center) (CNRS) for their collaboration. Since 1997, the CNRS is a World Health Organization and a Pan-American Health Organization AIDS Collaborating Center.

In the following sections, the main findings resulting from this qualitative material are shown. Most of the women interviewed had a low education level: only two had graduated from high school. Their ages ranged between 20 and 41 years old, being 29 the average age. Their profile was similar to that of a sample of women we interviewed in 2009 – as a baseline study – who attended the CNRS to perform their viral load tests or to test their babies. Among these last ($N=44$), which made up 26% of the women interviewed ($N=169$), 29 was the average age. Most of them had not gone beyond the elementary education level ($N=21$), a lower number had not finished their high school studies ($N=15$), and only a minority ($N=8$) had graduated from high school or higher level.

4 Findings

4.1 The Diagnosis and Its Impact

Most women we interviewed found out about their serology during a pregnancy control (four in the recent pregnancy and three in a previous pregnancy) (see also Chaps. 4, 15, 16, and 17 in this volume). Three other women, when their partners got sick or died, and one woman interviewed, who got the infection due to mother-to-child transmission, knew it "since forever."

Both among those who knew they were positive and those who ignored their serological status at conception, there were interviewees who had had wanted and unwanted pregnancies. Among the former, some women became pregnant without wanting it (either using a condom or because their partner refused to use it) and others willingly, to have children with their new partners.

The news of a positive diagnosis, Margulies and colleagues (2006: 292) contend, makes a difference as regards who the woman was until then and "opens a new way of living life which is more directly associated with death," and it is often processed not in the dichotomy of acceptance or denial but in feelings and actions that are ambiguous, even contradictory (see also Chap. 15 in this volume). The words of one of the women interviewed show those contradictions and ambiguities.

> I found out when I was almost six months pregnant. I couldn't believe it, because I have a stable partner, I've been married to him for fourteen years, I couldn't believe it. Many things were stirred up in our couple but well ... this showed up and well, we tried to overcome it the best we could, it was very hard for us, for our family, but well, thank God we tried to overcome it and thinking that a baby was to be born and that it was the most beautiful thing. I only wanted to have a baby and well this showed up. (33 years old, incomplete high school, 4 children)

Only the interviewee with the highest educational status (social work student, seronegative partner) clearly stated her feelings of self-rejection upon knowing her serology:

> When I came home all I did was look at myself in the mirror, it happened to me until recently, looking at myself in the mirror and feeling ... sick at the person I saw.

I[8]: Why?

Mainly because society judges and one is part of the society and until one understands that, one has to live with this … (22 years old, incomplete university, 1 son)

The rest of the women accepted the diagnosis without greater considerations as to their partners or themselves. Just one of them, whose husband knew about his HIV before they got married and did not tell her, reported having had fights with him, from whom she was already separated at the moment she received the news.

Regardless of the circumstances when they received the diagnosis, almost all women interviewed talked about that moment as an extremely difficult one, which aroused several emotions and worries: confusion, doubts about the means of infection, and various fears – specifically, (a) that the baby would be born with the infection or that her previous children would have it, (b) to transmit HIV to her children or partner (in case they are serodiscordant), (c) to the disease itself and to death, (d) that her children would become orphans, and (e) to relatives and friends' rejection and to social discrimination.

I: Tell me how and when did you find out about your HIV?
When I was 5 months pregnant.
I: And how was the experience upon finding out that you had HIV?
Awful, I wanted to die. I did not know what to do. I never imagined that it could happen to me. You never imagine that. I didn't want to tell my family, the only one who knew it was me, my husband (father of her first son and current partner) and the father of my baby. I felt I was hurting myself, because I did not tell anything, I cried every night, it hurt me and well little by little I began to tell. (24 years old, complete elementary school, 2 children)

In 1996 I found out … that I was HIV, when my husband died … he was a carrier. In 1995 one of my sons was born, (I got tested) but I was negative. And in 1996 I got tested again and it turned out positive and also one of my sons was positive. I have a thirteen year old son with HIV.
I: How did it feel to get that news?
A bomb, it is a bomb. Let's say…
I: Does it still feel like that?
Yes, it's been thirteen years and it is as if now you say … How do I go on? right? How do I explain this to …? He is now trying to find out, you know?, about relationships, girls who are after him. And that he …, he dreams about having eight kids. He tells me: "Mom, if I can have kids …" you know?, and it is quite an issue. It is painful. It is a backpack that you are going to carry for ever. It's that. (36 years old, high school, 4 children)

Some women report having received support when diagnosed; others, instead, were mistreated by some health professionals. Sometimes, the same woman underwent both experiences.

I found out and the doctor who told me … was a very good doctor who assisted me. It was in a small health care unit in Castillo. She was very kind, she told me very nicely, other people do not treat you that way, I went through other stages where I was not treated like that. But, she treated me nicely, she explained it to me very well, she told me to stay calm because there was a treatment. (…) Well, there, to tell you the truth, when they told me the second time, there was another doctor, who treated me badly. (…) She treated me badly, she

---

[8] Transcription note: I = Interviewer.

asked me how many partners I had. She told me: "How many partners do you have?" As if saying... (33 years old, incomplete high school, 4 children)

As regards the attitude of health professionals about these women's desire for motherhood or the "consummate fact" of a pregnancy, the experiences of the women interviewed confirm that while some physicians accompanied these desires, other discouraged them, and there were others who scolded them for getting pregnant (Oliveira and Junior 2003; Paiva et al. 2002; Weller et al. 2004; see also Chap. 2):

I: And how did you feel during the pregnancy?
Fine, I was as nervous as during my first pregnancy [she had two other grown up daughters)] and how it was going to turn out, but doctors relieved me a bit, they talked to me a lot, they calmed me down a lot. (32 years old, incomplete elementary school, 4 children)

(Husband[9]): Besides she (speaking about the doctor) said: "No more children." The same doctor. When she got pregnant for a second time, she scolded her.
Yes. (29 years old, incomplete high school, 2 children)

4.2 Pregnancy Experiences

The pregnancy and delivery experiences of the women interviewed varied considerably. On the one hand, some had experienced no inconveniences.

I: What was your pregnancy experience like knowing you had HIV?
The same as in the previous one. For me it was normal.
I: Well, it did affect you, this feeling that you say, that you felt sad.
Just the first weeks, the first month. After that, everything was normal, very nice.
I: And speaking about medical and hospital care did you live it a similar way in both pregnancies?
Fine, similar. (24 years old, incomplete elementary school, 2 children)
   (It was) a very beautiful delivery. I barely felt any pain. (22 years old, incomplete high school, 1 child)

On the other hand, some of them had complicated pregnancies and/or had to stay in bed or hospitalized for some time. In these situations, the contradiction between a "life-producing body" and a "life-threatening body" becomes more obvious, producing a psychic suffering frequently not acknowledged by health providers. A young woman who shared her hospitalization with women who were going through advanced stages of the disease expressed:

With his pregnancy I was sicker. I was hospitalized for almost a month and a half. And I also lied in bed a lot because I was thin, like this, I was very weak ... I was three weeks in the hospital. You see ugly things. I had never seen that, I had always been fine. But, you see thin girls, very thin, with diapers. (They were) in their last stages. And things like those made me think. I told my mom: "Take me out of here, because ..." I felt myself dying. I was discharged from the hospital and just then, during that week, I was hospitalized in a Maternal

---

[9] This was the only case in which the husband was present and insisted on participating of the interview.

and Child hospital because … because I kept vomiting and the baby had low weight, he weighted too little for seven months. And then I was referred to another hospital. (20 years old, incomplete high school, 2 children)

In most cases, the pregnancy had a positive meaning related to life and to the project of having a family. Two testimonies in which the women expressed that their babies "saved their lives" stand out:

For me, my pregnancy was difficult because of the disease, but at the same time it was beautiful, because my son saved my life. If I hadn't got pregnant I would have never known I had this. Because one is fine, you never go to the doctor, or at least I don't, I am a bit reluctant to doctors. (33 years old, incomplete high school, 4 children)

With this one I am suffering, I say oh! Please, let him not be positive. I also feel like paying for my sins. For me, he is a miracle, because if I hadn't got pregnant I would have not found out but on the other hand you know? I will feel guilty if he has it. (22 years old, incomplete university, 1 child)

This last testimony introduces a worry shared by all the women interviewed: the fear to have transmitted the infection to their babies.

I: And what was your pregnancy experience like knowing you had HIV?
Awful, always with fears, 24 hours a day.
I: Fear to what? What did you think?
With my daughter it was different because I was younger, I did not know about this, I did not know whether I could pass it on to her or not, but with him it was awful. I think that a big fear, very sad, from the day I saw him. And now that he is gaining weight is like I have a hope. (30 years old, see consent, 2 children)

I: Tell me, what was your pregnancy experience like knowing you had HIV?
It was complicated, and awful because you think many things, many things get into your head, you don't know whether your baby is going to be born, or not. Apart from the fact that I was alone, I spent the 9 months alone without sharing with anyone what I was going through. (41 years old, incomplete elementary school, 3 children)

Those fears, as shown in the last testimony, sometimes take place in a context of self- imposed loneliness due to the fear of the reactions that making the diagnosis known could provoke in their social environment.

4.3 *"Maternal Abnegation": Its Meanings and Implications*

Previous studies point out that parenthood, most often in women, influences adherence to treatment: having followed up all the medical, pharmacological, and routine indications to avoid vertical transmission, after delivery, women tend to have more flexible and unsystematic behavior as regards their own care and treatment in favor of their children (Pecheny et al. 2008). Biagini and colleagues' findings (2008) show something similar: the level of detail with which mothers spoke about the viral load and CD4 results and the treatments that their children receive deeply contrasted with the vagueness with which they often described their own health and follow-up.

The delay in seeking health care for themselves was also frequent among the women we interviewed. In most cases, their children's care or the need to go out to work made them abandon or postpone their own treatment.

I: And you, until when did you follow it (talking about the treatment)?
More or less two years, then I had to go out to work so I quit my treatment, because he was unemployed and I had to feed everyone (41 years old, complete elementary school, 3 children)

I: And then I had him by normal delivery. Because my load was low ... And now I have to get tested because I have not done so after my baby was born.
I: How old is he?
Nine months.
I: Well ... And why didn't you get tested?
Because no ... I don't know... (25 years old, incomplete high school, 2 children)

The same happened with other diseases or issues not related to HIV. The following story shows the paradoxical effect that delaying their own health care can have on their maternal capacities.

Then, two or three days later I had a gallbladder surgery. I was bent in pain when they took me to the hospital. As I didn't want to go ... because I didn't want to leave the girls and all that ... And finally, I could not stand the pain any longer, because I couldn't even look after them. (29 years old, incomplete high school, 2 children)

In other cases, instead, children act as an incentive to comply with the treatment. This behavior was also identified in other contexts: motherhood may strengthen the desire to go on living in order to take care of the children, indirectly promoting self-care (Castro 2001, cited in Gonçalves and Piccinini 2007), as the following testimonies reveal:

I: You have to go to the hospital, to get tested...
Well, that is what I was saying ... what for? But, then I started thinking, I have two kids, and they deserve that I do this. (24 years old, incomplete elementary school, 2 children)

Yes, I followed a treatment but you know I tried more to take care of the children, to take care of him, of the house, as he is unemployed now, he is "cartonero" (cardboard seller). As I began to work on my own, by the hour, I did not pay attention to myself, then well, now I try to take care of myself.
I: You did not use to go to the hospital?
Right. Now I do care about what is happening to me. Now I am interested. That's why now I am going to make all the tests.
I: And what changed?
Her (her baby daughter) (41 years old, complete elementary school, 3 children)

The priority given to the children, whether women postpone treatment or adhere to treatment "because of them," confirms the centrality motherhood has in the lives of these women. It could also indicate, as pointed out by Biagini and colleagues (2008: 123), "we are probably in the presence of an over-adaptation to the model of maternal abnegation, as a way to seek acceptance and exoneration, taking refuge in a socially accepted identity."

4.4 Birth Control Decisions and Practises

Most women interviewed reported that they do not want to have more children, and 5 out of 11 have already undergone a tubal ligation (and a sixth has asked for it without success).[10]

The option for a definitive method was essentially based upon the desire to avoid the possibility of mother-to-child transmission (expressions like "why do I have to take the risk?" and "it is a risk") and, to a lesser extent, in the tiredness or stress a pregnancy imposes on a woman with HIV or in the financial difficulties to be faced to support a new child.

Women, especially those who have a seronegative male partner, expressed their intention to use condoms, which is many times rejected by the male. These attitudes may be understood as a display of certain features of dominant male subjectivity (courage, taking risks, and so on) (Connell 2003; see also Chap. 2). Sometimes, as pointed out by Delvaux and Nostlinger (2007), unprotected sex was perceived as an expression of growing emotional intimacy.

No, he does not want to hear about that. No, because he says he has already had many partners before and he never used it, and then why would he use it with me, that we are … that in a short time we are going to get married. (29 years old, incomplete high school, 2 children)

I: Which was your partner's attitude?
Oh! Well, this, that's what I say, I fucked my life up, and he tells me: Do you think that I am going to leave you because of this? I don't care," he tells me, "I don't care," and I say: "You are facing the risk that, maybe, I may pass it on to you." One day we were about to have sex and we did not have condoms, and he told me: "I don't care" and I was the one who stopped him. (22 years old, incomplete university, 1 child)

…actually he does not want to use condoms, because of "love" he says. (33 years old, incomplete high school, 4 children)

Some women interviewed had to convince their partners of their decision to get sterilized. They used the HIV as a key argument.

First, I took the decision on my own, then I talked about it with him and he did not want it, but I said: "No. It's fine, you have two already, it's fine, why more? If we do not know we … Ok, we have this treatment that helps us but I do not know how much time it will prolong life" (32 years old, complete elementary school, 4 children)

First he said no (as regards the tubal ligation) … That maybe some time in the future…And I said no… And he said ok, do whatever you want … And he told me … "it's ok, do whatever you want to do." (20 years old, incomplete high school, 2 children)

The infection acts as an effective "negotiation strategy" also with health professionals, many of whom promote tubal ligation in this population.

I: How did it go?
I talked to the doctor who scheduled my cesarean section. She asked me if I wanted it (the tubal ligation). She explained that if I did not have the tubal ligation it was a kind of risky

---

[10] It should be taken into account that tubal ligation and vasectomy are legal in Argentina only since 2006.

to have another baby because he/she could be born with HIV. (33 years old, incomplete high school, 4 children)

They told me it was not allowed, that the law said I had to be over twenty one years old. But, as I have this (HIV/AIDS), I could … with my mother's signature … and with an order… yes, otherwise you cannot, you have to be older than twenty one years old. And in the last moment in the operating room, they asked me if I maintained my decision and I said yes. And they asked me … and said: "Well, if the chief here authorizes…Do you want to have the tubal ligation? And I said yes." (20 years old, incomplete high school, 2 children)

5 Conclusion

As the literature indicates (see, e.g., Sandelowski and Barroso 2003; Nelms 2005; Gonçalves and Piccinini 2007; see also Chap. 15), our findings show that getting an HIV-positive result, particularly during pregnancy, is a very difficult situation since it awakes strong and contradictory feelings, among which fear seems to be dominant. However, after the "initial shock," HIV infection becomes part of women's life and does not have a unique impact on their sexual and reproductive behavior (i.e., regarding condom use or reproductive intentions).

The fact that an offspring, whether wanted or unexpected, is associated with life counterbalances in some way the pain, fear, and/or shame that diagnosis elicits. The desire of women who already know their serological status to become mothers (especially when they do not have children or have a new partner) also indicates that motherhood is seen as part of women's lives and gives them strength to cope with the infection and/or adverse circumstances in their lives.

Still, the fear that the child might be infected haunts women during pregnancy and the process of the child's diagnosis and increases the tensions and contradictory feelings that pregnancy and motherhood inevitably entail.

As other authors have noted (e.g., Biagini et al. 2008; Pecheny et al. 2008), our interviewees complied with treatment to prevent vertical transmission as part of their responsibilities to their offspring but tended to postpone their own care (sometimes to provide income to the household and/or to take care of children or sick husbands). Though "abnegation" may be considered an essential feature of motherhood, it seems to be exacerbated among our interviewees: they cope with undesired effects of treatment they cannot put up with when nonpregnant, and they take all sorts of precautions, sometimes obsessively, not to infect other children, particularly other offspring, nephews/nieces, and friends' children.

Paraphrasing Biagini and colleagues (2008: 123), in spite of the emotional tensions and sufferings described, taking care of the children provides women who live with HIV, especially those who have had little access to material, cultural, symbolic, and/or emotional resources, a vital attachment and grants meaning and direction to their actions. The assertiveness that many of them have developed in their relation with health providers, not only regarding the prevention of vertical transmission, but also as regards their birth control wishes and needs, is a proof of the positive effects motherhood can bring about.

To sum up, we would like to highlight some implications of our findings for policy and service delivery that would benefit women undergoing similar situations. First, health services have to address male partners in various circumstances. It is crucial to offer the HIV test to male partners of women attending prenatal checkups since women who test negative at the beginning of a pregnancy may prove positive later on. In addition, partners of women who test positive for HIV need to be counseled regarding condom use to avoid infection (if negative or ignorant of their serology) or reinfection (if positive) and to adopt "double protection" to effectively avoid unwanted pregnancies. In general, men need to be targeted more systematically and effectively. If men knew their status earlier, treatment would benefit not only them but also, indirectly, their families and reduce women's risk of sexual transmission. Ob-gyns need to be targeted and sensitized as to the importance of bringing up and discussing with women and their partners both their contraceptive and reproductive intentions in order to prevent unwanted pregnancies and promote safer pregnancies.

Posttest counseling is also an area that definitely needs to be improved taking into account the emotional impact of diagnosis, especially during pregnancy. More information and support regarding babies' testing and diagnosis is also required to help women to cope with fear and anxiety.

Interventions aimed at developing women's abilities to communicate their status to relevant others, including their children, and to disclose their own status to positive kids, when necessary, are also needed in order to improve women's integral health and quality of life. Given the huge differences identified among women's personal resources, spaces in which positive women interact and share their experiences regarding contraception, reproduction, pregnancy, and motherhood would be an empowerment strategy worth pursuing.

References

Belmartino S (2000) The context and process of health care reform in Argentina. In: Fleury S, Belmartino S, Baris E (eds) Reshaping health care in Latin America. A comparative analysis of health care reform in Argentina, Brazil and Mexico. International Development Research Centre, Ottawa, pp 27–47

Bennetts A, Shaffer N, Manopaiboon C, Chaiyakul P, Siriwasin W, Mock P et al (1999) Determinants of depression and HIV-related worry among HIV- positive women who have recently given birth, Bangkok, Thailand. Soc Sci Med 49:737–749

Biagini G, Grigaitis L, Giri B (2008) Vivencias del proceso de salud-enfermedad-atención del VIH/Sida. Un estudio de casos de mujeres seropositivas embarazadas atendidas en efectores públicos seleccionados. Informe final. Instituto de Investigaciones Gino Germani, Facultad de Ciencias Sociales de la Universidad de Buenos Aires/UBATEC, Buenos Aires

Bianco M, Mariño M (2010) Dos caras de una misma realidad: Violencia hacia las mujeres y VIH Sida en Argentina, Brasil, Chile y Uruguay. Evidencias y propuestas para la reorientación de las políticas públicas. FEIM, Buenos Aires

Castro CM (2001) Os sentidos da maternidade para gestantes e puérperas vivendo com HIV. Dissertação de Mestrado em Enfermagem, Pontifícia Universidade Católica de São Paulo, São Paulo, Brazil

Connell R (2003) Masculinidades. Programa Universitario de Estudios de Género, Universidad Autónoma de la Ciudad de México, México DF

Coordinación Sida/GCBA (2010) Situación epidemiológica del VIH-Sida en la ciudad de Buenos Aires. Gobierno de la Ciudad de Buenos Aires, Buenos Aires, agosto de 2010

Delvaux T, Nostingler C (2007) Reproductive choice for women and men living with HIV: contraception, abortion and fertility. Reprod Health Matter 15(29):46–66

Fernández AM (1994) La mujer de la ilusión: Pactos y contratos entre hombres y mujeres. Paidós, Buenos Aires

García G (2009) Cuerpo y narrativa: Una aproximación etnográfica al proceso de atención del embarazo, parto y puerperio de mujeres viviendo con VIH en la Ciudad de Buenos Aires. Horizontes Antropológicos 15(32):247–272

Gianni MC (2006) Tiempo y narrativa desde la experiencia del tratamiento en VIH/SIDA. CEDES/FLACSO (Colección Tesis), Buenos Aires

Gogna M, Pecheny M, Ibarlucía I, Manzelli H, Barrón López S (2009) The reproductive needs and rights of people living with HIV in Argentina: health service users' and providers' perspectives. Soc Sci Med 69(6):813–820

Gonçalves TR, Piccinini CA (2007) Aspectos psicológicos da gestação e da maternidade no contexto da infecção pelo HIV/AIDS. Psicol USP 18(3):113–142

Greco A (2008) Las voces acalladas en la maternidad: Los controles prenatales ausentes o inadecuados en la perspectiva de las mujeres de sectores populares. CEDES/FLACSO (Colección Tesis), Buenos Aires

Grimberg M (2003) Narrativas del cuerpo. Experiencia cotidiana y género en personas que viven con VIH. Cuadernos de Antropología Social 17:79–99

Gruskin S, Ferguson L, O'Malley J (2007) Ensuring sexual and reproductive health for people living with HIV: an overview of key human rights, policy and health systems issues. Reprod Health Matter 15(29):4–26

Hebling EM, Hardy E (2007) Feelings related to motherhood among women living with HIV in Brazil: a qualitative study. AIDS Care 19(9):1095–1100

Kwalombota M (2002) The effect of pregnancy in HIV-infected women. AIDS Care 14(3):431–433

López E (2006) La fecundidad adolescente en la Argentina: Desigualdades y desafíos. UBA: Encrucijadas, Revista de La Universidad de Buenos Aires 39:24–31

Long C (2009) Contradicting maternity: HIV-positive motherhood in South Africa. Witwatersrand University Press, Johannesburg

Margulies S, Barber N, Recoder ML (2006) VIH-Sida y "adherencia" al tratamiento. Enfoques y perspectivas. Antípoda 3:281–300

Ministerio de la Nación (2010) Boletín sobre el VIH Sida en la Argentina. Dirección de Sida y ETS, Buenos Aires. Presidencia de la Nación. Año XIII, 27, noviembre de 2010

Nelms TP (2005) Burden: the phenomenon of the mothering with HIV. J Assoc Nurs AIDS Care 16(4):3–13

Oliveira LA, França Junior I (2003) Demandas reprodutivas e a assistência às pessoas vivendo com HIV/AIDS: Limites e possibilidades no contexto dos serviços de saúde especializados. Cad Saude Publica 19(2):315–323

Oosterhoff P, Nguyen TA, Pham NY, Wright P, Hardon A (2008) HIV-positive mothers in Viet Nam: using their status to build support groups and access essential services. Reprod Health Matter 16(32):162–170

Paiva V, Latorre M, Gravato N, Lacerda R, Enhancing Care Initiative – Brazil (2002) Sexuality of women living with HIV/AIDS in São Paulo. Cad Saude Publica 18(6):1609–1620

Pecheny M, Manzelli H, Gogna M, Binstock G, Rovner H, Barrón López S, Carioli N, Ibarlucía I (2008) Estudio nacional sobre la situación social de las personas viviendo con VIH en la Argentina. Libros del Zorzal/UBATEC, Buenos Aires. Available in Spanish. Retrieved 14 May 2011 from: http://www.ubatec.uba.ar/fondomundial/downloads/informeesspvs2006pecheny-manzellietal.pdf

Sandelowski M, Barroso J (2003) Toward a metasynthesis of qualitative findings on motherhood in HIV-positive women. Res Nurs Health 26(2):153–170

Sanders LB (2008) Women's voices: the lived experience of pregnancy and motherhood after diagnosis with HIV. J Assoc Nurs AIDS Care 19(1):47–57

Segurado AC, Paiva V (2007) Rights of HIV positive people to sexual and reproductive health: parenthood. Reprod Health Matter 15(29):27–45

Torres de Carvalho F, Piccinini CA (2006) Maternidade em situação de infecção pelo HIV: Um estudo sobre os sentimentos de gestantes. Interação em Psicologia 10(2):345–355

Weller S, Portnoy F, Gogna M (2004) Éxitos médicos, desafíos humanos. Reproducción y Anticoncepción en personas que viven con VIH. Buenos Aires: Coordinación SIDA-Secretaría de Salud, Gobierno de la Ciudad de Buenos Aires.

Zamberlin N (2005) Percepciones y conductas de las/los adolescentes frente al embarazo y la maternidad/paternidad. In: M Gogna (coord) Embarazo y maternidad en la adolescencia. Estereotipos, evidencias y propuestas para políticas públicas. CEDES/UNICEF/Ministerio de Salud de la Nación Buenos Aires, pp 285–316

Chapter 4
Making Decisions in Pregnancy About HIV Testing and Treatment: The Experience of Burmese Migrant Women in Northern Thailand

Pleumjit Chotiga, Kenda Crozier, and Michael Pfeil

1 Introduction

Poverty, lack of food, poor infrastructure, and inadequate education are persistent problems faced by those who live in the areas of Thailand that border Burma (also known as Myanmar) (European Commission Humanitarian Aid Office [ECHO] 2005). Due to the political and economic situation in Burma, people have had very little health education and health care. This creates a public health concern, as many undocumented, illegal migrants from Burma do not have access to health services, have increased morbidity, and present a number of public health risks (Ministry of Public Health 2006). HIV infection is one of the main health problems in the border regions (Celentano and Beyrer 2008).

There is an association between people movement and risk of HIV transmission, and borders are often considered as heightened HIV vulnerability areas (Shtarkshall and Soskolne 2000). It has been suggested that having various borders and population

P. Chotiga (✉)
Maternal and Child Nursing Department, Boromarajonani College of Nursing,
Chiang Mai, Don Kaew, Mae Rim, Chiang Mai 50180, Thailand
e-mail: P.Chotiga@gmail.com

K. Crozier
Faculty of Medicine and Health Sciences, University of East Anglia,
Norwich, UK NR4 7TJ
e-mail: k.crozier@uea.ac.uk

M. Pfeil
Children's and Young People's Nursing, Faculty of Medicine and Health Sciences,
University of East Anglia, Norwich, UK NR4 7TJ

NHS East of England, 2-4 Victoria House, Capital Park, Fulbourn,
Cambridge CB21 5XB, UK
e-mail: m.pfeil@uea.ac.uk

P. Liamputtong (ed.), *Women, Motherhood and Living with HIV/AIDS:*
A Cross-Cultural Perspective, DOI 10.1007/978-94-007-5887-2_4,
© Springer Science+Business Media Dordrecht 2013

subgroups led to the rapid spread of the HIV infection across Thailand. In Cambodia, Burma, and Thailand, HIV prevalence is higher among the provinces bordering with other countries (POLICY 2003; WHO 2004).

The Burmese who enter Thailand are primarily Karen, Karenni, Mon, and Shan people (Ekeh and Smith 2007). The largest population of Burmese migrants lives in the upper north of Thailand, and it is difficult to estimate how many of the migrants are living with HIV. Large numbers have come across the borders into Thailand in the last decade. These migrant populations are at higher risk of contracting HIV because of their sociocultural status. They have language difficulties that prevent them from accessing information about HIV and AIDS. Studies have reported that most immigrants have limited access to basic health-care services because they live and work illegally, and as Ekachai (2003) suggests, most HIV-positive immigrants have no access to health-care services in Thailand.

UNAIDS estimates adult HIV prevalence in Burma at between 1.3 and 2%, with up to 570,000 people infected in a population of 47.3 million and treatment largely unavailable (UNAIDS 2006). Although it has fallen to between 0.5 and 0.7% in 2009, it is still high (UNAIDS 2010). In Thailand, the HIV prevalence of migrant workers was 1.6 and 6.4%; HIV prevalence was very high in many regions, where it ranged between 1.0 and 1.6% (United Nation Development Programme 2004). However, there is no official report about the HIV prevalence among Burmese migrants both in Thailand itself and along the Thai-Burma border. Nevertheless, a study by Plewes et al. (2008) showed that HIV infection rates among pregnant Karen refugees living in one refugee camp in Tak Province, Thailand, increased from 0.2% in 1997 to 0.4% in 2005. Similarly, the HIV prevalence among Burmese pregnant women attending antenatal care in Mae Tao clinic located in Thailand near the Thai-Burma border also increased from 0.8 to 2.2% during the same time (Muang 2006).

Khin (2000) contends that a lack of HIV information, an inability to negotiate safer sex, and a lack of access to condoms have resulted in an increased vulnerability to HIV. Migrants also frequently lack access to basic educational and health services due to language barriers, financial problems, and illegal status. Most of the HIV education and information is provided in the Thai language. As second language speakers, education generally and HIV education in particular is therefore less accessible to Burmese. Moreover, in most health-care services, the health-care workers communicate only in the Thai language. While HIV prevalence in this migrant group is very high, their knowledge about HIV transmission is very low. Importantly, most female immigrant workers were found to lack necessary access to family planning and safe sex services, and many of them consequently suffer unplanned pregnancies and abortions (The Integrated Regional Information Networks 2007).

Although the minimum wage for workers is between 148 and 203 Thai Baht (£2–3 UK) per day (Office of Foreign Labor Migrant Commission 2008), most migrants receive less than this. The necessity to work to earn money means that they are more likely to go to hospital in an emergency rather than attend a health-care service for health prevention or promotion programs. Legal migrants have access to partial free health care, like the Thais, even if they do not access it for other reasons.

Illegal migrants, on the other hand, do not have any free health care. They therefore have to pay full costs when they visit hospital or health-care services.

At present, the Thai government is implementing a Universal Health Care Coverage policy where every Thai citizen is covered by at least one health insurance scheme. State officials receive free treatment under the Medical Welfare Scheme, while private employees are covered under the Social Security Scheme. Those Thais who are not government officials or have no social security insurance card must pay 30 Baht (about £0.50 or less than US$1) per visit when they receive care from government health facilities (Hughes and Leethongdee 2007; WHO 2007). Expensive treatments, including kidney dialysis and antiretroviral drugs for HIV/AIDS sufferers, are currently not being offered within this scheme. Other treatments under this universal health care include dental care.

Cross-border health is one of the major concerns of the Ministry of Public Health (MoPH) which is the main institution currently working on cross-border health issues. The activities involve disease surveillance, research, financial support for public health projects, short course training, and degree training for health workers or for migrant people (Wibulpolprasert et al. 2005). Currently, health service centers provide health care for non-registered migrants based on humanitarian grounds. However, these migrants often do not seek government services, partly due to the direct cost of health care that they have to pay for treatment. Moreover, there are indirect costs including transportation and loss of working time.

2   Maternal (Antenatal) Care Service in Thailand

The majority of maternal and child health services are delivered throughout the country by government agencies at all levels of the health-care system which are being provided by midwives at health centers or nurses at the hospitals. At village level, there is a primary health-care unit, where village health volunteers assist in providing advice and referring cases to health centers. The antenatal care service system at community level is complemented by the hospital component, made up of a network of community hospitals at district level, provincial, regional hospitals, maternal and child health hospitals, and university hospitals (MoPH 2006). All levels are linked together by an established referral system.

MoPH policy calls for at least four antenatal care visits, the first of which should be within the first 6 months of pregnancy (MoPH 2006). However, the number of antenatal visits varies depending on the woman and her health-care providers. In contrast, in the United Kingdom, the first appointment needs to be arranged before 12 weeks. In addition in the UK, a woman who is primigravid with a normal pregnancy is offered a schedule of ten appointments and for a woman who is multigravida without complications, a schedule of seven appointments (National Institute of Health and Clinical Excellence [NICE] 2008). Currently, the Thai MoPH reports that more than 90% of pregnant women receive at least 4 antenatal care visits (MoPH 2006). Commonly, a pregnant woman should seek to access an antenatal service to find out about her pregnancy (Liamputtong 2005, 2007). The woman will attend antenatal checkups every month until 28 weeks of gestation, then every fortnight from 28 to 36 weeks and every week after 36 weeks. Routine antenatal care services include taking medical history; physical examination; blood testing for anemia, blood group, hepatitis B antigen, syphilis, and HIV; urinalysis; diagnosis, treatment, and referral of women with high-risk pregnancies; tetanus toxoid vaccination; provision of vitamin and iron supplements; and education on health, nutrition, and self-care.

3   Prevention Mother-to-Child Transmission of HIV in Thailand

Before looking at how to increase the participation of these women, it is important to evaluate the quality and effectiveness of the program. The prevention of mother-to-child HIV transmission (PMTCT) program was launched as one of the national HIV programs in 2000 (MoPH 2006, 2007). It encourages early antenatal care and offers antiretroviral (ARV) therapy before, during, and after the labor period.

Pre- and posttest counseling with a voluntary HIV blood test is offered to pregnant women who attend the Antenatal Clinic (ANC). Voluntary HIV testing with consent is performed usually at hospital laboratories, using either rapid HIV tests or enzyme immunosorbent assays. Women whose test results are repeatedly positive are given posttest counseling at hospitals, generally the week following testing. If the test is positive, it is repeated, and if the second test is positive, the Western blot (WB) test is performed. Pregnant women who are found to be HIV positive will be offered treatment for prevention of maternal to child HIV transmission at this stage (MoPH 2006, 2007).

ARV therapy can be prescribed, usually zidovudine (AZT), one of the modern antiretroviral drugs which are highly effective at preventing HIV transmission during pregnancy, labor, and delivery. AZT is usually taken two or three times daily, starting after the first trimester sometime between 14 and 34 weeks of pregnancy until labor begins; during labor it is administered every 3 h. After birth, all babies who are born from HIV-infected mothers will receive AZT syrups initially. However, giving a single dose of nevirapine to mother and baby can cut the risk of transmission in half (Lallemant et al. 2004).

As previously mentioned, HIV prevalence among pregnant migrant women is more than twice as high as the prevalence among pregnant Thai women. In the northern part of Thailand, HIV prevalence among pregnant migrant women is estimated at 2.5% (UNDP 2004). Moreover, numbers of women found to be HIV-positive among the multigravida migrant pregnant women is higher than in multigravida Thais (Mae Sai Hospital 2006). Therefore, we need to find a way of targeting those most at need and identifying strategies to encourage them to accept testing and treatment aimed at preventing mother-to-child transmission. Moreover, understanding or clarifying these women's experiences in antenatal care service and HIV counseling was required to try to make improvements to services. The case studies that follow show some of the crucial decisions made by two Burmese migrant women who received positive HIV tests when they were screened in pregnancy.

4   The Study

The study adopted a grounded theory approach to develop an understanding of the needs of pregnant migrant women in relation to screening for HIV in pregnancy and the subsequent decisions needed. The participants included 26 health-care workers and 38 migrant women; however, this chapter aims only to describe the experiences of two women participants who discovered they were HIV-positive during the antenatal screening process and one woman with a negative HIV result. Thus, the research question that applied to this aspect of the study was what makes Burmese pregnant women accept or refuse to participate in the PMTCT program (HIV testing)?

The settings for this study were antenatal care units in hospitals run by the Ministry of Public Health in Chiang Mai, Chiang Rai, Tak, and Mae Hong Son, which are the Thailand-Burma border provinces in the northern parts of Thailand. Inclusion and exclusion criteria for participants are shown in Table 4.1.

Data collection was carried out by the first author, Pleumjit Chotiga, who had previous experience of working in these border areas of Thailand and was able to communicate effectively with the participants. They were interviewed in the Thai language, and all data was transcribed firstly in Thai and then translated into English in order to be coded and categorized.

The study took place with full consideration of the rights of human subjects; ethical approval was granted by the Faculty of Health Ethics committee of the University of East Anglia, UK, and local approval was gained for all the research sites in Thailand. All women gave consent either in writing or by thumb print. For those unable to read the information sheet and consent form, the researcher read the information to them and gave them a copy to take away so that a partner or friend could help them understand. Women who consented did so freely and in the knowledge that they could discontinue their involvement at any time without prejudicing their treatment or care. They were assured of confidentiality and that their data would be kept anonymous but could be used in reports that would help with service development and in academic publications. Although only 38 migrant women participants took part in interviews, two found that they were HIV-positive. The data from these two women are presented because they represent specific experiences of what it is like to know that a person has HIV when pregnant. They are useful in enabling us to understand some of the decisions that needed to be taken and ways in which they thought through their situations. Together with the data from the other women, they also provide insight into some of the specific health and information needs of this vulnerable group.

Table 4.1 Inclusion and exclusion criteria for participation in the study

Inclusion criteria	Exclusion criteria
Burmese migrant women living in Thailand	Acutely ill women (physical as well as in terms of mental health) or
Pregnant or had been pregnant and had either accepted or refused the HIV screening test and ARV prophylaxis in PMTCT (prevention mother-to-child transmission of HIV) program within the last year	Women with increased levels of vulnerability were not approached
Able to speak Thai sufficiently well to communicate with the interviewer	Women unable to speak enough Thai to communicate with the interviewer
20 years old and over (the legal age of consent in Thailand)	Women under 20 years old

5 The Case Studies

Two participants had gone through the HIV testing process and learned about their HIV-positive diagnosis.

5.1 *Case 1*

Pornpen, a Bamar-Burmese woman, was 25 years old and 20 weeks pregnant at the time of the study. She came to Thailand with her parents when she was 5 years old and could not remember the reason for migrating. She was illiterate in both Thai and her language, Burmese. She was married previously and had a child with her first husband, who was Thai and had died, and she claimed that she did not know the cause of his death. She had brought up her son alone and then met her second husband last year. He had left her after she told him she was pregnant and had never come back. She was now living alone with her son and running the small laundry in her first husband's house near the hospital.

Pornpen was diagnosed HIV-positive but did not know the HIV status of her husbands, and she could not tell which husband had infected her. She disclosed that her second husband had never stayed with her for long, and she supposed that he had had sexual affairs when he went away. Therefore, she decided to take a blood test because she wanted to know her HIV status and she knew that she had some risk factors. She was very scared of AIDS.

> I would like to know whether I have got AIDS or not. My husband never stayed with me for long and I did not know whether he slept with someone else. He left me when he knew that I was pregnant. My previous husband died a few years ago and I did not know why he died.

She evaluated her decision to take an HIV test as the right decision. She revealed that she was very fearful and concerned about her baby's health when she first knew about her HIV-positive result. She had been counseled by the nurse in the antenatal clinic, and she reported that she was informed about safe sex and the AZT drug. When she was offered AZT, she accepted it immediately because she was worried about her baby's future. She was worried that no one would be around to look after her baby and the other child if she died.

> After I knew that I had got AIDS, I decided to take the drug treatment because I feared that there would be no one to look after my children. I needed to take the treatment.

Thereafter, the doctor in HIV/AIDS clinic advised her about how to take AZT and when to take it. She knew that this AZT could prevent mother-to-child transmission of HIV, and she always asked for advice from nurses and doctors when she encountered any problems. She also reported that she had learned about the side effects of the treatment, and she had never had any problems with it. She intended to give her baby formula milk as advised by the health-care workers.

She told us that the health-care insurance was very useful and valuable for her because she did not have enough money to buy the drugs by herself. She usually paid only 30 Bahts [£0.50] per each hospital visit. Pornpen disclosed she felt unhappy and resentful particularly because she was alone. She revealed that her parents did not know her HIV status, and she thought that it was good that they now were living in Burma. Her 6-year-old child was HIV-negative.

She was hopeful that her baby would not suffer with HIV because the nurse had told her there was a strong possibility that treatment would prevent transmission of the virus to her unborn child. She felt very sure that her care was the same as Thai women in the same position.

5.2 Case 2

Nongnang, 28-year-old Burmese-Tai Yai woman, was diagnosed HIV-positive while her current husband received an HIV-negative result. She was told when she was 29 weeks pregnant (pregnancy usually lasts about 40 weeks).

She revealed that she had migrated to Thailand with her parents when she was very young and could not remember which area of Burma she came from. She did not have health insurance because her husband's employer told them that they did not have the right to apply, so she had never thought to apply for it. She had since learned that she could apply and intended to do so although this would be difficult for her with her low levels of literacy. Her husband was employed as a part-time laborer [house painter] in a small building site while she was a housewife and sometimes worked as a part-time housekeeper. Her husband could earn 170 Baht (£3 UK or US$6) per day. At the time of the study, she needed to pay the full cost for health care which was around 100 Bahts (£1.65 UK or US$3) and pay for transportation 40 Bahts (£0.70 UK or US$1.2). She always expressed concern about the payments she would face for the costing of giving birth in hospital. She reported that she faced financial problems and sometimes had to borrow money from other people. She was illiterate in both Thai and her language, Tai Yai, but her husband had learned to write and read Thai while he was a Buddhist monk.

She had agreed to take a blood test because she thought that it was one of the routine processes involved in attending antenatal clinic. She mentioned that she knew all pregnant women had been offered it. Moreover, she wanted to know her HIV status. But, when she knew her HIV-positive result and was informed about the treatment to prevent MTCT of HIV, she decided to participate in this prevention program because of concern for her baby's health and safety. And her husband encouraged her to receive the AZT drug because the treatment was free of charge.

In the post-counseling section, she was asked whether she could accept or not the coming result, and then she said that she could accept it. She told us that she was called to the private room and then she was asked by nurse that "will you be shocked or suicidal if I tell something to you" and then she answered that "why I need to do something like that" and confirmed that she would not do it because she thought that we have got just only one life.

She said she felt scared when talking about what happened when she first learned her HIV-positive result. She disclosed that at the early stage, she could not control her mind and had been stunned with fear. [She was crying when she reviewed her first emotion to the HIV-positive result.] She said to the health-care worker that she would like to tell the result to her husband by herself, but she did not tell him until he came to take the blood test.

When she knew that her husband was not HIV-positive like her, she was very sorry and surprised. After knowing the different results, her husband had never asked who she had been infected from. She assumed that it might be because he knew that she had never worked as a prostitute. She told how he took care of her and he always reassured and supported her. He usually reminded her when to take the treatment.

After she knew her HIV-positive result and was informed about the treatment to prevent MTCT of HIV, she decided to participate in this prevention program because of concern for her baby's health and safety. Her husband encouraged her to receive the AZT drug because the treatment was free of charge. However, she did it due to the hope of living longer.

> I did not know what it [the drug] is and what it can do for me. I took it because I hoped that I could live longer to look after my child.

She noted that she usually prayed for her baby to be safe, meaning HIV-negative the same as her husband, and said that "I got it [HIV] and that is enough."

The following two case studies are women who, although receiving HIV-negative result, demonstrated typical traits of understanding and decision making and therefore usefully illustrate the issues identified in the study as a whole.

5.3   Case 3

Ngamta, a Tai Yai woman, was 20 years old. She came to Thailand with her family when she was 7 years old. She had attended primary school in Thailand after her parents applied to be legal migrants. She could speak her own language, Tai Yai, while she was literate in Thai. Her husband is Thai and they lived together. She was a housewife and had health-care insurance. She paid 30 Bahts for each hospital visit and revealed that with her ability to speak Thai, she had never had any problem communicating with Thai health-care workers and Thai people. She had decided to attend for antenatal care at the suggestion of her neighbor.

This was her first pregnancy and she thought that attending antenatal care would be beneficial for her baby. She knew that AIDS was one of the diseases the blood tests were intended to screen for but could not explain the benefits of screening. She knew something about HIV/AIDS and its transmission. Her reason for taking the blood test was that she was at high risk of contracting HIV. She thought that there was the possibility she could be infected from her current husband.

> I took the blood test because I thought that I already had been infected. I had the risk. My husband already has AIDS and I fear I have got AIDS.

She revealed that she was fearful when health-care workers talked about HIV/AIDS screening. She said that it was very hard when she needed to ask her husband to take the blood test again as he already knew his HIV status. Her emotional feeling and stress were exposed by talking and crying only with her husband as she could not talk with other people, even within her family. However, her HIV status was negative. She said that health-care workers educated her about reducing her risk of HIV infection from her husband.

5.4 Case 4

Manee, a 24-year-old Tai Yai woman, had been in Thailand for 18 years. She had lived in a refugee camp with her parents when she was young and had been educated there until year 9. She revealed that she was taught Tai Yai language and English in the refugee camp but not Thai language. Therefore, she could not read or speak Thai well. She had left the refugee camp when she married and now lived in a Thai community.

She had learned about the hospital system and services since she was in a refugee camp. She had health insurance and paid 30 Bahts for each hospital visit. Expecting vaccines for her baby and medicine for herself and seeing a doctor every month made her come to the antenatal care clinic, and this gave her a feeling of safety. She revealed that at the first visit, it was difficult for her to communicate with Thai health-care workers as she could not speak Thai well. She experienced that sometimes doctors or health-care workers could not understand her questions, and she also could not understand their instructions.

She explained that sometimes she wanted to ask doctors about her health, but she thought that it was a bother to do that. She preferred to listen to their instructions without trying to ask anything. She compared her life and the quality of health care in Thailand with that which she had heard about in Burma.

> Health care in Thailand is good. It is better than the stories told by my parents in Burma. I never expected better care like this. My mother gave birth at home.

This was her third pregnancy and she had experienced one abortion. She revealed that she accepted the blood tests out of concern for her baby. She considered that her baby would receive benefits from this testing. However, she was unclear on what the benefit might be. She said that "I thought that it was useful for my baby." She also remarked that she did not identify any risks of contracting HIV. However, during counseling she said she was fearful when the nurse talked about mother-to-child-transmission. She feared that her baby would die if she was infected with HIV.

She still demonstrated misunderstanding about the diseases which were being screened in this pregnancy although she had undergone antenatal blood tests in three previous pregnancies.

Many diseases could be checked with this blood test such as Cancer, AIDS and Umm…I could not remember.

Moreover, she still did not see herself as having a choice when it came to the screening test as she thought that every pregnant woman needed to do it: "Everybody must take the test, mustn't they?"

Manee said that information about hospital services and antenatal care and knowledge about pregnancy and HIV/AIDS were very important and helpful for migrant women. However, she found that information leaflets were in Thai. It was difficult for migrant women who could not read Thai, and she would like to have had leaflets in Tai Yai.

6 Discussion of Themes Illustrated in the Case Studies

The vignettes presented in the previous section are illustrative of the themes that were generated from the data in the study (Table 4.2).

To understand the experience and lives of HIV-positive pregnant women, Pornpen's story provides a particularly clear example of an abandoned HIV-positive migrant woman who needed to live and look after herself alone. She did not have her family's support, but she had economic support from the health-care insurance system and her own business, and she felt capable of making her own decisions.

On the other hand, the experiences of Nongnang demonstrate the spirit of her husband who was HIV-negative [while she was HIV-positive]. Although she had an unstable financial status and faced financial problems without health insurance, she had a great deal of support from her husband.

The similarity in experience of these two women is that they decided to participate in the treatment program because of their babies. Both of them hoped to live longer and expected that this treatment could help them and their babies.

The prevalent themes which are illustrated in these two cases but which also spanned the data from the whole group of women were concern for their babies' health and fear and ignorance of HIV. Another themes illustrated in these cases are the lack of understanding about HIV testing and the acceptance of it as a generally routine

Table 4.2 Themes emerging from the women's stories

Theme	Category/coding
Lack of effective counseling	Lack of knowledge
	Missing the important information or step
Implications of migrant status	Facing financial hardships
	Limited health insurance
Barriers to gaining information	Avoiding shame
	Feeling uncomfortable
	Experiencing language difficulties
Social comparison	Comparing with Thai experience
	Comparing with Burmese experience
Self-efficacy	Seeking information
	Learning to survive

part of the process in antenatal clinic. This is highlighted across the data in the study as a whole with few women being offered one-to-one pretest counseling. The study highlighted the need for better quality information giving and the need to pay particular attention to the language used to ensure that women really understood. It is clear that women generally did not understand about the transmission of HIV, and some did not understand their own risk status. The health-care workers confirmed the view that the women did not have much knowledge but because of the pressures inherent in the system in which they were working, with a lack of resources to provide translated materials or adequate time for discussion, they felt powerless to change.

7 Conclusion

From the findings, we have been able to identify that Burmese migrant women experience limitations with communication, financial hardships, and complications with their migrant status while attending health-care services. The effective provision of health education, HIV counseling, and general care were hindered by communication barriers, time limitations, and health-care workers' workload.

These findings suggest that the pregnant Burmese migrant women need to be motivated to participate in health care including the prevention of mother-to-child transmission of HIV programs. However, they also need to be facilitated to access health care and accept HIV testing or participate in the prevention program with full and proper understanding. It is clear that motivating factors and influences should be started before they access health care and should be included at all levels from national policy to local practise level and individual level. There have been many supportive projects for migrants in Thailand. They have been run mainly by non-government organizations and also by government. However, not all migrants are aware of the projects; therefore, some thought needs to be given to improving access to the projects.

With language barriers and time limitations, health-care workers need to give health education or information effectively. The information about prenatal HIV testing and counseling should be given in different ways depending on individual clients. The findings suggest that health-care workers should apply appropriate techniques when giving information or counseling in order to meet individual needs. Information sheets in their own language should be prepared for take-home information.

These women hold a strong belief in the truth of what they are told by their husbands, Burmese friends, and employers. They also followed the people who were of the same nationality or ethnic group. Burmese women who can speak Thai fluently and have experiences with HIV testing or PMTCT program should be trained and employed as mentors to increase these women's trust and understanding. Peer support from women who have a sound knowledge of the health system and the health insurance schemes will enable information to be passed to women by someone they can trust.

The experience of these women allows insight into their decision making and knowledge about HIV testing and treatment in pregnancy. This should influence the way in which health-care workers individualize care to meet the needs of this vulnerable group. Recommendations for policy change to facilitate better access to health care and health insurance are made based on the findings. Changes to local practice that could provide a means of education to empower the women are also suggested. Further research is needed to identify the most effective way in which care and information can be provided to this vulnerable group to improve the health of mothers and babies.

Based on the findings of this study, it is recommended that policy makers and health professionals should

- Consider and target migrant pregnant women within their in HIV prevention projects
- Increase the awareness and understanding of HIV prevention and mother-to-child transmission of HIV among migrant women
- Provide easy access to health-care services, health-care insurance, and HIV prevention projects for all migrant women
- Improve the quantity and quality of health-care workers who deal with migrant women, including counseling and translation services

References

Celentano D, Beyrer C (2008) Public health aspects of HIV/AIDS in low and middle income countries: epidemiology, prevention and care. Springer, Baltimore

Ekachai S (2003) Immigrant workers: facts and figures. Bangkok Post, July 8, 2003

Ekeh C, Smith M (2007) Minorities in Burma. Minority Rights Group International, London

European Commission Humanitarian Aid Office (2005) Humanitarian assistance to the vulnerable populations in Myanmar and to Burmese refugees along the Thai-Myanmar border. http://ec.europa.eu/echo/files/funding/decisions/2006/myanmar_thailand_en.pdf. Accessed 31 Oct 2011

Hughes D, Leethongdee S (2007) Universal coverage in the Land of Smiles: lessons from Thailand's 30 Baht health reforms. Health Aff 26(4):999–1008

Khin A (2000) HIV/AIDS problem of migrants from Burma in Thailand. http://www.burmawatch. org/com-khin-hiv-aids-burmese-migrants-thailand.pdf. Accessed 15 Sept 2009

Lallemant M, Jourdain G, Le Coeur S, Mary JY, Ngo-Giang-Huong N, Koetsawang S et al (2004) Single-dose perinatal Nevirapine plus standard Zidovudine to prevent mother-to-child transmission of HIV-1 in Thailand. N Engl J Med 351:217–228

Liamputtong P (2005) Birth and social class: northern Thai women's lived experiences of caesarean and vaginal birth. Soc Health Illn 27(2):243–270

Liamputtong P (2007) The journey of becoming a mother amongst women in northern Thailand. Lexington Books, Lanham

Mae Sai Hospital (2006) Annual report: prevention mother-to-child transmission of HIV programme. Chiang Rai, Thailand

Ministry of Public Health (2006) Annual report on the AIDS situation in Thailand for the year 2005. Ministry of Public Health, Bangkok

Ministry of Public Health (2007) Towards Universal access by 2010: Thailand National HIV and AIDS Program. Ministry of Public Health, Bangkok

Muang C (2006) The Mae Tao clinic annual report 2005. Mae Tao Clinic, Tak

NICE (2008) Antenatal care routine care for the healthy pregnant woman. RCOG Press, London

Office of Foreign Labor Migrant Commission (2008) Minimum wage 2008. http://www.mapfoundationcm.org/eng/news/minimumwage_07_08.html. Accessed 2 Dec 2010

Plewes K, Lee T, Kajeechewa L, Thwin MM, Lee SJ, Carrara VI et al (2008) Low seroprevalence of HIV and syphilis in pregnant women in refugee camps on the Thai-Burma border. Int J STD AIDS 19:833–837

POLICY (2003) HIV/AIDS in the Mekong Region: Cambodia, Lao PDR, Thailand, & Viet Nam. POLICY Project for Bureau for Asia and the Near East, U.S. Agency for International Development. http://www.policyproject.com/pubs/generalreport/ACF1B3.pdf. Accessed 12 Jan 2010

Shtarkshall R, Soskolne V (2000) Migrant populations and HIV/AIDS. The development and implementation of programmes: theory, methodology and practice. UNESCO, Paris

The Integrated Regional Information Networks (2007) Thailand: migrant workers unprotected and uninformed. http://www.plusnews.org/Report.aspx?ReportId=75261. Accessed 28 Mar 2009

UNAIDS (2006) Report on the global AIDS epidemic. UNAIDS, Geneva

UNAIDS (2010) UNAIDS Report on The Global Aids Epidemic: 2010. UNAIDS, Geneva

United Nation Development Programme (2004) Thailand's response to HIV/AIDS: progress and challenges. UNDP, Bangkok

Wibulpolprasert S, Siasiriwattana S, Ekachampaka P, Wattanamano S, Taverat R (2005) Thailand health profile 2001–2004. Printing Press, Bangkok

World Health Organization (2004) HIV/AIDS in Asia and the Pacific region 2003. World Health Organization, Geneva

World Health Organization (2007) HIV/AIDS in the South-East Asia region. World Health Organization, New Delhi

Chapter 5
Motherhood, Infertility, and HIV: The Maasai Context of Northern Tanzania

Lauren K. Birks, Yadira Roggeveen, and Jennifer M. Hatfield

1 Introduction

In a culture emphasizing procreation and sexual relations as an integral part of everyday life and success in society, the Maasai of Northern Tanzania face a difficult task when confronting HIV/AIDS. Reproduction and motherhood are inextricably linked to prosperity and growth for the Maasai, which privileges sexual intercourse as a necessity of life related to good health, responsibility, and procreation (Talle 2007). In fact, Talle (2007: 355) asserts that "to produce children is life's (and marriage's) fulfillment" for both Maasai women and men. Thus, it is certain

L.K. Birks, PhD (✉)
Faculty of Nursing, University of Alberta, 116 St, Edmonton, AB, Canada, T6G 2R3

Population and Public Health, Community Health Sciences, Faculty of Medicine,
University of Calgary,TRW Building, 3rd Floor 3330 Hospital Drive N.W.,
Calgary, AB, Canada, T2N 4N1
e-mail: lkbirks@ucalgary.ca

Y. Roggeveen
Athena Institute for Research on Innovation and Communication
in Health and Life Sciences, VU University, De Boelelaan 1085,
1081 HV Amsterdam, The Netherlands
e-mail: y.roggeveen@vu.nl

J.M. Hatfield
Global Health and International Partnerships, Faculty of Medicine, University of Calgary,
TRW Building, 7th Floor 3330 Hospital Drive, N.W., Calgary, AB, Canada, T2N 4N1
Department of Community Health Sciences and Health and Society
Major and Global Health, O'Brien Centre for Bachelor of Health
Sciences Program, University of Calgary, TRW Building,
7th Floor 3330 Hospital Drive, N.W., Calgary, AB, Canada, T2N 4N1
e-mail: Jennifer.hatfield@ucalgary.ca

P. Liamputtong (ed.), *Women, Motherhood and Living with HIV/AIDS:*
A Cross-Cultural Perspective, DOI 10.1007/978-94-007-5887-2_5,
© Springer Science+Business Media Dordrecht 2013

that a woman without children is to be pitied, thereby receiving license to "go to sexual extremes" to cure her affliction of so-called infertility (Talle 2007: 355). HIV/AIDS becomes of particular concern when infertility is a factor for Maasai women trying to achieve motherhood. These concerns arise from increased exposure to the disease through a great number of sexual partners – as a result of culturally unique sexual practises – as well as cultural expectations to produce many children (see also Chap. 6 in this volume).

The purpose of this chapter is to describe HIV in the Maasai context in Northern Tanzania and to link Maasai women's experiences of motherhood and fertility with the risk of HIV. We will examine the juxtaposition between the desire of Maasai women to experience motherhood and the risk to get infected with HIV in their attempt to become a mother. We will highlight and discuss challenges of achieving motherhood in the face of infertility, HIV, and specific cultural practises, like polygamy. We conclude the chapter by articulating the implications of our findings, which can help to inform HIV policy makers and to develop effective HIV prevention strategies, while maintaining respect for Maasai cultural practises that seek to mitigate infertility and achieve motherhood.

2   The Maasai: Social and Cultural Contexts

2.1   Maasai Culture and History

The Maasai are a seminomadic, pastoralist population of approximately 840,000 people living in Northern Tanzania and Southern Kenya. Until the late 1800s and early 1900s, the Maasai functioned largely as an egalitarian society with distinct and separate gendered and age-related roles where *both* men and women occupied sections of the domestic and public (i.e., economic and political) spheres (Hodgson 1999a, b). Women maintained the Maasai production system by functioning as traders of surplus milk, hides, donkeys, and small livestock with groups of non-Maasai women traveling through their homesteads or with other permanent trading settlements for goods such as grains and other foodstuffs (Hodgson 1999a, b). By trading with other groups, women were "crucial intermediaries in the extensive and active trade networks that enabled the Maasai to sustain their specialized production strategy by linking them to commodities of regional and global commerce" (Hodgson 1999a, b: 48). Hodgson (1999a, b) asserts that while men were more central in the political sphere, women occupied a more central role in the sphere of ritual.

Contemporary Maasai social structure is governed by such age and gender distinctions that were in place prior to German colonialism in the late 1800s. Although German colonialism (1890–1910) had an influence on the Maasai, it was inconsistent and had limited long-term impacts on Maasai social, economic, and political structures. Following World War I, British colonialism in Tanzania significantly altered Maasai society with profound implications for Maasai gender roles. British colonial leadership designated Maasai men as the "authorities" in communications between Maasai communities and the British colonists (Hodgson 1999a, b). British fears of unpredictable young male Maasai "warriors" motivated colonialists to reinforce the power of elder male authorities while disregarding the vital social roles of both young men (moran) and women in guiding and governing Maasai society (Hodgson 1999a, b). At once, the British eroded Maasai women's economic power as traders and caregivers of livestock, political power as ritualistic leaders, and social currency as a valuable part of the Maasai identity by relegating women to domestic duties (Hodgson 1999a, b). Men became the dominant and most important members of Maasai society, which is now understood by Maasai themselves as "being a pastoralist and a warrior: a dominant masculinity forged in "modernity" and sustained by certain economic and social interventions" introduced and propagated by British colonists (Hodgson 1999a, b: 122).

For Maasai women, the consequences of the colonial-induced shift in Maasai society from an egalitarian system to a patriarchal structure are far-reaching. Most notably, Maasai women have been affected in terms of their rights to livestock, property, ritualistic roles (i.e., facilitating rites of passage for both men and women), and political participation. By and large, Maasai women have been marginalized by being limited to domestic duties with little to no power beyond that sphere, which has further emphasized an already existing stress on female reproduction.

2.2 Gender, Social Constructs, and Sexuality of the Maasai

As mentioned previously, Maasai society is governed by "distinct social, developmental and social-sexual phases according to age-gender sets" (Birks et al. 2011: 585). Primary to the age-set system is the division of the male population into hierarchal age groups, which also govern sexual and gender relations in this patriarchal society (Talle 1994). Each male age-set is marked by a rite of passage, starting with circumcision between the ages of 16–18 years, upon which time Maasai men become "warriors" (moran or the preferred term is *ilmurran*) (Talle 1994). Morans are under the authority of elders, are recognized as protectors of people and livestock, and must refrain from marrying, reproducing, or associating sexually with married women (Talle 1994). During the 7–8 years that Maasai men are part of the moran age-set, they are viewed as "separate" from the rest of society and engage in ritual practises of solidarity such as slaughter, physical togetherness, and commensality, which aim to build their physical and sexual strength (Talle 1994). While building physical strength is important for the protection of people and livestock, the building of sexual strength is an essential part of moranhood and Maasai social structure because moran sexuality is considered to be directly linked to female fertility. In fact, female fertility is a culturally mediated process that does not occur naturally (Talle 1994).

Female fertility is developed over a period of time with the help of morans, who start engaging with young girls in a process of gradual coital penetration, which is ultimately consummated when the girl's mother and moran agree that she is sufficiently mature (Talle 1994). The early sexual debut of Maasai girls is based on the cultural idea that semen of the morans promotes the development of young females' breasts and sexual "health," thus making the "services" of the moran imperative for women's physical development and attainment of fertility (Talle 1994). Once young women have fully developed physically, have attained fertility through regular sexual interactions with morans, and have been circumcised, they are considered to be ready for childbearing and are married to men 10–15 years their senior (Talle 1994). The implications for women's sexual and reproductive health are seen in their elevated risk of exposure to sexually transmitted infections, such as syphilis, and more recently HIV. That Maasai gender roles threaten women's sexual and reproductive health is largely due to the subordination of women and the value ascribed to them as vehicles for propagating as many children as possible.

3 Theoretical Framework: Introducing Participatory Action Research and the Study

We used participatory action research (PAR) methodology to gather data in a culturally sensitive manner, to emphasize a participatory approach, and to encourage action – based on research findings. By combining participation with action, research is made contextually relevant. In order to foster an understanding of people's problems, the roles of the researchers and the researched are interchanged to promote communication and encourage mutual development of knowledge and learning (Swantz 2008). The PAR approach enables ordinary people (i.e., Maasai women) to directly engage the research process rather than remaining at arm's length (Swantz 2008). Greenwood and Levin (2007) refer to this process of direct engagement as *cogenerative inquiry*, where knowledge is cogenerated through collaborative communication between the researcher and the coresearchers. Fundamentally, the knowledge and experiences shared between researchers and coresearchers coalesce to reveal new knowledge about the investigated phenomenon (i.e., Maasai women's knowledge about, and experiences of, motherhood, (in)fertility, and HIV/AIDS). PAR methodology ensured that our inquiry into Maasai women's experiences of motherhood, (in) fertility, and HIV/AIDS would encourage action for social change, relevant to the local context and local knowledge, the very essence of PAR (Greenwood and Levin 2007). Central to the PAR approach is a critical assessment of social experiences that drives both participants and researchers toward identifying social needs and achieving social transformation. Employing cogenerative inquiry and corresponding iterative critical interpretation generates knowledge that then calls for the new ideas or new ways of such knowledge to be translated into new practise (Wadsworth 2006: 330).

In addition to direct engagement that was culturally sensitive, we acknowledged the historical impact that previous research has had on many Maasai communities. Although Maasai have been the subject of much social sciences-based research and are familiar with the concept of research, they have rarely been asked to participate in studies that seek to include them as coinvestigators. Rather, like other researched populations, they are more familiar with traditional research methods that take people as objects of research (Swantz 2008). Therefore, by emphasizing participation of both the researchers and the local people in the research process, a bidirectional exchange of existing knowledge fostered an enriched understanding of motherhood, infertility, and HIV. In this way, PAR became the mechanism by which Maasai women codirected our study and formulated solutions to the problems they identified through the research process.

Participants were selected after seeking advice from local hospital staff familiar with women that would be consistently participatory during the research sessions and were from villages within walking distance to the local hospital (maximum 2 h). In order to respect cultural and community hierarchies, we sought to involve traditional birth attendants (TBAs) and women representing a cross section of the local community while still holding separate meetings to request permission from and inform local community leaders about our research topic and process.

4 Principle Issues

4.1 Examining HIV Prevalence and Risk in the Maasai

The primary hospital serving the Ngorongoro Conservation Area population is a faith-based (Roman Catholic) hospital, and is the only hospital in the area that offers HIV/AIDS care and treatment (CTC), voluntary counseling and testing (VCT), provider-initiated counseling and testing (PICT), and prevention of mother-to-child transmission (PMTCT) services, as regulated by Tanzanian government policy. Aside regular outreach clinics for Mother and Child Health (MCH), special outreach camping trips are done. During these special trips, hospital staff sets up camp in remote corners of the catchment area for 2 weeks at a time to offer these services locally (funded by the Elizabeth Glaser Pediatric AIDS Foundation). Around 80% of the catchment population of the hospital is Maasai.

To date, data on HIV prevalence among Tanzanian Maasai remains sparse. Local hospital surveillance estimates HIV incidence at approximately 1.7% as compared with the national prevalence at 6.5% (UNAIDS 2009; Hospital Records 2010). While HIV prevalence among Maasai seems notably low, hospital surveillance reflects only an estimated 12.4% of the total NCA population (i.e., 10,040 people from 2007 to September 2010, out of an estimated population of 81,071) (Census Report Ngorongoro District 2010). Hence, surveillance of HIV may not be reflective of the actual incidence and prevalence of HIV among these Maasai communities. The limited number of people tested for HIV can be explained by several factors including a remote and dispersed population located far from the hospital (the area of the NCA is approximately 8,300 km^2), limited access to services, limited medical outreach capacity, stigma associated with both HIV testing and diagnosis, and lack of knowledge and understanding about HIV/AIDS.

Lack of access to healthcare, combined with unique sexual practises, places Maasai at greater risk for health-related problems, including high rates of HIV transmission (Morton 2006). Such risk factors include the cultural practise of polygamy, the widespread perception that HIV is not a Maasai or a rural problem, a reluctance to use condoms due to the belief that fertility and masculinity can be negatively impacted by condoms, as well as difficulties around translating and interpreting the concept of HIV (Coast 2006; Coast 2007; TACAIDS 2008).[1] Additional factors that may amplify the impacts of HIV/AIDS for the Maasai women include the slow decrease in female HIV infections – in Tanzania, 6.6% of women in reproductive age are HIV positive as compared to 4.6% of men (TACAIDS 2008) – Maasai cultural practises (discussed in detail below), exclusion from health education, food insecurity, gendered divisions of labor and decision making, and urban migration (Morton 2006). These factors, linked with the Maasai viewpoint that achieving motherhood is an integral element of successful womanhood, create high risk for HIV infection in Maasai women of childbearing age (approximately ages 14–40 years). Thus, understanding the local cultural setting and applying culturally appropriate prevention and relevant testing and treatment strategies are essential to attenuating the risk of HIV infection in pregnant mothers. The importance of reproduction and children in Maasai culture must be acknowledged as a priority, as the role of mandatory motherhood adds significant complexity to achieving HIV prevention. Therefore, while considering the status of a potential HIV epidemic among these communities, we employed a culturally sensitive research methodology to investigate this emotive topic.

4.2   Emergence of (In)Fertility and Motherhood as Salient Factors in Risk of HIV Infection

Initially, we set out to examine women's knowledge and experience of HIV/AIDS and how such knowledge relates to prevention of mother-to-child HIV transmission. Our questions focused on defining HIV, establishing local knowledge of HIV, discussing HIV transmission (vertical and horizontal), and pregnancy. According to the participatory and collaborative tenets of PAR, these questions were posed in conversational style sessions that enabled women to introduce their own experiences of motherhood and pregnancy, beyond the topic of HIV and HIV transmission. Such experiences of motherhood and pregnancy included birthing practises, hospital care, obstetrical difficulties, sexually transmitted infections, family planning, and fertility issues.

As the research progressed, fertility concerns became increasingly apparent. This realization required us, as researchers, to adjust our research approach and to

---

[1] In KiMaasai, the Maasai language, *biitia* is the word used to refer to HIV/AIDS. *Biitia* is used to represent multiple diseases that are associated with significant weight loss, as its meaning is literally "to shrink." Consequently, multiple meanings for HIV and other diseases with similar external symptoms lead to confusion about how to define HIV, as well as how to address causation, prevention, and treatment.

focus on including an in-depth examination of Maasai maternal health, traditional birthing practises, and (in)fertility-related cultural practises. The emergence of safe motherhood issues and fertility concerns signified that participants began to feel comfortable enough to bring up issues such as infertility and its associated risks (both socially and physically) as a major concern that extended beyond HIV. By being open to their identified concerns, our approach to formulate HIV prevention and treatment strategies became more relevant to their aims of achieving fertility and becoming a mother. By incorporating hospital staff, knowledge about sexual and reproductive health from a medical perspective was contributed throughout the research process. Thus, stakeholder interaction was amplified by the PAR approach, as questions and answers of Maasai women, as well as the hospital staff about pregnancy, infertility, and STI prevention were considered. Both women and hospital staff, to improve maternal health, could immediately use knowledge gained from our interactions with the women.

Reproduction and motherhood are inextricably linked to prosperity and growth for the Maasai. This linkage privileges sexual intercourse as a necessity of life related to good health, responsibility, and procreation (Talle 2007). In fact, Talle (2007: 355) asserts, "to produce children is life's (and marriage's) fulfillment" for both Maasai women and men. Because "fertility is linked to clan or ethnic or family name continuation," Maasai culture emphasizes the importance of reproduction (Coast 2007: 389). The success of Maasai men is directly proportional to the number of children they father; similarly, successful Maasai women are those who are able to bear children. Hence, motherhood can be seen as mandatory in Maasai culture. In other words, it is not socially acceptable for Maasai women to *choose* not to have children.

The implications of mandatory motherhood are far-reaching, both in terms of social ramifications and in terms of biological effects. The maternal mortality ratio among women attending antenatal clinics in the Ngorongoro area is estimated at 642 per 100,000 live births (Magoma et al. 2010). Moreover, the local hospital has no blood bank and relies on local transfusion services only. Thus, pregnancy poses a fatal risk to Maasai woman. For these women, working toward fertility and motherhood starts with the very first sexual contact. Maasai girls start having sexual relationships prior to puberty with young male adults (*ilmurran*) (Talle 1994). Talle (1994) describes how young Maasai girls are gradually introduced to sexual contact with young men, mostly under supervision of an older woman. Further, Talle (1994: 281) describes that once girls are considered to be mature enough, they "comply to be penetrated, but not without fear or anger sometimes, because they know that the making of their "hole" opens their way to birth giving and finally social adulthood." Girls choose male sexual partners, announcing their choice through a milk-drinking ritual (*Inkipot*)[2] (Talle 1994). Coast (2007) and Talle (1994, 2003) describe how

---

[2] *Inkipot* is a milk-drinking ritual initiated by Maasai girls, where each girl "publicly" selects moran boyfriends (usually three). The girl provides the selected morans with milk, and then each reciprocates with semen (Talle 1994). Before the girl presents the milk to the moran and his age-mates, it must be clean and prepared well. This ritual is seen to be the exchange of two bodily fluids that symbolizes a complimentary although not equal relationship between Maasai men and women (Talle 1994).

exposure to sperm and semen from the *ilmurran* helps young Maasai girls to become full-grown, fertile females. Because the development of physical puberty traits (i.e., growth of breasts) and achievement of female fertility (i.e., menstruation) are believed to be enhanced by male sperm, female contact with sperm must be direct (i.e., without a condom) for the sperm to stimulate fertility and female sexual development (Talle 1994; Coast 2007). Once a woman is fertile, the role of sperm transitions to that of procreation and maintenance of sexual health (Coast 2007).

Though female circumcision is illegal in Tanzania, it is still practised among Maasai communities. Traditionally, when considered sexually mature and ready for marriage, the girl is circumcised in order to "[…] avoid pre-marital pregnancy" (Coast 2007: 391). Furthermore, Talle (1994: 282) asserts "clitoridectomy and marriage transfers the sexually "free" girl into a potential childbearer." Female circumcision involves excision of the clitoris (clitoridectomy) and labia minora, which results in the female genitals getting a more "open look" (Talle 1994: 282). The clitoris is removed to prevent continued growth that may not only obstruct childbirth but also male sexual penetration (Talle 1994). Our findings confirmed that female circumcision is recognized by the local community as a risky practise for HIV infection, particularly because the same knife is often used for various circumcisions, thus potentially leading to cross infection of HIV (Birks et al. 2011). In addition, if a woman is infected with HIV and becomes pregnant, female circumcision increases the risk of mother-to-child HIV transmission during childbirth, as usually the joined labia tear during labor and delivery (personal communication with hospital staff).

4.3 Toward Motherhood by Enhancing Fertility: Planning a Family

In our discussions with Maasai women, it became clear that the cultural practices discussed above are not only an integral part of developing sexual maturity but also in achieving fertility and ultimately motherhood. By giving birth and becoming a mother, Maasai women meet social norms and attain social adulthood. What also became clear was that in the absence of motherhood, Maasai women live on the margins of their society and, in some cases, can be ostracized by other women. Motherhood is, by and large, considered to be a mark of success, thus making mothering somewhat mandatory. As our understanding of the Maasai female experience of mandatory motherhood began to expand, we were privileged with questions from our coresearchers about family planning, contraception, and birth spacing. At the same time, similar questions from local women were beginning to manifest in the outpatient department (OPD) at the hospital. Therefore, we decided to directly address these questions in our research sessions, as well as with local hospital staff. We discovered that, in the past, Maasai had perceived family planning approaches as offensive. Although we were unable to confirm reasons for such offense, we suspect that it is because contraception and the idea of avoiding reproduction and motherhood fly in direct contradiction to traditional Maasai beliefs. Furthermore, NGOs practicing in the area had been using "family planning" as a synonym to contraceptive use, which is in line with common use of this term, although family planning according to (inter)national definitions includes infertility care (WHO 2010). Of particular note is that while the Maasai people have had little interest in preventing conception, they have had an interest in *planning a family*. In planning a family, infertility plays a particularly distressing role. Our coresearchers clearly linked the need for planning a family to the cultural norm of mandatory motherhood, not only in terms of appropriate birth spacing, but also in terms of addressing the concerns of infertile women. Bringing the discussion back to how HIV influences family planning, we were also able to address questions and concerns about adequate HIV prevention, in spite of the desire and requirement of motherhood. For example, we emphasized the importance of testing for STIs and HIV prior to pregnancy or upon conception, as well as the rationale of a hospital delivery under skilled attendance (increased care in case of complications for all women, availability of medication to prevent PMTCT in case of HIV infection).

Infertility is a major concern for Maasai women, and contraception is rarely considered. Women who are unable to conceive due to infertility face potential social isolation and judgment. Although circumstances occur where families who are close to one another will "share" children with women who are unable to conceive by gifting a child to the afflicted woman, infertility is still an embarrassing and difficult experience (Talle 2004). A woman without children is to be pitied and licensed to "go to sexual extremes" to cure her affliction (Talle 2007: 355). Women who try to achieve motherhood through increased sexual activity are subject to increased risk of HIV infection. Concerns about HIV infection related to infertility and motherhood stem from two principle factors: (1) the exposure to greater numbers of sexual partners correlates with greater exposure to STIs, including HIV (Talle 1994; Birks et al. 2011); and (2) societal norms regarding development of female fertility and mandatory motherhood compel females to perform sexual practices from an early age. A protracted period of sexual activity combined with the encouragement to have sexual intercourse with multiple partners situates these women closer to HIV infection.

As mentioned, Maasai culture has many unique practises around sex and sexual development. In case of infertility, women seek help from local traditional healers, who mostly attribute infertility to social imbalances. Women organize separate meetings with women only at local spiritual places, to ask for blessing from Engai, the Maasai god (Johnsen 1997). Men can ask friends from the same age-set to help his wife get pregnant, to strengthen their friendship (Talle 1994). For infertility, once every couple of years, a big ceremony is organized: the *Olamal,* meaning "blessing ceremony." The ceremony is officially announced and can be attended by Maasai women from anywhere, even across borders. It therefore mostly is a far and ritual journey that Maasai women undertake to enhance their fertility and/or to address infertility. Central concept in the ceremony is the cleansing of any sin that can cause infertility and to be cleansed of the sin that infertility is itself. During Olamal, a traditional healer or important elder facilitates rituals and prayers to overcome infertility (Johnsen 1997; Llewelyn-Davies 1985). The film "The Women's Olamal" gives an insight on Olamal practises by Kenyan Maasai women (Llewelyn-Davies 1985). It is well known, and anecdotally confirmed by our research, that

Tanzanian Maasai women also engage in the fertility practises of Olamal. While it is not openly discussed in public, it is widely understood that when practicing Olamal, women are engaging in sexual intercourse with multiple sexual partners to enhance existing female fertility and/or to overcome infertility by increasing the likelihood of pregnancy (male infertility issues aside). Consequently, the risk of STI infection, especially HIV, becomes exponential.

Maintaining cultural sensitivity during our research process required us to challenge our own ideologies and assumptions about what is more important: prevention of HIV or fertility and achievement of motherhood. We necessarily acknowledge that shifting our emphasis from HIV transmission toward infertility posed a considerable digression from our original research objective. Still, our experiences with these women provoked us to accord our original research agenda with the needs of our coresearchers. Ultimately, the way to improve HIV prevention is through better understanding the needs of this community. We thus see primary prevention of HIV in (to be) mothers, as a strategy in PMTCT. The rationale then is that a reduction of HIV infection in (to be) mothers leads to less HIV-infected pregnant women and leads to a decreased risk of mother-to-child transmission, thus less HIV-infected children.

We suggest that our decision to reorient our research objectives is persuasively illustrated by one of our coresearchers/participants:

> Children are the most important to us, Maasai. When we become a mother, and have children, we feel the blessing of God. We have the burden of life. Being a mother helps us to tighten our relationship with the children's father. We can also ensure that the cattle will be inherited by our children. So, then we will always have cattle and income to take care of us mothers.

By establishing an in-depth cognizance of the role of infertility, as related to mandatory motherhood in the Maasai, we come to comprehend why women are not willing to use protective measures, such as condoms, to protect against HIV and other STIs. Essentially, sex with multiple partners and exposure to diseases are, on balance, worth the risk if it means successful conception and the achievement of motherhood. As illustrated by a quote from Coast (2007: 396):

> Even if a young girl gets this disease, she will still have a baby, so it is Enkai (God) telling you to have children, but just die sooner.

Our participants expressed concern about HIV infection, trying different sexual partners in an attempt to conceive. They requested to learn more about infertility, and we realized there was more to learn about the Maasai perspective on infertility.

4.4 Infertility Causes: The Maasai Perspective and the Medical Perspective

Maasai women recognize different reasons for infertility. For example, syphilis (*emireka*) is known to cause internal boils that may "harm the womb" (Johnsen 1997: 271–272). Sins and a "bad look" of particular individuals are documented as potential reasons for infertility (Johnsen 1997). The "softness" of children and "the child in the back" are also important concepts relating to infertility. A child that is born is considered a "soft child," which is a child that first needs to prove its existence by surviving the first years of life (Johnsen 1997). Similarly, in the first trimester of pregnancy, Maasai women regard the conception "not ready" or as "being in a fluent state that gradually becomes solid under the influence of semen [from intercourse] in the first three months of pregnancy" (Johnsen 1997: 271–272). This might not be surprising, as when a miscarriage occurs in the first 3 months, the fetus is undifferentiated amidst blood clots.

Strange cravings of a mother with a *young* pregnancy are seen as the "blood" desire of the fetus. When something goes wrong in this blood flow, the fetus can "dry out...leaving only an empty child" (Johnsen 1997: 263), thus becoming a "child in the back." The vital role of sperm to resolving this condition is conveyed by Johnsen (1997: 263): "The condition is only terminated when the dry, undeveloped fetus once more becomes filled with blood, with life that is, after having met with men."

Therefore, it becomes clear that semen, which Maasai men and women refer to as blood (*sangre*), is important in establishing fertility and in addressing infertility (Coast 2007). For Maasai, the importance of semen not only plays a role in fertility and conception but also plays a role in a community-wide aversion to condom use. The Maasai culture views collection of sperm in a condom, whether it is for contraception or for STI prevention, as wasting semen (Coast 2007). Wasting semen, either with condom use, oral sex, or masturbation, is viewed as less than desirable in the Maasai culture because every sperm is seen as a potential life and therefore valued above all else, including protection from STIs (Coast 2007). Coast's assertions regarding condoms and the corresponding wasting of semen have significant implications for HIV prevention. Furthermore, observations during ultrasounds at the outpatient department of the local hospital, which were confirmed in research discussions with participants, confirm the existence of the cultural concept of "the child in the back" in the local community. When women with infertility have an ultrasound, many of them ask if "the child in the back" can be seen. If not aware of the importance of this child in the back (being able to conceive, but just having a child inside that does not grow), one could easily reply "no." More cultural sensitive in this case is to reply that the machine that is used (ultrasound) is not able to display such a dry child in the back. This is actually true and respecting the status of the woman as possibly having "conceived" in another meaning than medical.

Factors that are known in the etiology of infertility are many, among which are tubal pathology (after ectopic pregnancy, pelvic inflammatory disease, STIs), endometrial granuloma (tuberculosis, schistosomiasis), ovulation defects, a history of spontaneous abortion, complications after delivery, STIs, semen pathology, and higher age (Larsen et al. 2006). Though no research on causes of infertility is conducted in the local community, several of these factors are present at the local hospital: it is located in a tuberculosis endemic area; STIs and pelvic inflammatory disease are frequently diagnosed at the outpatient department and wards. Syphilis incidence at antenatal controls is 3–4% (Endulen Hospital data 2009). Of deliveries in the district, only 7% take place with skilled attendance (Magoma et al. 2010). Complications/illness during pregnancy covered 15% of the annual female hospital admissions in 2008 (Endulen Hospital data 2009). Most couples attending OPD with infertility had a history of STIs, most notably of syphilis. Syphilis is a frequent diagnosis, mostly in the top ten of Endulen Hospital diseases among adults. Although it is understood that the disease can be prevented through barrier methods, the preference of Maasai to refrain from condom use remains unchanged. Hospital staff reports the Maasai value antibiotic treatment with injections as a "good therapy," thus decreasing the perceived need for prevention of infection. In addition, Maasai men lack motivation for partner treatment when their wife is the symptomatic case, thus allowing for reinfection and a ground for both infertility and HIV superinfection. The Maasai's familiarity with syphilis treatment may have contributed to the local idea that HIV can be cured as well, therefore encouraging a lack of condom use. Moreover, hospital staffs have consistently reported difficulties in explaining to patients that antiretroviral medication does improve health, but does not cure HIV. Therefore, while there is a significant overall understanding of HIV in the Maasai community, such complete understanding does not extend to knowledge about prevention and effective treatment.

Although we did not collect quantitative data on infertility in the community, prevalence of infertility cases in consultations by the medical officer started at zero and increased to approximately 25% of the female consultations in the outpatient department (OPD). We suspect that the increase in numbers of women experiencing infertility presenting at the OPD was due to word spreading through the community that infertility was an acceptable medical topic and that potential treatment could be provided at the hospital. In fact, couples attending the OPD mentioned their increased trust to discuss the topic of infertility and increased awareness of services in counseling on infertility in the hospital. At the same time, hospital staff became more aware that infertility is a concern and referred couples to the medical officer for review. During counseling, aside full medical history and physical examination, diagnostic and treatment options are discussed, including referral possibilities. It is made clear that no successful outcome, a pregnancy, can be guaranteed. After basic diagnostics, counseling, and treatment at the hospital, five couples chose to be referred to a larger hospital outside the NCA for more comprehensive diagnostics and treatment of infertility, after which two couples had a successful pregnancy. One led to hospital-based delivery in collaboration with the traditional birth attendant, who made explicit that because of great infertility care, she had more trust in the hospital institution as a whole. There is anecdotal evidence on satisfaction with the infertility service, even when not leading to a pregnancy. At the same time, more fertile couples presented at OPD with questions on birth spacing (both natural and contraceptives). Creating successful stories in a narrative culture, as the Maasai, is a strategy that is not to be underestimated.

4.5 Implications for HIV Prevention and Care and Treatment in the Face of Infertility

When conception is the goal of sexual contact, as is the case in infertility, use of condoms is contradictive. Vaginal application products that reduce STIs/HIV transmission risk could be a solution to the STI/HIV risk that semen contact brings, while keeping the procreative function and cultural appreciation of semen. Recent research shows promising but also ambiguous results (Mc Cormack et al. 2010; McCoy et al. 2010). Two different applicants, one with and one without contraceptive effect, would be ideal for the Maasai setting, allowing women to make own reproductive choices.

In addition to this background not in favor of condom use, culture-sensitive education on and availability of condoms are low throughout Ngorongoro district. In a local village, an advert sign by a condom provider was put in the center of the village, showing a happy non-Maasai couple, a man and one woman (and no cattle). This picture does not reflect the ideal Maasai family picture at all. Although condoms are on sale at the local shops, our participants felt not in charge of the decision to use them and find them expensive. This makes accessibility to condoms low, in addition to remote and dispersed populations and religious beliefs (Catholic hospital service only). Interestingly, the women denied that the condom would not fit the Maasai male genitals, something believed by outsiders due to the specific male circumcision technique, which leaves the foreskin hanging loosely aside the glans penis.

However, it is also futile to push HIV prevention in the face of cultural practises that emphasize mandatory motherhood, enhancement of fertility, and sexual practices that attempt to mitigate infertility when such practises are an essential cultural norm. By neglecting the importance of cultural practises, HIV prevention efforts are likely to be unsuccessful. Moreover, a lack of cultural respect discourages the community from discussing infertility issues. By incorporating Maasai knowledge of fertility and infertility with knowledge of HIV prevention, we are more likely to maintain the respect and engagement of the community in biomedically derived strategies that seek to mitigate HIV transmission while relieving major concerns about infertility.

The action and knowledge translation from this research has led to the adaptation of maternal health services, including infertility care at the local hospital. Attention to infertility at OPD and awareness of traditional practises can lead to an open discussion of treatment options and the application of basic diagnostic tools (physical examination, laboratory investigation, and ultrasound).

The research discussed in this chapter has been collected over the course of 2 years, between 2008 and 2010 in the Maasai community of the Ngorongoro Conservation Area (NCA) in Northern Tanzania. Although the original research purpose was to examine women's knowledge and experience of HIV/AIDS and how such knowledge relates to pregnancy, motherhood and prevention of mother-to-child HIV transmission, safe motherhood issues, and fertility concerns emerged during the research process as equally significant matters for Maasai women. It is notable that the emergence of safe motherhood issues and fertility concerns in the context of this research signifies differences in perceptions of salient cultural interests between the researchers and the Maasai women. Participatory action research is a useful tool in overcoming such barriers and can be used in any local setting.

5 Conclusion

Mandatory motherhood has significant implications for risk of HIV infection in women. In particular, the Maasai women living in the Ngorongoro Conservation Area of Northern Tanzania face not only the expectation of procreation and motherhood but also the expectations associated with other unique cultural and sexual practices of the Maasai as potential risk factors for contracting HIV. Most notably, these unique cultural practices include polygamy, fertility-inducing sexual practices, female and male circumcision, extramarital sexual practices, and traditional birth outside hospital circumstances. Ultimately, our exploration of HIV and motherhood in the context of the Maasai of Northern Tanzania has showed us that mandatory motherhood leads to significant distress when women experience infertility because of failure to achieve womanhood and social isolation. Therefore, it is notable that when Maasai women experience infertility, the imperative nature of motherhood leads them to pursue sexual practices that will increase their risk of HIV infection. The risk of HIV infection is not without acknowledgment; however, HIV infection is less important than the experience of motherhood and ability to procreate within the Maasai context of social norms and cultural expectations.

Acknowledgments Fieldwork was possible in collaboration with the University of Bugando, the Catholic Archdiocese of Arusha, local village authorities, the Ngorongoro Conservation Area Authority, all Endulen Hospital staff, and the University of Calgary. We would like to acknowledge the open and active participation of all men and women involved in the research, as well as our local translator, Mr. Saning'o Godwin Ole Mchuma. A part of the results was presented at the International Conference on Family Planning: Research and Best Practices, Kampala, Uganda, 16th November 2009. Comments by conference participants and collaborative efforts to increase access to infertility care in remote communities are acknowledged. The Bill and Melinda Gates Foundation sponsored Y. Roggeveen's attendance to this conference. Ethical approval was obtained from the University of Calgary and NIMR, Tanzania, under NIMR/HQ/R.8a/VolX./876 (Developing complex interventions: A multidisciplinary project that integrates a holistic pastoralist-centered approach to education, prevention, and treatment of HIV/AIDS and other coinfections, Hatfield, Manyama, et al.). Local approval was obtained from Tanzanian authorities and the Catholic Archdiocese of Arusha as legal owner of Endulen Hospital. At the beginning of each session, participants were reminded of the research context after which oral consent was requested. Participants were informed they could end their participation at any time.

References

Birks LK, Powell CD, Thomas AD, Medard E, Roggeveen Y, Hatfield JM (2011) Promoting health, preserving vulture: adapting RARE in the Maasai context of northern Tanzania. AIDS Care 23(5):585–592

Coast E (2006) Local understanding of, and responses to, HIV: rural-urban migrants in Tanzania. Soc Sci Med 63:1000–1010

Coast E (2007) Wasting semen: cultural context of condom use among the Maasai. Cult Health Sex 9(4):387–401

Endulen Hospital (2009) Patient statistics report. Ngorongoro Conservation Area, Tanzania

Greenwood DJ, Levin M (2007) Introduction to action research: social research for social change. Sage, Thousand Oaks

Hodgson DL (1999a) "Once intrepid warriors": modernity and the production of Maasai masculinities. Ethnology 38(2):121–150. http://www.jstor.org/stable/3773979. Accessed 5 July 2010

Hodgson DL (1999b) Pastoralism, patriarch and history: changing gender relations among Maasai in Tanganyika, 1890–1940. J Afr Hist 40(1):41–65. http://www.jstor.org/stable/183394. Accessed 25 June 2009

Hospital Records (2009, 2010) Patient statistics report. Endulen Hospital, Ngorongoro Conservation Area, Tanzania

Johnsen N (1997) Maasai medicine: objectifying iloibonok and fertility – the interrelationship of bodily perfection, morality and magic. In: Practicing health and therapy in Ngorongoro Conservation Area, Tanzania. PhD dissertation. Institute of Anthropology, University of Copenhagen, Denmark

Larsen U, Masenga G, Mlay J (2006) Infertility in a community and clinic-based sample of couples in Moshi, Northern Tanzania. East Afr Med J 83(1):10–17

Llewelyn-Davies M (1985) The Women's Olamal (1985), film via Documentary Educational Resources. www.der.org. Accessed 30 June 2010

Magoma M, Requejo J, Campbell OMR, Cousens S, Filippi V (2010) High ANC coverage and low skilled attendance in a rural Tanzanian district: a case for implementing a birth plan intervention. BMC Pregnancy Childbirth 10(13):1–13

Mc Cormack S, Kamali A, Rees H, Crook AM, Gafos M, Jentsch U et al (2010) PRO 2000 vaginal gel for prevention of HIV-1 infection (Microbicides Development Programme 301): a phase 3, randomized, double-blind, parallel-group trial. Lancet 376:1329–1337

McCoy SI, Watts CH, Padian NS (2010) Preventing HIV infection: turning the tide for young women. Lancet 376:1281–1282

Morton J (2006) Conceptualising the Links between HIV/AIDS and pastoralist livelihoods. Eur J Dev Res 18(2):235–254. http://www.tandfonline.com.ezproxy.lib.ucalgary.ca/doi/pdf/10.1080/09578810600708247. Accessed 22 Feb 2008

Ngorongoro District (2010) Census report. Ngorongoro Conservation Area, Tanzania. Ngorongoro Conservation Area Authority

Swantz ML (2008) Participatory action research as practice. In: Reason P, Bradbury H (eds) The Sage handbook of action research: participative inquiry and practice, 2nd edn. Sage, Thousand Oaks, pp 31–48

TACAIDS (2008) Tanzania Commission for AIDS – Tanzania HIV/AIDS and malaria indicator survey 2007–2008. http://www.tacaids.go.tz/hiv-and-aids-information/current-status-of-hiv-and-aids.html. Accessed 19 Nov 2010

Talle A (1994) The making of female fertility: anthropological perspectives on a bodily issue. Acta Obstet Gynecol Scand 73:280–283

Talle A (2004) Adoption practices among the pastoral Maasai of East Africa: enacting fertility. In: Bowie F (ed) Cross-cultural approaches to adoption. Routledge, Oxfordshire/New York, pp 64–78

Talle A (2007) 'Serious games': licenses and prohibitions in Maasai sexual life [Electronic version]. Africa 77(3):351–369

UNAIDS & World Health Organization (2009) 2009 – AIDS epidemic update. http://www.unaids.org/en/HIV_data/2007EpiUpdate/default.asp. Accessed 20 Nov 2009

Wadsworth Y (2006) The mirror, the magnifying glass, the compass and the map: facilitating participatory action research. In: Reason P, Bradbury H (eds) Handbook of action research, Concise paperback edition. Sage, Thousand Oaks, pp 322–334

Chapter 6
"I Will Give Birth But Not Too Much": HIV-Positive Childbearing in Rural Malawi

Sara Yeatman and Jenny Trinitapoli

1 Introduction

Demographic and public health research on the sub-Saharan African AIDS epidemic has centered on its mortality and morbidity consequences; however, there is growing interest in the potential implications for the region's notoriously high rates of fertility. HIV/AIDS affects the fertility of people who are infected in two distinct ways. First, both symptomatic and asymptomatic infections have physiological consequences for reproductive age adults, compromising fecundity (the ability to have children) and lowering child survival rates, particularly for those born to infected mothers (Zaba and Gregson 1998; Casterline 2002; Nguyen et al. 2006). HIV can also affect fertility in volitional ways through altering the reproductive goals and behaviors of people who know they are infected. In this chapter, we examine evolving social norms around HIV-positive childbearing in a town in southern Malawi and explore the childbearing desires of young HIV-positive women in order to better understand why some women want to continue having children while others do not.

S. Yeatman (✉)
Department of Health and Behavioural Sciences, University of Colorado Denver,
P.O. Box 173364, Campus Box 188, Denver, CO 80217, USA
e-mail: sara.yeatman@ucdenver.edu

J. Trinitapoli
Department of Sociology, Penn State University, 500 Oswald Tower,
University Park, PA 16802, USA

Population Research Institute, Penn State University, 500 Oswald Tower,
University Park, PA 16802, USA
e-mail: jat28@psu.edu

P. Liamputtong (ed.), *Women, Motherhood and Living with HIV/AIDS:*
A Cross-Cultural Perspective, DOI 10.1007/978-94-007-5887-2_6,
© Springer Science+Business Media Dordrecht 2013

2 HIV and Fertility Preferences in Sub-Saharan Africa

Early in the epidemic, studies suggested that there was little relationship between HIV status and fertility preferences (Casterline 2002). This was understandable given that access to HIV testing was poor and rarely used; only a small proportion of HIV-positive individuals were aware of their status, and there was probably little deliberate attempt to limit pregnancies in response to AIDS (Setel 1995). With the spread of HIV testing over the past decade, however, a number of recent studies have considered how being HIV-positive influences the desire to have children in a wide variety of contexts across sub-Saharan Africa. This body of research shows that women who know they are HIV-positive are more likely than other women to want to stop having children, but there is considerable variation in their desires (Cooper et al. 2007; Hoffman et al. 2008; Yeatman 2009; Taulo et al. 2009).

Qualitative research has uncovered a number of reasons why women may not want to have children when they are HIV-positive. Despite the relatively widespread reach of prevention of mother-to-child transmission programs, some women still fear transmitting HIV to their children (Cooper et al. 2007). Others worry about having children that will become orphans in the future (Grieser et al. 2001; Feldman and Maposhere 2003). And, women from across eastern and southern Africa report concerns that childbearing will worsen a woman's HIV infection and hasten the onset of AIDS symptoms (Rutenberg et al. 2000; Cooper et al. 2007; Nduna and Farlane 2009; Yeatman 2009). Indeed, while conducting interviews in rural Malawi in 2006, this was the most common reason we heard for why HIV-positive women (mostly in their 30s) wanted to stop having children. It was a widespread belief shared by women and men, infected and uninfected alike, that pregnancy and childbirth were actually physically dangerous to HIV-positive women (Yeatman 2011). Nonetheless, some of the HIV-positive women we interviewed expressed the desire to have more children, even while simultaneously acknowledging the physical risks they would face if they did.

Indeed, every study of HIV and fertility preferences in sub-Saharan Africa has found that a sizeable proportion of HIV-positive women still report desires—frequently intense—to have children (e.g., Cooper et al. 2007; Nduna and Farlane 2009; Yeatman 2009). This is common in, but not exclusive to, communities where antiretroviral therapy (ART) is readily available and is understood to be effectively preserving the health of many community members. Across the region, many HIV-positive women want to pursue the commonly shared goal of motherhood. Smith and Mbakwem (2010) described HIV-positive women they interviewed in Nigeria as particularly sensitive to the social pressures around marrying and having children, viewing these as opportunities to lead "normal" lives and reduce stigma associated with their illness. Cooper et al. (2007) found a diversity of reproductive intentions among HIV-positive women in urban South Africa: While many women did not want to get pregnant, others felt strong desires to experience parenthood. And some wanted to stop childbearing but felt social pressure to have more children because others did not know they were positive. A study from Kenya found high rates of pregnancy among HIV-discordant couples suggesting that the desire for pregnancy superseded concerns about infecting one's partner or becoming infected oneself (Guthrie et al. 2010).

These studies demonstrate that even as HIV reduces the fertility desires of HIV-positive women on the aggregate, it does not do so universally. But what explains the variation in responses within a given context? Why do some HIV-positive women choose to stop having children, while others still strongly desire them?

One important consideration is the number of children a woman has. Of course, the desire for more children decreases with parity (number of children), and while most survey research acknowledges this by statistically controlling for parity, it fails to satisfactorily consider the role that reproductive experience may have in moderating the relationship between HIV and fertility. A few recent studies provide motivation to focus on parity more specifically in attempting to understand how HIV status influences fertility desires, intentions, and behaviors. First, a study from Nigeria found that HIV-positive women without children universally expressed a desire to get pregnant (Oladapo et al. 2005). Second, a study from Zimbabwe found that all the HIV-positive pregnant women in their sample who admitted to having wanted the pregnancy ($n=7$) were childless or had recently entered a new relationship (Feldman and Maposhere 2003). Other evidence suggests that there might be a parity threshold effect—HIV-positive women in Rwanda with more than four children were less likely to become pregnant during the follow-up period than HIV-positive women with fewer children (Allen et al. 1993). The relationship was unique to HIV-positive women and persisted net of other sociodemographic characteristics. We interpret this finding as an indication that women who learned they were positive still wanted to have children but that the strength of the motivation depended on how many children they already had.

In this chapter, we combine survey data and in-depth interviews with a subsample of survey respondents to explore how parity moderates the relationship between HIV and childbearing desires. We posit that considering a woman's stage of life, and in particular, her past reproductive success, is critical for understanding the relationship between HIV and childbearing in the context of Malawi—and indeed, across sub-Saharan Africa. Although many fear the consequences of pregnancy and childbirth given an HIV-positive status, the desire for children—in and of itself and also for maintaining regard in the community and "normalcy"—is paramount. By extension, this consideration informs a secondary argument that at this point in the epidemic, a broader social consensus about HIV-positive childbearing is emerging.

3 The Childbearing Imperative in Sub-Saharan Africa

Our study's framework draws from a wide literature on the importance of childbearing in sub-Saharan Africa. In particular, we focus on the intrinsic values of childbearing, which we see as rooted in three domains in the Malawian context: achieving full adulthood, maintaining the moral order, and cementing a relationship. We argue that while women's HIV status is, indeed, a component of the childbearing calculus, it is balanced with many other components, some of which supersede AIDS in importance and relevance.

For Westerners, the demotion of AIDS as a key factor in childbearing decisions may be a hard pill to swallow. Those of us who do research on AIDS are familiar with statistics about the magnitude of the devastation the disease has brought and the increasing numbers of orphans, and we often describe it as the most pressing health crisis of our time. For many, it seems obvious that AIDS would be among the most important factors (if not the single most important one) a woman living amidst a generalized AIDS epidemic would consider. However, this perspective is simply not shared by most of our research participants—positive and negative alike. We argue that the careful consideration of these three factors, which, at least in the Malawian context, considerably outweigh HIV in importance, allows greater insight into the childbearing desires of HIV-positive women.

The first perspective on childbearing situates the act as a step on the path towards achieving full adulthood in most sub-Saharan African societies. It is difficult (and potentially unwise) to generalize about the precise importance of childbearing and the consequences of infertility across a region as diverse as sub-Saharan Africa. Nonetheless, we will do so cautiously in an attempt to illustrate just how powerful a force childbearing is to women and how loathsome barrenness is perceived to be. Across Africa, infertile women are often unable to attain full womanhood (Lesthaeghe 1989; Suggs 1993; Hollos 2003; Dyer 2007; Hollos and Larsen 2008; Hollos et al. 2009). Meyer Fortes (1978: 125) describes the transition to parenthood as the "*sine qua non* for the attainment of the full development as a complete person to which all aspire." In Cameroon, Jennifer Johnson-Hanks (2004) argues that it is often not until a woman's second birth that she attains full female adulthood. So, while women may fear exacerbating their HIV infection or transmitting HIV to a child, these perceived "risks" are unlikely to be sufficiently strong to offset the alternative, where that involves assuming the role of perpetual adolescent or electing membership in some "third" (not male, not female) category.

A second, less obvious perspective is rooted in moving beyond the vision of childbearing merely as a demographic act and sees it as part of the moral order, where moral orders are defined as "intersubjectively and institutionally shared social structuring of moral systems that are derived from the larger narratives and belief systems" (Smith 2003:10). While many demographers discuss childbearing in Africa as a "normative behavior," the moral order framework sees childbearing as far more than that. Political scientist, Patrick Chabal (2009), identifies the "cycle of life" as one of the three components of the African ethical framework. And demographers and anthropologists, John and Pat Caldwell (1987: 419, 412), hint at this very fact when they write: "To a great extent, African religion is essentially the reproduction of the lineage" and that "barrenness is a matter of fundamental social and theological significance." Throughout much of Africa, the moral order is framed around one's duty to have a child. To not do so violates shared standards and expectations for what it means to be a "person." See also Chap. 5 in this volume.

Christian Smith (2003: 25) argues that "one of the best ways to reveal the moral character of social institutions…is to violate moral norms and observe the reactions."

For a woman, to choose not to have children would be to fundamentally violate the moral order of her society and face the consequences—stigma, divorce, ostracism—of doing so. While women may fear the consequences of having a child while HIV-positive, disrupting the moral order is a much more egregious—and transcendental—violation. This fear is likely to be particularly acute among women who have yet to become mothers and for those with a conspicuously insufficient number of children (e.g., two, in a context where the average is close to six).

The third, often overlooked, perspective on the childbearing calculus focuses on its importance to a relationship. In African contexts, marriage is often described—and understood—as a process involving many steps and many actors (Meekers 1992). Childbearing is a critical step along the path to a complete marriage. Sharing a child cements a relationship between the two members of a couple and provides them with respite from the intense pressure from relatives to procreate (Grieser et al. 2001; Boerma and Urassa 2001; Hollos and Larsen 2008). In our previous qualitative research in rural Malawi, marriages that had failed to produce children were described as "not marriage" or "disturbed." Couples who have yet to have children are aware of the discussions and gossip around them and are usually subject to intense pressure from relatives to have children or to leave their partner so that they may have children elsewhere (Yeatman 2008). As a result, the failure to have a child (whether physiological or volitional) is a leading cause of relationship instability and divorce (Dyer 2007; Dyer et al. 2002; Hollos et al. 2009).

Of course, in relatively high-fertility societies, having one child may not be sufficient. There is no universal acceptable number of children; rather, it varies by context and particular situation—related to the local standard, age of the couple, children from previous relationships, and the length of the union. Work by Hollos and Larsen (2008) and Hollos et al. (2009) in Nigeria and Tanzania illustrates how context mediates the pressures faced by those struggling to have children. They find that in urban areas where fertility is substantially lower than in rural areas, women with secondary infertility (i.e., a period of infertility that occurs after having one or more children) face less pressure even if they have had only one or two children compared to their counterparts in rural areas. In both contexts, however, primary infertility (i.e., childlessness) generates considerable stigma. The findings highlight what the authors describe as "the absolute necessity for a woman to have a child," even in an urban context (Hollos and Larsen 2008: 170). Rather than the number of children a woman has, the crucial point is that she has a child—achieving the status of mother. In rural areas, the threshold is likely to be higher, particularly where childhood mortality is high and where normative fertility is high and less variable. There is a three-tiered hierarchy of sorts that places childless women, particularly those who have never conceived, at the bottom, followed by subfertile women, and those who have produced a respectable "minimum" number of offspring at the top (Hollos and Larsen 2008; Hollos et al. 2009; Larsen et al. 2010).

Research from across sub-Saharan Africa has established that primary infertility is relatively rare (~3%) but that secondary infertility is considerably more common due mainly to the high burden of sexually transmitted infections (5–23%). This is true in Malawi where primary infertility is as low as 2% but secondary infertility affects 17% of women (Larsen 2000). In other words, not having any children is a rare event, but stopping—whether because of biology or choice—is common.

Relative to the three fundamental considerations for childbearing—attaining full adult status, maintaining the moral order, and cementing relationships—HIV status belongs to a set of secondary factors that influence a woman's fertility goals, her intentions, and ultimately, her behaviors. It is only after considering the primary forces outlined above that the risk-reward balance between childbearing and stopping begins to shift with respect to secondary factors like HIV. John Bongaarts (2001) argues that competing preferences explained some of the dissonance of intentions for women who had not yet achieved their ideal family size but also indicated they did not want to have more children. We hypothesize that the desire to protect one's own health and one's future children from infection is a *competing preference* that becomes more pronounced for HIV-positive women as their number of living children increases.

4 The Studies

4.1 Study Context

Twelve percent of reproductive age individuals are estimated to be HIV-positive in Malawi, making its epidemic among the most severe in the world (NSO and ORC Macro 2005). As elsewhere in the region, HIV prevalence in Malawi rose throughout the 1980s and early 1990s before stabilizing in the late 1990s due to a decline in incidence (Bello et al. 2006; White et al. 2007; Bongaarts et al. 2008). Nonetheless, the number of infected individuals continues to increase because of population growth and the spread of ART, which increasingly allows infected individuals to live longer than they would have otherwise.

Beginning in the mid-1990s, media and public health campaigns disseminated information about the epidemiology of HIV, the major sources of transmission, and common opportunistic infections associated with AIDS and their symptoms. To prevent the spread of HIV, interventions encouraged premarital abstinence, marital fidelity, and condom use. By the late 1990s, awareness of HIV was widespread, and rural Malawians regularly talked about the disease (Watkins 2004). As early as 2004, most district hospitals began to offer nevirapine to HIV-positive pregnant women in order to limit the vertical transmission of HIV from mother to child. Early on in the program, uptake of HIV testing at antenatal clinics was low, as was the use of nevirapine. With the spread of HIV testing across the country and a policy change to opt out testing in antenatal clinics, the use of nevirapine increased, but coverage remains below 50% of HIV-positive pregnant women (Moses et al. 2008; Malawi Ministry of Health 2009; UNICEF 2010).

HIV testing and counseling was not readily available outside of urban areas in Malawi until 2005 when it spread to all district hospitals and limited rural health clinics (UNAIDS/WHO 2006; Malawi Ministry of Health 2007). The provision of free ART was expanded to district hospitals in 2006 and has been scaled up since then. The initial eligibility criteria for ART required that infected individuals be clinically staged as WHO Criteria 3 or 4[1] before initiating treatment, meaning that most infected individuals wait until they are very sick to begin treatment. More recently, CD4 machines have spread to some district hospitals and private clinics permitting more people to be eligible for ART based on their low CD4 count rather than only on external symptoms (Malawi Ministry of Health 2009). Nonetheless, waiting lists, limited availability of treatment, and the distance to district hospitals still constrain many rural Malawians' access to ART. In 2004, there were approximately 11,000 (urban) Malawians on ART. By December 2009, a total of 270,000 people had ever begun treatment and 200,000 people were actively on ART (Malawi Ministry of Health 2009).

Our studies are based in and around Balaka, Malawi, a growing town in the country's southern region, approximately 90 km from the city of Blantyre. The southern region has the highest HIV prevalence in the country (18% in 2004; NSO and ORC Macro 2005). Women in this region reported a mean ideal family size of 4.1 children although the average was lower for young women (women 15–24 reported a mean of 3.4 children; NSO and ORC Macro 2005).

4.2   Data

Our analyses draw on two sources of data. First, we use two waves of data from Tsogolo la Thanzi (TLT),[2] a panel study of young adults in southern Malawi. Our analyses use Waves 1 and 5, which were collected between June and August 2009 and October and December 2010, respectively. The TLT sample was drawn from a complete household listing of young adults aged 15–25 living within a 7-km radius of Balaka town. Approximately 1,500 women and 600 men were randomly selected from the household listing and recruited into the study. Additionally, the male romantic and sexual partners of female respondents were recruited into the study using respondent-driven sampling. Since we are predominately interested in women's beliefs around HIV-positive childbearing, we limit the present study to female respondents. All interviews were conducted in private rooms at the TLT research center in order to better protect confidentiality. Ninety-six percent of contacted and eligible women were successfully interviewed at Wave 1. The project also involved the offering of HIV testing and counseling to a random sample of respondents following completion of the survey. By Wave 4, two-thirds of the sample had been

---

[1] The WHO provides a clinical staging system for assessing the advancement of HIV disease in the absence of a CD4 count. Stage 3 refers to external symptoms indicative of advanced HIV disease, and Stage 4 refers to symptoms of AIDS (WHO 2005).

[2] Tsogolo la Thanzi is a research project designed by Jenny Trinitapoli and Sara Yeatman and funded by grant R01-HD058366 from the National Institute of Child Health and Human Development.

Table 6.1 Sociodemographic characteristics of TLT sample

Age, mean (SD)	19.5 (3.3)
Years of education, mean (SD)	7.7 (2.8)
Marital Status, %	
Married	42.2
Never married	50.1
Formerly married	7.7
Number of living children, %	
0	50.6
1	26.4
2	16.8
3+	6.2
Sample size	1,497

Source: Tsogolo la Thanzi, Wave 1, 2009

offered testing through TLT, although at any point respondents could use the free testing services available elsewhere in the town.

We use the data from Wave 1 because this survey contained a unique set of questions designed to gauge social norms around HIV-positive childbearing. Using a series of vignettes, the interviewer asks the respondent how she would advise a set of women on their childbearing given a set of varied conditions. We additionally use data on fertility preferences from Wave 5 because approximately two-thirds of the sample had recently learned their HIV status through testing that took place the previous wave.[3] We restrict our analyses of HIV status to those respondents who were tested through TLT because we can confirm their status and that they received their test results. Table 6.1 presents a basic descriptive overview of the female TLT sample.

The second source of data comes from a qualitative project nested within TLT.[4] The project was designed to examine how household or personal experience with HIV infection affects the way people think about HIV. In total, 44 interviews were conducted with a subsample of TLT respondents who either lived with someone who was HIV positive and not on ART, lived with someone who was on ART, had HIV themselves, or had no direct household contact with someone with a known HIV infection. Respondents were recruited based on their responses to TLT questions at Wave 6. The analyses presented here focus on respondents who acknowledged they were HIV positive ($n = 16$; 10 women, 6 men).[5] Apart from questions on

---

[3] 57 women (4.5% of the Wave 5 sample) were offered testing and refused; 7 of these women were pregnant and would have been excluded from the analyses with Wave 5 data for that reason.

[4] Young Adults' Responses to ART is funded by grant R03 HD067099 from the National Institute of Child Health and Human Development (PI Yeatman).

[5] The quotes used are exclusively from HIV-positive women, but the men's data were similar and helpful for clarifying our thinking as we developed our argument.

their experience with HIV and ART, interviewers asked about respondents' plans for the future with particular emphasis on their childbearing plans and whether and how these plans were affected by their disease.

5 Results

5.1 Social Norms Around HIV-Positive Childbearing

We begin by describing social norms around HIV-positive childbearing. At their first interview, respondents were asked how they would advise a series of hypothetical female friends about their childbearing in a set of slightly altered vignettes. The commonality across the scenarios is that the female friend in question would like to have another child. In other words, the friend's desire for another child does not vary across the three vignettes.

In the first scenario, a friend named Lucy and her husband are both HIV-positive. They have four children but would like another child. Only 11% of women in the TLT sample reported that they would advise Lucy to have another child. The second friend, Agnes, is similar to Lucy in all respects except that she does not yet have any children. In this case, 30% of respondents said they would advise her to have children. In the last scenario, respondents are asked about Emily, a woman who has four children and both she and her husband are HIV-negative. This last scenario was designed to assess general norms around childbearing. Fifty-eight percent of respondents reported that they would advise her to have more children if she wanted them. What these vignettes tell us is that 42% of young women in Balaka think that people should not have more than four children even if they want them and are not infected with HIV. Once we introduce HIV into the picture, the story changes. Respondents are much more likely to advise their HIV-positive friends to stop having children regardless of the number of children they already have. But that is not the complete story. Almost three times as many women report a willingness to advise a friend to have children even if she is HIV-positive if she has no children as would advise a friend who already has four. In other words, norms around HIV-positive childbearing are contingent on the specific situation and, in particular, the number of children a woman already has.

At Wave 1, there are only a small number of women ($n = 19$) who acknowledge in the survey that they are HIV-positive. With such a small number, we must be cautious in drawing conclusions, but nonetheless it is informative to look at their responses to these same questions. How do women who are positive themselves view HIV-positive childbearing? Their responses to childbearing are very similar to the sample at large for women who have four children, regardless of their HIV status. However, when asked whether an HIV-positive woman should have children if she has none already, 74% of these women reported supporting the decision—more than twice as many as the rest of the sample (Table 6.2).

Table 6.2 Vignettes: women who would advise their friend to have a/another child

	LUCY:	AGNES:	EMILY:
	both HIV+, 4 children	both HIV+, 0 children	both HIV-, 4 children
Women who are not HIV-positive (or do not know they are) ($n = 1,478$), %	11.2	29.8	57.9
Women who know they are HIV-positive ($n = 19$), %	10.5	73.7	52.6

Source: Tsogolo la Thanzi, Wave 1, 2009

5.2 The Fertility Preferences of HIV-Positive Women

Using the TLT Wave 5 data, we are able to examine the personal fertility preferences of HIV-positive and -negative women. Approximately 60% of respondents were offered (and accepted) testing by the end of Wave 4.[6] We examine Wave 5 responses to the question on whether or not respondents want to have a/another child by the number of children respondents currently have. Although the question on fertility preferences was also asked at Wave 4, we use Wave 5 responses because it is important to our inquiry that respondents are aware of their status at the time they answered the question.

Figure 6.1 shows the desire to continue childbearing by HIV status and parity for the 628 HIV-negative and 72 HIV-positive women in our sample who were reinterviewed at Wave 5 and not currently pregnant ($n = 128$ for excluded due to pregnancy). Among women without any children, there is no difference in the desire to continue childbearing between those who are HIV-positive and those who are HIV-negative—they essentially all want to have children. Moving to examine women who already have one child, a gap emerges—while the vast majority of women want to have more children, HIV-positive women are less likely than HIV-negative women to report wanting more. This gap continues to grow—in a nonlinear fashion—as parity increases. By the time we get to women who have three or more children, just over one-fifth of HIV-positive women express a desire to continue childbearing compared with approximately three-quarters of women who recently tested negative. T-tests confirm that the differences between the two groups are significant beginning at women with one child (p-value <0.01).

The reported preferences of women based on their HIV status and number of children mirror the reported social norms with one notable difference. HIV-positive women with no children universally expressed ($n = 16$) a desire to have children. When asked to advise a friend, only three-quarters of HIV-positive women reported advising a friend to have children in this circumstance. Still, the

---

[6] As described earlier, the respondents who were offered testing were a random two-thirds subsample of the entire TLT sample.

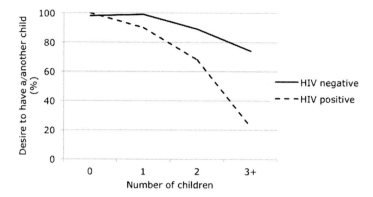

Fig 6.1 Desire to continue childbearing by HIV status and parity (*Source*: Tsogolo la Thanzi, Wave 5, 2010)

actual preferences of HIV-positive women with no children are more similar to the hypothetical advice of HIV-positive women than to that of HIV-negative women, only 30% of whom would advise a friend to have children if she was HIV-positive and had no children.

5.3   The Voices of HIV-Positive Women

The survey findings offer a good picture of social norms around HIV-positive child-bearing and the fertility desires of HIV-positive and -negative women by parity. However, they fall short in aiding our understanding of how HIV-positive women themselves articulate their childbearing desires. Here, we use the qualitative data to explore women's own voices, focusing on how they explain their fertility desires through the lens of their own particular situation.

Young people in Balaka are generally aware of the resources available for HIV-positive women to have children. Virtually, everybody we interviewed made some reference to existing hospital services that help prevent transmission of HIV from mother to child. Not all women knew the details of the program, and fewer still knew the name of the exact medicine (nevirapine), but they all, HIV-positive and -negative alike, seemed to know that it was important for HIV-positive pregnant women to go to antenatal clinic earlier than usual and to take certain medicines. Respondents expressed concerns about breastfeeding and the risk of a child "sucking" the disease. Many were aware of the current recommendations that HIV-positive women should stop breastfeeding after 6 months to limit the likelihood of passing the virus on, but they also expressed doubts about the feasibility of this strategy given that there are few realistic alternatives in this setting. See also Chaps. 10 and 11 in this volume.

When asked about their childbearing plans, most HIV-positive women voiced desires to have children in the future. This was particularly true of those with no or few children. Janet, a 25-year-old HIV-positive woman with no children, responded the following when asked about her childbearing plans:

> J: ...though I was found with the virus but still I want to have only one child.
> I: Why do you want to have one child only?
> J: Just that...(laughing)....
> I: ...(laughing)...how many children does your mother have?
> J: My mother has 7 children.
> I: So you want to have one child only?
> J: Because, the problem is that since I was found with it, we rushed...(both laughed) Yes, the problem is that we rushed...(laughing).

The interviewer clarified that the woman meant that she and her husband "rushed" to get this disease because they contracted it so young in life. Later in the interview, she added:

> J: ...what I get anxious most is about the child because I don't have a child, yes, where I get anxious so much is there.
> I: Actually what are your anxieties?
> J: I want to, I already said that I want to have at least one child right. [Pause.] But the child, I want to try my best so that the child should not contract it also.

Despite being 25 and married, Janet does not yet have children. She makes it clear to the interviewer that she is anxious about not having a child and that she strongly desires one. At the same time, she states that, because she and her husband have HIV, she will stop at one child.

The absolute number of children a woman has is only part of her decision of whether or not to have more. Equally, in a context where divorce and remarriage are extremely common, and children are needed to cement a relationship, having children within new unions is vital to their stability. Grace, a 25-year-old HIV-positive woman, provides a good example of this. She and her ex-husband have two children together, one of whom has full blown AIDS. She recently remarried a man who is aware of her status.

> G: I have said that I have two children. This husband has just married me recently, it cannot be possible for him. Had it been that maybe he is the husband who gave me the children and I am staying with him, while I know that I have given birth for him the two children and then been found with that kind of problem, then we could have agreed that we should stop giving birth... here, but for the person who has just married me recently, him too will want that, since we have been found with this kind of problem. I too am supposed to have my one child. I should be having courage when staying where, staying here. So those are what can cause that maybe I will give birth because of that kind of problem. Yes but if I can give birth to one child maybe that will be the end because the husband will know that, "I have given birth, this is my child", but we have this kind of problem, for us to protect ourselves, or that we should stay, we should be staying that we should stand still we are supposed not to give birth again.

For women who are HIV-positive but already have a number of children with their current partner, the thought process differs. Mercy, a 26-year-old woman, learned she was HIV-positive when she attended an antenatal clinic during the pregnancy of her fifth, and most recent, child. She describes how learning she was HIV-positive led her to get a tubal ligation after the birth, but she also speculates that if she had a small number of children, her calculation would have differed.

I: What role do you think HIV will take on the part of your having other children?

M: Currently?

I: Yes.

M: I cannot say that things will be like this because when this one [infant with her] had just been born, I said that "I do not need to continue, no. I should just stop right here." And I stopped from this one.

I: Are you telling me that you stopped giving birth?

M: I followed contraception methods of never giving birth.

I: You followed contraceptive methods of never giving birth?

M: Yes.

I: Why did you follow contraceptive methods of never giving birth?

M: The reason for my following contraceptive methods of never giving birth is that I realized that the way things are, most people say that a person if you have that problem, it is not advisable to continue giving birth. Besides, had it been that I had not given birth enough as to what I was thinking at that time, if the problem was found I could try to keep on giving birth. Because at that time, I could have two children or only one and I could say that "I am not satisfied". And I could want to go forward. But the way I could see things, and the way I could see myself and the way I could think, I said that "aah, the way things are right now, I just have to stop. Those [the children] that I have are enough."

Following the birth of her last child, Mercy sought a tubal ligation, a relatively uncommon contraceptive method in this context (e.g., used by fewer than 1% of Malawian women under 30; NSO and ORC Macro 2005). The fact that she elected this permanent method of contraception in a context where the possibility of *continued* childbearing is so highly valued emphasizes how important it was for her to not put herself or her children (current or future) at future risk. At the same time, she acknowledges that she made the decision to do so because she already had a sufficient number of children. If she had only one or two children, she would have continued to have children regardless of her concerns about infection.

6 Conclusion

People in Balaka, Malawi, are very familiar with HIV. They have lived with it, worried about it, and dealt with its consequences for over two decades. And while its effects have been transformative, they have never upended the larger cultural mores of childbearing. HIV-positive women confronted with the decision of whether or not to have children think carefully about the consequences of doing so. But researchers, policy makers, and lay people must keep in mind the relative unimportance of HIV when weighed against these larger forces shaping how childbearing is understood and evaluated. We err when we assume that HIV is—or is even among—the most fundamental considerations.

The question of HIV-positive childbearing is not limited to HIV-positive women themselves; every woman (and man) considers what having HIV means for young people. They form opinions, and from these emerge a broader consensus about HIV-positive childbearing we describe here. The social norms surrounding HIV-positive childbearing are being continually reevaluated. Today, the social acceptability of HIV-positive childbearing hinges on the number of children a woman already has. In Malawi, achieving sufficient family size is constitutive of being a full person, having a good life, and fulfilling one's social responsibilities. While there is no universally accepted sufficient number of children in Balaka, our analyses suggest that it likely falls somewhere between one and four. The murkiness of the minimum threshold for HIV-positive women (as different from other women) is articulated most clearly by an HIV-negative respondent with a sister on ART. During the in-depth interviews, we asked HIV-negative women whether a hypothetical HIV infection in the future would affect their childbearing plans. These data were not part of our formal analysis, but this 19-year-old's response merits attention. She said that these days people are having children while HIV-positive. When the interviewer probed and asked her to think about what she herself would do if she became infected, she responded: "I will give birth but not too much...even two children. That's all. Then just stay." We think this appropriately encapsulates women's opinions of HIV-positive childbearing in Balaka—it is essential for a woman to have children, but if she is HIV-positive, she should not have "too much."

Our results carry a few policy implications. First, it is important for health practitioners to recognize and accept that many HIV-positive women want and are going to have children. In fact, new evidence suggests that both HIV-positive women and those who are uncertain about their HIV status are likely to accelerate their childbearing plans in order to take advantage of limited window of sufficiently good health (Trinitapoli and Yeatman 2011). Today, HIV-positive persons are more likely to receive counseling on effective methods of contraception to avoid childbearing altogether than they are to receive advice about safe ways to have children (Agadjanian and Hayford 2009). Advice on how to safely achieve their reproductive goals will almost certainly be better received than recommendations on how to avoid having children—which young women (even HIV-positive ones) are likely to ignore completely. Although the young adults in our sample knew broadly about hospital services to prevent vertical transmission, the majority of HIV-positive pregnant women in Malawi are still not fully taking advantage of such resources (UNICEF 2010). Every young woman in Malawi who tests positive for HIV will have questions about what it means for childbearing and what her options are. It is critical that HIV testing counselors address these issues during counseling since many women may be too afraid to ask themselves. Providing a welcoming environment where HIV-positive women feel comfortable discussing their reproductive goals is critical to ensuring that HIV-positive women get the care they need to keep them and their children safe.

Second, not all HIV-positive women will want to have children and unwanted pregnancies can be avoided by more fully integrating HIV and family planning services. There has been a movement to do so in the region (Mayhew 1996; Rutenberg and Baek 2005), but these resources too often remain isolated from one another. To date, efforts to integrate HIV prevention with family planning in Malawi have moved almost exclusively in a single direction: mandating testing for pregnant women (in antenatal clinics) and making medicine to prevent the vertical transmission of HIV accessible to pregnant HIV-positive women. Some family planning clinics also provide basic information about HIV to women who are seeking contraception. Since concerns about childbearing and HIV go hand in hand in this context, integrating discussions about family planning into established HIV testing programs would well serve those who are concerned about their status. HIV counselors frequently do not discuss family planning options—apart from condoms—with their clients, and condoms will never be a long-term method of birth control in Africa, particularly within marriage. The desire to completely stop childbearing is historically uncommon in much of the region; spacing was the most common reason for women to seek out family planning services (Caldwell et al. 1992; Tabutin and Schoumaker 2002). Increasingly, however, women do want to stop having children entirely—for HIV-related and unrelated reasons. Providers should offer women (and men) complete information about permanent options, even while also encouraging condom use among discordant couples.

We may refer to this subgroup of young women in our study as HIV-positive women, but perhaps it would be helpful to remember that first and foremost they are young African women. They just happen to be living with the virus that causes AIDS. When HIV status is framed as a secondary consideration compared to factors like obtaining adult standing, solidifying a relationship, and maintaining the moral order, the fact that infected women feel a drive to have children should not surprise. In this chapter, we hope to have shed some light on the heterogeneity of fertility desires among HIV-positive women in Malawi. We cannot develop a model to precisely predict the conditions under which a woman will want to have children, but that was never our goal. Rather, we argue that without considering the larger forces motivating childbearing in high-fertility settings like Balaka, we will never understand the childbearing patterns of HIV-positive women. In Balaka, women who are HIV positive are more likely to want to stop childbearing than uninfected women. But their reproductive goals are still shaped by a desire to be a mother, to be a complete person, and to be a contented wife.

References

Agadjanian V, Hayford SR (2009) PMTCT, HAART, and childbearing in Mozambique: an institutional perspective. AIDS Behav 13:S103–S112

Allen S, Serufilira A, Gruber V, Kegeles S, Vandeperre P, Carael M, Coates TJ (1993) Pregnancy and contraception use among urban Rwandan women after HIV testing and counseling. Am J Public Health 83(5):705–710

Bello GA, Chipeta J, Aberle-Grasse J (2006) Assessment of trends in biological and behavioural surveillance data: is there any evidence of declining HIV prevalence or incidence in Malawi? Sex Transm Infect 82:I9–I13

Boerma JT, Urassa M (2001) Associations between female infertility, HIV and sexual behaviour in a rural area in Tanzania. In: Boerma JT, Mgalla Z (eds) Women and infertility in sub-Saharan Africa: a multidisciplinary perspective. Royal Tropical Institute Press, Amsterdam, pp 176–187

Bongaarts J (2001) Fertility and reproductive preferences in post-transitional societies. Popul Dev Rev 27:260–281

Bongaarts J, Buettner T, Heilig G, Pelletier F (2008) Has the HIV epidemic peaked? Popul Dev Rev 34(2):199–224

Caldwell JC, Caldwell P (1987) The cultural-context of high fertility in sub-Saharan Africa. Popul Dev Rev 13(3):409–437

Caldwell JC, Orubuloye IO, Caldwell P (1992) Fertility decline in Africa – a new type of transition. Popul Dev Rev 18(2):211–242

Casterline JB (2002) HIV/AIDS and fertility in sub-Saharan Africa: a review of the recent literature. United Nations, New York

Chabal P (2009) Africa: the politics of suffering and smiling. Zed Books, London

Cooper D, Harries J, Myer L, Orner P, Bracken H (2007) "Life is still going on": reproductive intentions among HIV-positive women and men in South Africa. Soc Sci Med 65(2):274–283

Dyer SJ (2007) The value of children in African countries – insights from studies on infertility. J Psychosom Obstet Gynecol 28(2):69–77

Dyer SJ, Matthews N, Hoffman M, van der Spuy ZM (2002) 'Men leave me as I cannot have children': women's experiences with involuntary childlessness. Hum Reprod 17(6):1663–1668

Feldman R, Maposhere C (2003) Safer sex and reproductive choice: findings from 'positive women: voices and choices' in Zimbabwe. Reprod Health Matters 11(22):162–173

Fortes M (1978) Parenthood, marriage and fertility in West Africa. J Dev Stud 14(4):121–149

Grieser M, Gittelsohn J, Shankar AV, Koppenhaver T, Legrand TK, Marindo R, Mavhu WM et al (2001) Reproductive decision making and the HIV/AIDS epidemic in Zimbabwe. J South Afr Stud 27(2):225–243

Guthrie BL, Choi RY, Bosire R, Kiarie JN, Mackelprang RD, Gatuguta A, John-Stewart GC et al (2010) Predicting pregnancy in HIV-1-discordant couples. AIDS Behav 14(5):1066–1071

Hoffman IF, Martinson FEA, Powers KA, Chilongozi DA, Msiska ED, Kachipapa EI, Mphande CD et al (2008) The year-long effect of HIV-positive test results on pregnancy intentions, contraceptive use, and pregnancy incidence among Malawian women. JAIDS-J Acquir Immune Defic Syndr 47(4):477–483

Hollos M (2003) Profiles of infertility in southern Nigeria: women's voices from Amakiri. Afr J Reprod Health 7(2):46–56

Hollos M, Larsen U (2008) Motherhood in sub-Saharan Africa: the social consequences of infertility in an urban population in northern Tanzania. Cult Health Sex 10(2):159–173

Hollos M, Larsen U, Obono O, Whitehouse B (2009) The problem of infertility in high fertility populations: meanings, consequences and coping mechanisms in two Nigerian communities. Soc Sci Med 68(11):2061–2068

Johnson-Hanks J (2004) Uncertainty and the second space: modern birth timing and the dilemma of education. Eur J Popul [Revue Europeenne De Demographie] 20(4):351–373

Larsen U (2000) Primary and secondary infertility in sub-Saharan Africa. Int J Epidemiol 29(2):285–291

Larsen U, Hollos M, Obono O, Whitehouse B (2010) Suffering infertility: the impact of infertility on women's life experiences in two Nigerian communities. J Biosoc Sci 42(6):787–814

Lesthaeghe RJ (1989) Reproduction and social organization in Sub-Saharan Africa. University of California Press, Berkeley

Malawi Ministry of Health (2007) 6-Monthly report from the HIV Unit, Ministry of Health, Malawi: January–June 2007. Malawi Ministry of Health, Lilongwe

Malawi Ministry of Health (2009) Malawi antiretroviral treatment programme: quarterly report with results up to 31st December 2009. Malawi Ministry of Health, Lilongwe

Mayhew S (1996) Integrating MCH/FP and STD/HIV services: current debates and future directions. Health Policy Plan 11(4):339–353

Meekers D (1992) The process of marriage in African societies: a multiple indicator approach. Popul Dev Rev 18(1):61–78

Moses A, Zimba C, Kamanga E, Nkhoma J, Maida A, Martinson F, Mofolo I et al (2008) Prevention of mother-to-child transmission: program changes and the effect on uptake of the HIVNET 012 regimen in Malawi. AIDS 22:83–87

National Statistical Office, and ORC Macro (2005) Malawi demographic and health survey 2004. NSO and ORC Macro, Calverton

Nduna M, Farlane L (2009) Women living with HIV in South Africa and their concerns about fertility. AIDS Behav 13:S62–S65

Nguyen RHN, Gange SJ, Wabwire-Mangen F, Sewankambo NK, Serwadda D, Wawer MJ, Quinn TC, Gray RH (2006) Reduced fertility among HIV-infected women associated with viral load in Rakai district, Uganda. Int J STD AIDS 17(12):842–846

Oladapo OT, Daniel OJ, Odusoga OL, Ayoola-Sotubo O (2005) Fertility desires and intentions of HIV-positive patients at a suburban specialist center. J Natl Med Assoc 97(12):1672–1681

Rutenberg N, Baek C (2005) Field experiences integrating family planning into programs to prevent mother-to-child transmission of HIV. Stud Fam Plann 36(3):235–245

Rutenberg N, Biddlecom AE, Kaona FAD (2000) Reproductive decision-making in the context of HIV and AIDS: a qualitative study in Ndola, Zambia. Int Fam Plan Perspect 26(3):124–130

Setel P (1995) The effect of HIV and AIDS on fertility in East and Central Africa. Health Transition Rev 5(Suppl):179–189

Smith C (2003) Moral, believing animals: human personhood and culture. Oxford University Press, New York

Smith DJ, Mbakwem BC (2010) Antiretroviral therapy and reproductive life projects: mitigating the stigma of AIDS in Nigeria. Soc Sci Med 71(2):345–352

Suggs D (1993) Female status and role transition in the Tswana life cycle. In: Suggs D, Miracle A (eds) Culture and human sexuality. Brooks Cole Publishing, Pacific Grove, pp 103–117

Tabutin D, Schoumaker B (2002) The demography of Sub-Saharan Africa from the 1950s to the 2000s: a survey of changes and a statistical assessment. Population 59(3):455–555

Taulo F, Berry M, Tsui A, Makanani B, Kafulafula G, Li Q, Nkhoma C et al (2009) Fertility intentions of HIV-1 infected and uninfected women in Malawi: a longitudinal study. AIDS Behav 13(1):20–27

Trinitapoli J, Yeatman S (2011) Uncertainty and fertility in a generalized AIDS epidemic. Am Sociol Rev 76(6)

UNAIDS and WHO (2006) AIDS epidemic update: December 2006. UNAIDS and World Health Organization, Geneva

UNICEF (2010) Malawi: PMTCT. http://www.unicef.org/AIDS/files/Malawi_PMTCTFactsheet_2010.pdf. Accessed 15 Sept 2011

Watkins SC (2004) Navigating the AIDS epidemic in rural Malawi. Popul Dev Rev 30(4):673–705

White RG, Vynnycky E, Glynn JR, Crampin AC, Jahn A, Mwaungulu F, Mwanyongo O et al (2007) HIV epidemic trend and antiretroviral treatment need in Karonga District, Malawi. Epidemiol Infect 135(6):922–932

World Health Organization (2005) Interim WHO clinical staging of HIV/AIDS and HIV/AIDS case definitions for surveillance: African region. World Health Organization, Geneva

Yeatman S (2008) Childbearing in an AIDS Epidemic. Unpublished PhD thesis, Department of Sociology, University of Texas at Austin, Texas, USA

Yeatman S (2009) HIV infection and fertility preferences in rural Malawi. Stud Fam Plann 40(4):261–276

Yeatman S (2011) "HIV is an enemy of childbearers": the construction of local epidemiology in rural Malawi. Cult Health Sex 13(4):471–483

Zaba B, Gregson S (1998) Measuring the impact of HIV on fertility in Africa. AIDS 12:S41–S50

Part II
Motherhood, Infant Feeding and HIV/AIDS

Chapter 7
"I Always Wanted to See My Babies Grow Up": Motherhood Experiences for Women Living Longer than Expected with HIV/AIDS

Donna B. Barnes

1 Introduction

For women living longer than expected with HIV/AIDS, the opportunity to see their "babies grow up" becomes possible with access to improved medical care. Likewise, motherhood offers women with HIV/AIDS a reason for living, a valued position, and a social status (see also Chap. 1 and chapters in Part I in this volume).

Women with HIV/AIDS initially were not expected to live a long life. By 1991, HIV/AIDS was predicted to be one of the five leading causes of death in women of reproductive age (Chu et al. 1990). With the advancement of medical treatments (Connor et al. 1994; Anastos et al. 2004), AIDS-related mortality declined (Cohen et al. 2002). Use of antiretroviral therapy assisted in the prevention of mother-to-child transmission (Sperling et al. 1996). These discoveries and treatments offered women opportunities of motherhood and for mothers to participate in their children's growth, education, family, and social experiences.

Several longitudinal studies followed women's clinical and social conditions examining the possibilities of a longer life with adherence to medications (Cook et al. 2004; Siegel et al. 2004; Ahdieh-Grant et al. 2005; Ickovics et al. 2006). While no evidence was found that highly active antiretroviral therapy (HAART) improved psychological health for women (Siegel et al. 2004), others cautioned that without therapy for depression, there was an increased likelihood of AIDS-related deaths among women with chronic depressive symptoms on HAART (Cook et al. 2004). Psychological resources defined as positive emotions, positive HIV expectancy, and finding meaning in life contributed to the physical health of women with HIV and possibly protected against HIV-related mortality (Ickovics et al. 2006). Other longitudinal studies (Anastos et al. 2005; Kapadia et al. 2005; Kohli

D.B. Barnes (✉)
Women's Studies, California State University East Bay, Hayward, CA, USA
e-mail: donnabarnes1@gmail.com

P. Liamputtong (ed.), *Women, Motherhood and Living with HIV/AIDS:*
A Cross-Cultural Perspective, DOI 10.1007/978-94-007-5887-2_7,
© Springer Science+Business Media Dordrecht 2013

et al. 2006) examined the clinical and sociodemographic factors of depression, drug use, race and aging, and women's disease process with HIV/AIDS, suggesting for aging adults there were unknown long-term effects of HAART on physical and emotional health.

While these quantitative and longitudinal studies add to the knowledge of HAART and women with HIV/AIDS living longer, longitudinal qualitative studies of women's experience of longevity and motherhood (Sandelowski and Barroso 2003; Barnes 2008; Murphy et al. 2010) suggest further examination linking longevity, illness status, social conditions, and motherhood.

In this chapter, I report on a longitudinal study using qualitative methods focusing on how women with HIV/AIDS from two northern United States cities construct motherhood. The study is based on participants' everyday experiences of motherhood who had lived with HIV/AIDS an average of 14 years.

2 Theoretical Frameworks

The perspectives of grounded theory (Charmaz 2006; Glaser and Strauss 1967; Glaser 1978; Strauss 1987; Strauss and Corbin 1998) and feminist theory (Smith 1987; Collins 2000; Olesen 2003) guided the data collection and analysis and demanded the avoidance of preconceived categories. The purpose of grounded theory is to explain variations in human activity. Theory is developed by conceptualizing the interacting elements in the situations under study. Grounded theorists generally adopt the social constructionist's viewpoint of "defining the situation" as real as if it were real (Thomas and Thomas 1970/1928) and social construction of reality as subjective processes (Berger and Luckmann 1967). The symbolic interactionist's perspective on social processes includes interpreting the microlevel analysis of interaction (Mead 1962/1934) simultaneously with the macro-level analysis of social contexts (Strauss 1959).

As a feminist, I emulate Smith (1987: 10) by listening to "women's experience from the woman's standpoint and explore[ing] how it is shaped in the extended relations of larger social and political relations." Women's constructed knowledge of their life experiences was regarded as unique, in agreement with Olesen (2003). Participants were respected as central to and experts about their own stories (Collins 2000). The approach foregrounds the women's perspectives on their social realties in depicting essential dynamics of their experiences of motherhood.

3 The Study

3.1 Design and Recruitment

Fifty-nine women living with HIV/AIDS, from Oakland, California ($n=30$) and Rochester, New York ($n=29$), participated in an initial study on reproductive decisions between 1995 and 2001 (Barnes and Murphy 2009). In this follow-up study, between 2005 and 2009, of the original 59 participants, 51 women were living and 8 had died. Each death (Oakland $n=5$; Rochester $n=3$) was corroborated by two pieces of evidence, verbal information from recruiters based on medical records or personal information, and newspaper obituaries or death certificates.

Of the 51 potential participants, 2 declined to participate. One woman canceled two scheduled appointments and informed me by telephone "she had two jobs and did not have time to participate." The other woman declined informing the recruiter that she did not want to participate.

Of the 49 remaining original participants, the recruiters informed me that they were unable to locate 13 women for the following reasons:

1. Lack of contact information ($n=6$) (Oakland $n=5$, Rochester $n=1$)
2. Women had "disappeared" (Oakland $n=3$)
3. Were "still on the streets" (Oakland $n=1$)
4. Moved with no forwarding address ($n=3$) (Oakland $n=1$, Rochester $n=2$)

I worked with 29 recruiters from Oakland ($n=14$) and Rochester ($n=15$) attempting multiple times to contact the original study participants over a period of 4 years (2005–2009). In addition, I utilized Internet searches for information and contacted vital statistics departments of California and New York for death certificates.

I completed face-to-face interviews with women ($n=36$) from Oakland ($n=16$) and Rochester ($n=20$) for a final follow-up rate of 70.6% (36/51). The contact and recruiting protocol was designed on a person-by-person basis using the determinant of what was best for the potential participants. Original recruiters or friends, who had an established, trusted relationship made the initial contact. Training sessions were conducted with recruiters. They were paid $20 for training sessions and for each participant recruited and scheduled.

Written informed consents were reviewed in participants' native language and signed by participants prior to the interview. The original translator was utilized during the interviews for two Spanish-speaking women. Participants were given $50 honorarium for their time and expertise. The interviews ranged in length from 90 to 120 minutes. The data were collected between June 2005 and February 2009. Interviews were conducted in a private setting of participants' choice, often their home.

Data collection was focused on topics concerning living with HIV long term, participants' reflections on their life choices since learning of their HIV status, and sharing the ways in which their histories affected their choices. The interviews were audio-recorded, transcribed, and analyzed using grounded theory qualitative methods. Data analysis was a collaborative, constant comparative, and systematic process that began with the first interview and continued throughout data collection. The process continued in regular meetings with consultants at both sample sites and with research associates for shared data coding, memo writing, and diagramming. As analysis progressed, core concepts were validated by participants and social and outreach workers from both sample sites.

An interviewer-administered structured questionnaire, pretested with four women, was conducted at the end of the interview. The Institutional Review Board of California State University, East Bay, approved the study protocol.

The mean time between the initial interview and the follow-up was 8.5 years with a range of 5–11 years. The lower range represents participants who had sporadic use of health care, were homeless, or were not expected to live. The mean time between participants' first positive HIV test and the follow-up interview was 14.8 years with a range of 8–25 years.

3.2   Participants Characteristics

The sample ($n = 36$) was predominantly women of color (29/36), with a mean age of 42.6 years and a range of 26–62. There were diverse levels of income with half (18/36) reporting an annual household income of less than $15K. Participants were equally currently employed (16/36) and not employed (17/36) with a few never employed (3/36). Half (18/36) were in the same income category in both the initial and follow-up interviews. Over one-third (36.1%, 13/36) went from a lower to a higher income category. And for a small percentage (13.9%, 5/36), their income was lower. Forty-two percent (15/36) of the participants had completed some additional education since the initial interview.

The majority (25/36) reported their current relationship status as single ($n = 14$), divorced ($n = 4$), separated ($n = 5$), or widowed ($n = 2$). Six ($n = 6$) were married. Five ($n = 5$) reported either being engaged or having a fiancé, boyfriend, or domestic partner. More than half (21/36) of the participants had children living with them. The majority (21/36) reported their current HIV status as asymptomatic. Less than a quarter reported as symptomatic (8/36) or a diagnosis of AIDS (7/36). Almost two-thirds (23/36) reported having "ever had a problem with addiction to drugs or alcohol." Eight (8/23) reported current drug or alcohol addiction problems.

4   Motherhood Experiences and the Challenges for Women Living with HIV/AIDS Longer than Expected

Participants' expectations of a premature death significantly influenced their motherhood choices and experiences, which had lingering effects. When participants received their HIV test results, they assumed that they had a shortened life span.

> I was never told how long I would live but statistics had us at the time (1990) about 2 years you would drift into full-blown AIDS (Living with HIV/AIDS. (LWH) 18 years)

Participants had lived through the evolution of the AIDS epidemic in the United States from a death sentence to living with HIV with the discoveries and availability of medications and treatments. The majority of participants had children prior to learning their HIV status. Thus, longevity gave them the unexpected time to see their children grow up.

I never thought that I would be around to be able to see my babies grow up, and next year my daughter is graduating. I never thought that. (LWH 14 years)

For participants who chose abortion prior to or when HIV-positive, living longer came with mixed feelings about their reproductive decisions.

When I was twenty-six, and I'm now forty-four, I didn't see my life going that far, so I would have made different choices. I think my main thing would have been my choice of having children. I was caught in the middle of the epidemic then. I regretted not having that child. And, you know, as life went on, I still regret it. (LWH 18 years)

Longevity with HIV/AIDS was a double edge sword for women who had chosen abortion, had given up children for adoption, or avoided motherhood for fear they would not be alive to care for their children.

I present motherhood experiences for women living with HIV/AIDS longer than expected in three categories.

4.1 Participants who had children living, unexpected longevity offered opportunities of fulfilling dreams of seeing their children grow up with unique challenges influenced by their HIV status.

4.2 Participants' longevity offered the possibilities of attempting to regain contact with children who had been given up for adoption, were or had been in foster care, or with family members.

4.3 Participants living longer offered the possibilities of becoming mothers through pregnancy, but opportunities were complicated with reconciling past reproductive experiences and choices.

4.1 Fulfilling Dreams of Seeing Their Children Grow Up

For those women (31/36) who had children, the unique challenges of mothering included "lost mothering" opportunities and attempts to make up for the lost time and disclosure of their HIV status to their children. The loss of mothering time included being physically, but not emotionally present to being physically separated from their children. In recounting their experiences of initially learning their HIV status, participants typically referred to their assumptions about dying and how this affected their mothering.

You're going to a state of panic, of fear. . . . It's big and you want to do what you can do to be able to teach them [children], pour into them, do all of this in a short period of time because that's what you're thinking. I have a short period of time so I need to take all of this and throw it at 'em. (LWH 17 years)

Years after women were told their HIV status, the effects of their diagnosis on their mothering practises shaped their relationships with their children into adulthood.

I really needed to be healed for the way I reacted with my daughters. . . . And now with [daughter's name], we're working it out. . . . It's a little harder for us because she got the brunt of it. She was five when I was first [diagnosed]. (LWH 17 years)

Mothering time was lost during separations from children because of illness, both acute episodes that involved hospital stays for such illnesses as pneumonia and also chronic conditions of fatigue, malaise, and depression. Hospital stays could involve days, weeks, or months. When participants were released to their homes or convalescent facilities, they would have recovery time and therapy that further added to loss mothering time. It was a reoccurring concern for participants.

> I have a really bad fear of me ending up back in the hospital. Because when I was in the hospital, I missed Christmas, I missed New Year's, and I missed my baby's birthday. (LWH 14 years)

Chronic conditions and illnesses influenced women's decisions to give up the care of their children to family members, or in other instances children were mandated to child protective services (CPS) with consequential foster care and potential adoption. These physical separations varied from months to years, to a child's lifetime. In the following example, a woman had a long cyclical battle with depression and substance abuse.

> I had pneumonia and the reason I had pneumonia 'cause I was doing drugs, and the reason why I was doing drugs 'cause I was depressed. My parents took care of my son… They've been scraping me off the pavement for 25 years and that's not fair to them. And it's time for me to be a mother. (LWH 17 years)

The consequences of loss mothering time often came with lasting and unresolved guilt.

> I feel I could have done better. It's always, the guilt, in the back of my head. (LWH 21 years)

It also influenced how participants mothered their children.

> I think I'm still tryin' to make up for the time I took away from them. I know I am. I try too hard to please, to make up for what I did. (LWH 12 years)

The process of forgiving themselves was reported as being a long, continuing journey. When possible, being present in relationships with their children was important, but for some this was not possible, as we will examine later.

Another challenge of mothering was the disclosure of their HIV status to their children. Participants spoke of protecting their children and maintaining their trust.

> I was afraid people were going to go to the girls and say something that was meant to be helpful, but that would be really hurtful like, "Gosh, I'm so sorry that your mommy's dying of AIDS".... I can't let them hear this from somebody else. So, to maintain trust they need to hear it from me first. (LWH 18 years)

Disclosing to children could necessitate that they maintain secrecy to protect themselves and the family. For women who had not disclosed to their children, the following exemplifies the mothering dilemma and fear of the consequences if their child told others.

> I think when they're really young they don't know. Like even if my daughter is like, "Oh my mom's got HIV", the kids don't know what it is. But, then the kids will go home and the parents will put something in their head that's probably not true. And then it blows up from there. (LWH 9 years)

Negative consequences of disclosure did happen to another participant who spontaneously disclosed her HIV status to her 8-year-old son one morning when she was counting out his asthma pill and her medications when he questioned why she took so many pills.

> And I told him, "That's between me and you and the family. I hope you don't tell teachers, your schoolmates, and you don't tell friends". And ironically enough last year, my son, his friend, and his mother were driving in her car. Somehow it got brought up and my son goes, "My mommy has HIV." So, the lady calls me up freaking out. She said, "Is this true? Your son says you have AIDS." I go, "Really I wonder where he got that from." She goes, "Oh, what a relief." My heart was pounding and I felt bad 'cause I'm calling him a liar, but I had to do it to protect him. So, I had to tell my son "you shouldn't have said anything." I go, "From here on out you don't tell nobody." (LWH 17 years)

At what age could children understand the consequences of telling others that their mother has HIV? The burden of children maintaining a family secret is daunting and has potential for negative results perhaps beyond their understanding. One mother who had disclosed her HIV status to her 7- and 9-year-old children attempted to educate them about potential stigma from living with HIV.

> I made an effort to explain about the stigma and about some of the ways people got HIV, and how those people were stigmatized. They didn't really want to hear about that part and they still don't. (LWH 18 years)

The additional challenge of mothering for women with HIV/AIDS includes educating, advising, and protecting children from potential stigmatization from HIV. It also demands that children maintain their mother's secret to protect her, themselves, and family members. If the participants were not physically present for mothering, someone else had these responsibilities.

4.2   Attempting to Regain Contact with Children

Unexpected longevity allowed women who had been separated from their children the opportunity to attempt to regain contact. More than a third of the women (14/36, 39%) had their children taken away by child protective services (CPS) or in foster care ($n=8$), gave children's custody to family ($n=6$), and signed termination of parental rights for adoption ($n=4$). There were women ($n=4$) that had children in more than one of these situations. Three women (3/14) had teenage sons who were taken by CPS or were incarcerated, while these three participants mothered their other children living with them.

The process of attempting contact with children outside of participants' custody was complicated with mixed outcomes. In the following example, the participant had three sons. Her story exemplifies three different processes of attempted reunification. Her oldest son, age 16, had been raised by her sister-in-law. At the time of the interview, he was in a locked group home facility. Unexpectedly, he contacted her, and after phone conversations, the mother visited him. She last saw him when he was nine.

> I knew my son was in a group home, but I didn't know where he was. It was exciting and nice because he wanted to find out who his biological mother was. He wanted his mama back in his life. (LWH 12 years)

To locate her second son, age 14 years, she initiated contact with CPS. She learned that he was living with a foster family. Through contact with the foster mother, a telephone call was arranged. The participant received a call from her son, and within a month he came for a visit. Her son was seven when she last saw him. At the time of the interview, she had phone contact and planned monthly visits.

She had given up her third son as an infant for adoption and she had no further contact. She knew the adoptive parents, but said,

> I know once you sign the adoption papers, you no longer a part of that child's life. But, I'm gon' call one day and see how he's doin' cause he's thirteen now, and the other brothers want to see their brother. (LWH 12 years)

Reunification of siblings is another complicating and guilt-producing aspect of "lost mothering" when children are separated from their mother and their siblings.

Reunions are further problematic when mothers have no contact information. The following participant started the process of reunification because her long held goal was to contact her child when he became an adult. She had stumbled onto an agency while looking for a job on Craig's List, an Internet network of online communities, featuring jobs, housing, and services. Instead of calling the agency for a job application, this mother contacted a woman who suggested that she came in and signed a release of information.

> The woman said, "I'll try to go open the file and see if he left anything. If not, your information will go into the file in case he does come lookin." I told her, "Well he's not even 18 yet, how would he be able to put something in the file?" She says "Well, if he knows he's adopted, and with the parental consent from his adopted parent, he will be able to do that." I'm hoping that's the case, but she said, "Don't get your hopes up high."

The results were unknown at the time of the interview. She reflected on her past decision to give her son up for adoption.

> This child got taken [adopted] because of my drug addiction in 1988. And at that time, you know it wasn't the right time. But, that's something I still deal with, because I feel a lot of guilt, behind that and I want to see him really bad. (LWH 15 years)

Another complexity of reunification is seen in the next example. The participant's three daughters were in the care of her grandmother. When her youngest was born, he was "taken" at the hospital by CPS. The participant signed the termination of rights documents in order for her aunt, her mother's sister, to adopt her son. The participant last saw her son when he was 12 years old. When she visited him he called her "Auntie" and referred to his great aunt as "Mommy." The participant suspected her son knew that she was his mother.

> He looked at me like people say the blood will call you. . . . 'cause he looked like me, my dark complexion. You know, my aunt is light, my uncle too. And 'cause my son has green eyes, and his real father got green eyes. . . . I'm gonna talk to my aunt straight and I'm gonna let her know, if you don't talk, I'm gonna talk. Cause he got 16 years, and I think at that age he will understand. (LWH 17 years)

The tension between the child understanding without being told, the possibility that her son could have overheard the adults talking about his biological mother, or perhaps the great aunt telling the child some information about his mother all add to the multiple layers and emotional costs of maintaining family secrets. It also influences the process and probability of reunification. Who tells the child and how he is told could have ramifications both for the child and the familial relationships.

The last example of attempting reunification and its consequences are depicted in this participant's reuniting with her 18-year-old son. She had moved from her country to the United States and left her son with her family when he was 2 and ½ years old. She had visited him once when he was 12 years old. More visits were not possible, because if she left, she would have been prevented from reentering the United States. She was divorced from her American husband, and she had to qualify for citizenship. Through the mother's initiative, as a recent citizen, her son had secured a visa and would soon be living with her and attending community college. Learning to mother an adult child, making up for lost time, and fearing disclosure of her HIV status made her challenge overwhelmingly stressful and painful. When her son told her he wanted to study to be a nurse, she said he was worried about working with HIV-positive people. She shared what he said to her:

> The only care I'm doing is what about those HIV-positive people. I don't want to be around them and get infected. . . . Well, Mommy, if it is like that, a job is a job. I'm not gonna take them with me to my house.

She was surprised and hurt to learn his negative feelings about people with HIV/AIDS. She spoke of the effects of her "lost mothering" opportunities.

> I never be with my son with him daily. I never did stuff as a mother to show him love. That bothers me because someone else was doing that job. He's a man now. To show him the love he was not getting from me all these years, it's lost. I feel lost. It's gone. . . . I cried, I cry, I cry. While even when I'm walking I just shed tears. I'm like I have no one today I can really fellowship. (LWH 11 years)

Her sadness, loss of mothering, and fear of rejection left her lonely and isolated.

The outcomes of contacting children that have been given up for adoption, foster care, or family member care are interwoven with issues of "lost mothering" opportunities, guilt, fear of disclosure, and social isolation. Bureaucratic procedures and lack of contact information add to the complexities of reunification.

4.3 Possibilities of Becoming Mothers Through Pregnancy

None of the women in this study (2005–2009) gave birth for the first time; however, there were six women who had children since the initial study (1995–2001). All children ($n = 7$) were negative for HIV. These six women had had children prior to learning their HIV status, except one who learned she was HIV-positive when she was pregnant. Four women were raising all their children. One woman was raising her youngest child, and her adult child was also living with her. Her middle child was in foster care. One participant had birthed four children who were in foster care. She had refused to sign parental rights termination documents.

Five participants (5/36) had never given birth. Three of these women had been pregnant while HIV-positive, two had had abortions, and one ended in a miscarriage. One woman had been pregnant prior to the AIDS epidemic and had an abortion. One had never been pregnant but still thought she wanted children after she completed more education, paid off her car, and saved for a house with her fiancé.

Past decisions to terminate pregnancies were reexamined in the light of participant's unexpected longevity. The sadness and regret they reported from previous decisions to terminate and miscarriage were addressed in a variety of ways, often with spiritual or religious rituals. One participant had chosen a name for her child when she was pregnant, prior to her subsequent abortion. Sometime after, the participant found comfort from a psychic's message. She said the psychic told her, "He's with you. He said it wasn't his time to be here." Some years later her nephew was given the chosen name. His parents knew nothing of the participant's name selection. She shared the following:

> And my nephew is like this fireball of a soul. He was gonna come, regardless, and be part of our family. And so, that's the way I look at him. He's extra special to me because of that. It's my way of being spiritual about it and being able to deal with it. (LWH for 16 years)

Another woman said that sharing in the births of her partner's children brought her joy. But, the sadness still lingered from her abortion.

> When the kids were born I could have seen myself when I had my baby, but I didn't. Right now my baby would be eleven years old. (LWH for 24 years)

She remembers the day she had the abortion, "that's the date that for me that she was born and that she died." On the anniversary of her abortion, she lights a candle at her home altar where she keeps religious symbols and photos of her family.

4.4 "Lost Mothering"

Women with HIV/AIDS with increased longevity had different mothering challenges compared to HIV-positive women's mothering, who prepared for their untimely deaths in the early 1990s. In a previous paper (Barnes et al. 1997), we analyzed HIV-positive women's videotapes made from 1991 to 1993 for their children. We developed the concept of "eternal mothering" suggesting that mothering does not end with death. By leaving videotapes, these women provided explanations, advice, warnings, secrets, and words of love in a visual legacy.

Instead of facing a presumed death sentence, women with HIV/AIDS with increased longevity (hereafter referred to as women) found living meant reconciling past reproductive and mothering decisions that had ramifications for the present and future. The disbelief of living longer than expected that women expressed as "I'm still here" (Barnes 2008) competed with regrets for decisions made in their earlier stages of HIV for abortion, child custody arrangements, and mothering actions that had far reaching effects.

Women's diverse conditions and decisions influenced their mothering, resulting in mixtures of physical and emotional separations from their children of varying lengths of time. Their mothering circumstances were linked to their initial response to HIV, episodic HIV-related illnesses, reactions to antiretroviral therapy, other illnesses including depression, and for some, substance abuse and activities resulting in incarceration. Some of these separations ended in participants' children living with family members, being in foster care, and, in some cases, adopted. In addition, some women were reevaluating choices of previous abortions and uncertainties of becoming a mother related to their HIV condition, relationship status, and age. I examined the interconnectedness of these constructs of social life to illustrate how mothering is contextualized, focusing on (1) opportunities of seeing their children grow up, (2) attempting to regain contact with children, and (3) possibilities of becoming mothers through pregnancy. I labeled this concept "lost mothering."

How women managed their "lost mothering" opportunities, as they defined loss, is interrelated with their attitudes about how mothers should care for their children and how mothers' related HIV stigmatization may affect their children, similar to "eternal mothering." Distinctions in the two concepts are (1) the reconciliation of past reproductive and mothering choices given women's longevity with (2) the historical unfolding of AIDS changing from a death sentence to a chronic disease. Similar to "eternal mothering," women's multiple marginalization of social conditions emanated from gender, race, ethnicity and class, family relations, child custody issues, acute and chronic episodes and stages of illness, substance use, and incarceration.

I analyzed women's multiple perspectives and the numerous possible versions of their world arising from their experiences building on "eternal mothering." "Lost mothering" is the construction of everyday knowledge to inform participants' realities based on their experiences and the social conditions not necessarily of their choosing.[1] HIV/AIDS illness is not a choice. Potential stigma associated with HIV/AIDS is not a choice. The rendition of the everyday world as problematic (Smith 1987) is illustrated by the women in this study being active participants in their everyday mothering work, including attempting to regain contact and reconciling past reproductive choices, within the limits of their social capital.

Participants yearned to see their babies grow up, whatever the "lost mothering" opportunities, be that abortion, children taken by CPS or given up for adoption, or children they raised from birth. Those women who had the opportunities to mother their children faced challenges specific to their HIV status because of "lost mothering" time in adjusting to their diagnosis assumed to be a death sentence and of potential stigma to themselves and to their children. These women hoped to live long enough to guide their children to adulthood.

> They keep me going. I keep thinking to myself each and every day. Because if I'm not here who's gonna do it for 'em? I know there's people that live for 15, 20 years and I'm just hoping that I can get to this point when he's of age. (LWH11 years)

---

[1] "Men make their own history, but they do not make it just as they please; they do not make it under circumstances chosen by themselves, but under circumstances directly found, given and transmitted from the past." Karl Marx (1978/1852: 595).

In circumstances where this had not been possible, such as abortion, women depended on spiritual and religious rituals for support, particularly when the abortion was kept secret. For those women who had never had children, or who birthed children but had not mothered them, spiritual rituals and beliefs brought them comfort though the sadness and, for some, regret stayed.

> I draw a lot on my beliefs and my strengths, and hoping and praying. I know that you don't get what you always want, but you do get what you need. I mean I wanted something else but, I guess I didn't need it. I needed something else. I'm drawn to things using sage and smudging and that's all very Native American. My spiritual animal that I feel really close to is a wolf. Like my dogs are very close to the wolf family, so I mean I'm drawn to things like that. (LWH 17 years)

For women who had reunited with their children and adult children and had not disclosed their HIV status, mothering brought isolation, with few resources for comfort. For those women who attempted and made initial contact with their children, there was joy in learning their children wanted to find their biological mother. For the mothers who were raising their children, they believed that everyday experiences of mothering were a strong motivator for staying alive. Mothering sustained hope for living with HIV. This hope was more fragile particularly for those women seeking to find and reconnect with children. They credited God for their longevity and their motivation for living.

> That's God doin', no mine. I have nuttin' to do wit' it. He has a plan for me to tell my story. I'm here to tell my story to other people, to pass it on, my inspirations, my struggles, my triumphs, my success, my failures, everything. (LWH 12 years)

"Lost mothering" suggests women embrace longevity with disbelief for being alive while reconciling past mothering and reproductive decisions and actions.

5 Conclusion

In this study, I systematically examined women's perspective and experiences of mothering post-HAART regime and conceptualized a framework of "lost mothering." I argue that although women in this study did not face immediate mortal threat as they did in the earlier stages of the epidemic, the conceptualization of "lost mothering" is unique and builds on earlier conceptualization of mothering work as eternal, defensive, and redefined for women with HIV/AIDS (Barnes et al. 1997; Ingram and Hutchinson 1999; Van Loon 2005). My research is complementary to Murphy et al. (2010) expanding their idea of missed activities for mothers with HIV to include mothers who had relinquished their children and attempted reunification.

While this study provides an important glimpse of mothering, it has limitations. First, the sample size limits the generalizability of the results. Second, data collections rely on retrospective recall of sensitive information that the participants choose to share. What are the elements of women's living with HIV/AIDS that they are not talking about or that they have not yet found the words or means of expressing? For example, one participant kept "silent" about her daughter's suicide. The participant spoke of her children in detail, including sharing photographs of them, but not her deceased daughter. The point is well taken that "The voice of suffering and the void of silence alert us to the perils of imposing narratives on often fragmented, elusive stories participants struggle to tell" (Charmaz 2002: 323).

Future studies could explore children's experiences of missed and disruptive mothering. Studies of biological fathers, foster and adoptive parents' perspectives could be informative. I encourage larger qualitative longitudinal studies on mothers and women living long term with HIV/AIDS from diverse communities and countries to examine mothering including empirical investigations of children and family perspectives.

I wish to underscore the importance of listening to women with HIV/AIDS and supporting the strategies that prove useful for them for living longer lives. The findings have implications for developing novel programs on mothering skills for women reuniting with children and assistance in the policies of finding, contacting, and reuniting families. Support groups focusing on helping women with HIV/AIDS reconcile past reproduction and custodial decisions could be supportive. I agree with Sandelowski and Barroso (2003) that such programs acknowledge the centrality of mothering for women with HIV/AIDS and minimize the burdens of motherhood for women and for their children.

Studies on mothering for women with HIV/AIDS suggest that the uniqueness is providing care and protection for their children from issues of stigma by association (Clark et al. 2003; Sandelowski and Barroso 2003; Sandelowski et al. 2004, 2009). I add to that notion proposing that participants reported fears of discrimination speaks to the issue that stigma continues to exist for women living longer lives with HIV/AIDS for themselves and their children in these two United States cities.

Acknowledgements This research was funded by the National Institutes of General Medical Sciences grant GM 48135. The content is solely the responsibility of the author and does not necessarily represent the official views of the National Institute of General Medical Sciences or the National Institutes of Health. I wish to thank the women who shared their experiences and their reflections; also the consultants Sheigla Murphy, Margaret Kearney, Susan Taylor-Brown, Monica Bill Barnes, and Craig Sellers for their contributions to data analysis and valuable feedback; and Audrey Alforque Thomas for statistical analysis, and Parul Baxi and Tim Smith for statistical support, and Parul Baxi and McCoy Burford for research support.

References

Ahdieh-Grant L, Tarwater PM, Schneider MF, Anastos K, Cohen M, Khalsa A, Minkoff H, Young M, Greenblatt RM (2005) Factors and temporal trends associated with highly active antiretroviral therapy discontinuation in the Women's Interagency HIV Study. J Acquir Immune Defic Syndr 38(4):500–503

Anastos K, Barron Y, Cohen MH, Greenblatt RM, Minkoff H, Levine A, Young M, Gange SJ (2004) The prognostic importance of changes in CD4+ cell count and HIV-1 RNA level in women after initiating highly active antiretroviral therapy. Am Coll Phys 140:256–264

Anastos K, Schneider MF, Gange SJ, Minkoff H, Greenblatt RM, Feldman J, Levine A, Delapenha R, Cohen M (2005) The association of race, sociodemographic, and behavioral characteristics with response to highly active antiretroviral therapy in women. J Acquir Immune Defic Syndr 39(5):537–544

Barnes DB (2008) I'm still here: a 10 year follow up of women's experiences living with HIV. In: Kronenfeld JJ (ed) Research in the sociology of health care. JAI Press, Bingley, pp 123–138

Barnes DB, Murphy S (2009) Reproductive decisions for women with HIV: motherhood's role in envisioning a future. Qual Health Res 19:481–491

Barnes DB, Taylor-Brown S, Wiener L (1997) "I didn't leave y'all on purpose": HIV-infected mothers' videotaped legacies for their children. Qual Sociol 20(1):7–32

Berger PL, Luckmann T (1967) The social construction of reality: a treatise in the sociology of knowledge. Doubleday, Garden City

Charmaz K (2002) Stories and silences: disclosures and self in chronic illness. Qual Inq 8(3): 302–328

Charmaz K (2006) Constructing grounded theory: a practical guide through qualitative analysis. Sage, Thousand Oaks

Chu SY, Buehler JW, Berkelman RL (1990) Impact of the human immunodeficiency virus epidemic on mortality in women of reproductive age, United States. J Am Med Assoc 264(2):225–229

Clark HJ, Lindner G, Armistead L, Austin B (2003) Stigma, disclosure, and psychological functioning among HIV-infected and non-infected African-American women. Women Health 38(4):57–71

Cohen MH, French AL, Benning L, Kovacs A, Anastos K, Young M, Minkoff H, Hessol NA (2002) Causes of death among women with human immunodeficiency virus infection in the era of combination antiretroviral therapy. Am J Med 113:91–98

Collins PH (2000) Black feminist thought: knowledge, consciousness, and the politics of empowerment, 2nd edn. Routledge, New York

Connor EM, Sperling RS, Gelber R, Kiselev P, Scott G, O'Sullivan MJ, VanDyke R, Bey M, Shearer W, Jacobson RL, Jimenez E, O'Neill E, Bazin B, Delfraissy JF, Culnane M, Coombs R, Elkins M, Moye J, Stratton P, Balseley J (1994) Reduction of maternal infant transmission of human immunodeficiency virus type 1 with Zidovudine treatment. N Engl J Med 331(18): 1173–1180

Cook JA, Grey D, Burke J, Cohen MH, Gurtman AC, Richardson JL, Wilson RE, Young MA, Hessol NA (2004) Depressive symptoms and AIDS-related mortality among a multisite cohort of HIV-positive women. Am J Public Health 94(7):1133–1140

Glaser BG (1978) Theoretical sensitivity: advances in the methodology of grounded theory. The Sociology Press, Mill Valley

Glaser BG, Strauss AL (1967) The discovery of grounded theory: strategies for qualitative research. Aldine De Gruyter, New York

Ickovics JR, Milan S, Boland R, Schoenbaum E, Schuman P, Vlahov D (2006) Psychological resources protect health: 5-year survival and immune function among HIV-infected women from four US cities. AIDS 20:1851–1860

Ingram D, Hutchinson SA (1999) Defensive mothering in HIV-positive mothers. Qual Health Res 9:243–258

Kapadia F, Cook JA, Cohen MH, Sohler N, Kovacs A, Greenblatt RM, Choudhary I, Vlahov D (2005) The relationship between non-injection drug use behaviors on progression to AIDS and death in a cohort of HIV seropositive women in the era of highly active antiretroviral therapy use. Soc Study Addiction 100:990–1002

Kohli R, Klein RS, Schoenbaum EE, Anatos K, Minkoff H, Sacks HS (2006) Aging and HIV infection. J Urban Health Bull N Y Acad Med 83(1):31–42

Marx K (1978/1852) The eighteenth Brumaire of Louis Bonaparte. In: Tucker RC (ed) The Marx-Engles reader, 2nd edn. W.W. Norton & Co, New York, p 595

Mead GH (1962/1934) Mind, self, and society. The University of Chicago Press, Chicago

Murphy DA, Robert KJ, Herbeck DM (2010) HIV disease impact on mothers: what they miss during their children's developmental years. J Child Family Stud OnlinefirstTM, 24 July 2010. http://www.springerlink.com/content/?k=Murphy%2c+D.+A.%2c+Roberts%2c+K.+J.+and+Herbeck+D.+M. Accessed 24 Jan 2011

Olesen V (2003) Feminisms and qualitative research at and into the millennium. In: Denzin NK, Lincoln YS (eds) The landscape of qualitative research: theories and issues. Sage, Thousand Oaks, pp 332–397

Sandelowski M, Barroso J (2003) Motherhood in the context of maternal HIV infection. Res Nurs Health 26:470–782

Sandelowski M, Lambe C, Barroso J (2004) Stigma in HIV-positive women. J Nurs Scholarsh 36(2):122–128

Sandelowski M, Barroso J, Voils CI (2009) Gender, race/ethnicity, and social class in research reports on stigma in HIV-positive women. Health Care Women Int 30(4):273–288

Siegel K, Karus D, Dean L (2004) Psychosocial characteristics of New York city HIV-infected women before and after advent of HAART. Am J Public Health 94(7):1127–1132

Smith DE (1987) The everyday world as problematic: a feminist methodology. In: Smith DE (ed) The everyday world as problematic: a feminist sociology. Northwestern University Press, Boston, pp 105–145

Sperling RS, Shapiro DE, Coombs RW, Todd JA, Herman SA, McSherry GD, O'Sullivan MJ, Van Dyke RB, Jimenez E, Rouzious C, Flynn PM, Sullivan JL (1996) Maternal viral load, Zidovudine treatment, and the risk of transmission of human immunodeficiency virus Type 1 from mother to infant. N Engl J Med 335(22):1621–1629

Strauss A (1959) Mirrors and masks: the search for identity. Free Press, Glencoe

Strauss AL (1987) Qualitative analysis for social scientists. Cambridge University Press, New York

Strauss AL, Corbin J (1998) Basics of qualitative research: techniques and procedures for developing grounded theory, 2nd edn. Sage, Thousand Oaks

Thomas WL, Thomas DS (1970/1928) Situations defined as real are real in their consequences. In: Stone GP, Farberman HA (eds) Social psychology through symbolic interaction. Ginn-Blalsdell, Waltham, pp 154–155

Van Loon RA (2005) Redefining motherhood: adaptation to role change for women with AIDS. In: Turner F (ed) Social work diagnosis in contemporary practice. Oxford University Press, New York, pp 110–119

Chapter 8
Do You Tell Your Kids? What Do You Tell Your Kids? When Do You Tell Your Kids? How Do You Tell Your Kids? HIV-Positive Mothers, Disclosure and Stigma

Karalyn McDonald

1 Introduction

HIV-positive mothers face the complex and challenging decision of whether to disclose their HIV status to their children. Not only do HIV-positive mothers worry about the potential emotional burden this disclosure may impose on their children, but there is also the risk of unwanted disclosure by children and the possibility of ensuing stigma (see also Chap. 1 in this volume).

When thinking about the disclosure of one's HIV status to another, stigma is implicit. HIV is still a much stigmatized illness with the prevalence of HIV/AIDS-related stigma and discrimination widely documented (Sontag 1989; Alonzo and Reynolds 1995; Bennetts et al. 1999; Herek 1999; Ciambrone 2001; Sandelowski et al. 2004; Scambler 2009). HIV-positive women have a unique experience of stigma due to their ability to bear children and therefore place "innocent" children at risk. Furthermore, the stigmatization of HIV-positive mothers has been intensified because of the assumed association of HIV-positive women with drug use and promiscuity (Sandelowski and Barroso 2003; see also Chap. 9 in this volume). This has resulted in the canonical narrative of motherhood within Western society rejecting HIV-positive women's worthiness as mothers (Carovano 1991; Patton 1993; Sherr 1993; Baylies 2001; McDonald 2002, 2006a). Like other marginalized women such as women in prison, drug-using women and teenagers, HIV-positive mothers have mothered against the odds, and many women have found it difficult to escape the prevalent idea that they were either bad mothers or even bad women for desiring motherhood (Coll et al. 1998; McDonald 2012; see also Chap. 9).

K. McDonald (✉)
Department of Infectious Diseases, Monash University,
VIC 3004, Melbourne, Australia
e-mail: karalyn.mcdonald@monash.edu

P. Liamputtong (ed.), *Women, Motherhood and Living with HIV/AIDS:*
A Cross-Cultural Perspective, DOI 10.1007/978-94-007-5887-2_8,
© Springer Science+Business Media Dordrecht 2013

Today, more than 33 million people are estimated to be infected with HIV/AIDS and women make up around half of that figure. However, Australia's rate of HIV is relatively low. By the end of 2012, more than 31,000 people had been diagnosed with HIV and women make up only 9% of the total population of people living with HIV/AIDS (The Kirby Institute 2012). Due to Australia's vast geography and relatively small population, the 1,994 women living with HIV are widely dispersed, and many women are therefore isolated and often not visible within the epidemic in Australia. Nevertheless, the consequences of an HIV-positive diagnosis for women are highly significant (McDonald 2002, 2006a, 2006b, 2011; McDonald and Kirkman 2011) as most women are diagnosed during their reproductive years, with the median age of diagnosis 30 years (NCHECR 2006).

In this chapter, I explore HIV-positive women's accounts of disclosure and how women construct both public and private accounts of living with HIV as a way of deriving meaning from their diagnosis as well as a way of managing disclosure and its potential ramifications. I also examine the role of stigma in the decisions made about disclosure, including disclosure to children.

2 Theoretical Frameworks

The analysis presented draws upon narrative identity theory and Goffman's theory of stigma. Narrative identity refers to the stories we tell about ourselves (both to ourselves and to others). By telling stories about ourselves, we tell others who we are and who we would like to be: "We express, display, make claims for who we are – and who we would like to be – in the stories we tell and how we tell them. In sum we perform our identities" (Mishler 1999: 5).

Individual narrative identities are developed within the cultural influences, dominant discourses and canonical narratives available to the individual. Narrative identity formation requires individuals to either position themselves within, or in opposition to, these available stories. This is an ongoing process and something we do all of our lives. As Riessman (1990b: 1195) put it, "we are forever composing impression of ourselves, projecting a definition of who we are, and making claims about ourselves and the world that we test and negotiate in social interaction."

Other researchers have written about the ontological assault of chronic illness (see, e.g., Charmaz 1991; Garro 1992; Frank 1995; Mathieson and Stam 1995) and the disruption caused by the inability to perform previous social roles and identities (Williams 1987), as well as the strategies employed to maintain some semblance of normality or adjustment (Strauss and Glaser 1975). Chronic illness fundamentally disrupts the taken-for-granted world of everyday life (Berger and Luckman 1966; Garro 1994; Crossley 1998) and in turn calls for a new narrative to be told or an existing narrative to be revised. Women who are diagnosed as HIV-positive are usually both devastated and traumatized. Their existing identities and imagined futures are shattered, and they must learn to incorporate a new identity into their life story, as a woman and a mother, with a chronic and potentially life-threatening illness

(Davies 1997; Doyal and Anderson 2005). Furthermore, they must do this within a society that both stigmatizes and ostracizes them because of the disease with which they live (McDonald 2006a).

HIV/AIDS-related stigma has been widely documented (Sontag 1989; Alonzo and Reynolds 1995; Bennetts et al. 1999; Herek 1999; Ciambrone 2001; Sandelowski et al. 2004; Scambler 2009; Liamputtong 2013). (see also other chapters in this volume). Stigma is complex and multilayered (Campbell and Gibbs 2009); however, for the purpose of this chapter, I utilise Goffman's theory of stigma (Goffman 1963), in particular, to examine the ways in which HIV-positive women resist a spoiled identity and present accounts of themselves as informed and responsible within their sexual relationships with HIV-negative men and, ultimately, as "normal" women living "normal" lives.

Goffman (1963: 45) noted that "persons who have a particular stigma tend to have similar learning experiences regarding their plight, and similar changes in conception of self – a similar 'moral career'". Career, as defined by Goffman (1961: 119), refers to "any social strand of any person's course through life". A similar moral career could be identified for the women in my study. All of the women in this study were acutely aware of the stigma attached to an HIV-positive diagnosis and the stereotypes that are associated with HIV-positive women. The first stage of their "plight" or journey included making decisions about disclosure. HIV-negative people often positioned HIV-positive women as "discreditable" by warning them to refrain from telling many people in the first few weeks of their diagnosis, thereby confirming their spoiled identity. Denise, one participant in my study, remembered that, "the other thing that the STD clinic said when we were diagnosed was, 'don't tell anyone'". Even family members tried to limit women's disclosure, fearing ramifications. When another participant, Helen, disclosed to her mother, "she didn't want me to tell my two sisters", and "the first thing" Brooke's mother said was, "don't tell Dad; whatever you do, don't tell Dad", because he had cancer and her mother was "concerned it would make him worry and make him sicker". So, the fear of stigma was ever-present even if it was not actually experienced.

3 The Study

This chapter is based on my doctoral thesis examining the impact of an HIV diagnosis on women's thoughts and feelings about motherhood including experiences of disclosure, stigma and discrimination (McDonald 2008). Thirty-four HIV-positive women who were diagnosed during their childbearing years were interviewed around Australia. Participants volunteered after seeing a notice about the research distributed among AIDS Councils and organizations that support and provide services to HIV-positive women or after being told about the research by another participant.

Initial in-depth interviews (lasting on average one hour) were conducted in 2001 by myself at a location of the participant's choice, usually her home but occasionally at an organization that offered peer support to HIV-positive people. Interviews were recorded, with the women's permission, and transcribed. An interview schedule was developed from an extensive literature search and previous research I had been involved in (McDonald et al. 1998). The interview schedule had six main themes: diagnosis, motherhood, identity, partners, disclosure, power and control, and passage of time. Each had a variety of prompts (if required) to explore these areas according to each woman's individual circumstances and experience. I began each interview with the question, "can you please tell me your story of how being diagnosed with HIV has influenced your thoughts and feelings about motherhood?" By asking for a story, I was encouraging a plot and sequence of events (Kirkman 1997). This question and subsequent probes also helped provide the "scaffolding" for the women's stories to be told (Cazden 1983; Bruner 1986, 1987).

Participants were sent copies of their own transcript and asked to verify and update the account. Intermittent contact was continued for six years to enable participants to update information and validate interpretations of their accounts, including the resource book, *Common threads: women stories of pregnancy, parenting and living with HIV* (McDonald 2006c), that was developed in consultation with the participants and the support organization, Positive Women Victoria Inc.

La Trobe University Human Research Ethics Committee approved the research. Participants gave written consent. Their confidentiality is protected by the use of pseudonyms and the concealment of identifying details in reporting results. Information about counseling and referral services was offered to each participant.

Of the 34 women, 28 women were mothers to 51 children. Sixteen women had given birth to 23 children since their diagnosis. All but two of these children were born after 1994 and the introduction of the Paediatric AIDS Clinical Trials Group (PACTG) 076 protocol (which significantly reduced the likelihood of mother-to-child transmission). Only one child, born in 1994, was HIV-positive. Two women were pregnant with their first child at the initial interview and updated details about their birthing and mothering experiences in postnatal interviews. Four women had been diagnosed during a pregnancy; all proceeded to term.

4   Disclosure

4.1   *Private Accounts and Disclosure*

The women in my study had constructed a private account of their HIV infection to help understand and gain meaning from being diagnosed with a disease most knew little about and certainly did not expect. Women's private accounts often included how they contracted HIV, how devastated they were by their diagnosis and how, over time, they dealt with this shocking news. Stigma was at the forefront of most women's minds when first diagnosed, and they often faced the dilemma of wanting to share the most significant event of their lives contrasted with the need to protect themselves from rejection and stigma.

Consequently, most women refrained from telling very many people. Women differed in their approaches to protecting themselves (and any children) from stigma. Avoiding disclosure and thereby keeping one's status a secret was the surest way not to attract stigma and discrimination and ensured that women could "pass" as normal (see also Chap. 15 in this volume). Person and Richards (2008) also found that non-disclosure was key to normalcy amongst a heterosexual sample of people living with HIV/AIDS (PLWHA) in Australia. Disclosure was also recognized by many women as a part of their life they could control when so much of the rest of their lives seemed chaotic and out of control. Laura explained:

> I think one of the few things that you feel that you have left when you are first diagnosed is whom you tell. There are a whole lot of things that seem to be taken away from you but one of the few things that you do have left, that you have some control over, is whom you tell.

It is not surprising then, that most women chose to tell only a few people, usually immediate family and a few friends. Two women told only their sexual partners. Monica had disclosed to her sexual partners and two friends, whom she told because she "was in an emotional upheaval but now I don't feel any need to disclose." She had not told any members of her family because she did not "feel the need to and I also think it's a bit difficult now because it's been a long time." Carol also had not told any members of her family "because it didn't really become an issue for them to know." She believed that she was "close" to her family but that "if it was a different diagnosis … if it was cancer or if it was something else, would I say? And I don't really think I would." The common theme in the accounts of women who had not disclosed to their families was preventing unnecessary "worry." Women could also be understood to be protecting their families by avoiding disclosure. They were protecting them from the worry of knowing a loved one was living with a life-threatening illness, and they were also protecting them from the possibility of stigma from their association with someone with HIV.

Even when women were comfortable with their wider family and friends knowing their HIV status, some found it necessary to control information given to others by concealing certain details and constructing an account that was acceptable. The father of Miranda's first child was also HIV-positive, so there was no perceived need for them to be practising safe sex. However, the father of her second child, and current partner, was HIV-negative and when they announced their pregnancy, friends and family asked her, "how could you risk Allan's life like that?" Miranda believed others would find it more acceptable if she told them "it was just the once", explaining that "people can't deal with it and it's not like how can *he* risk his life, it's how can *you* risk his life?" Miranda went on to say that she had her "tubes done during the cesar" and "even now occasionally we will have unprotected sex":

> And that's really hard; I am telling you because you're doing the research but I'd never tell anyone other than another positive women that we do that, because people can't understand that we don't wear a condom. But, that's his choice. He knows what he's up against and I'm really worried about it.

By having a tubal ligation, Miranda has removed the risk to any potential child but, whilst she knew female-to-male transmission was a lower risk than male-to-female transmission, she still had to bear the burden of having to participate in an activity in which she was a danger to her partner, knowing that others would blame her if her partner did seroconvert. Others have also found that condom use within the relationships of HIV-positive women is often fraught (Lawless et al. 1996a; Lather and Smithies 1997; Gurevich et al. 2007) and that women's focus on protecting others can impede their own sexual fulfilment (Gurevich et al. 2007).

4.1.1 Private Accounts and Children

Maintaining a private account ensures the protagonist protects herself as well as the ones she loves (Kirkman 1997, 2001). This is particularly important for HIV-positive women who are mothers. Many of the stories women told me revealed a great deal of energy consumed by worrying about their children and the impact that HIV would have on their children's lives. Potentially, motherless children, a frail or ill mother unable to carry out duties that well mothers are able to, or discrimination directed at their children were scenarios that played out in the minds of many women. Denise explained how, in the early years of her diagnosis, she spent many hours worrying that someone might discover her HIV status. During this time, she worked in her children's school canteen. Evident in her account is perceived stigma and worry:

> I thought, oh God, what if someone finds out that I'm positive and I'm making lunches? I know that there is no risk but it's their reaction and then what their kids will hear them say, and then they'll come to school and say something to my kids. Then I'll have to go up there and deal with it. All that emotional energy is just incredible. And it has to impact on your health.

4.1.2 Disclosure to Children

Several studies have examined HIV-positive mothers' disclosure to their children and all concluded that it was a difficult and complex decision (Moneyham et al. 1996; Draimin et al. 1999; Marcenko and Samost 1999; Tompkins et al. 1999; Ingram and Hutchinson 2000; Schrimshaw and Siegel 2002; Sowell et al. 2003; Sandelowski et al. 2004; Tompkins 2007; Murphy 2008). Studies have found that up to 40% of mothers had disclosed to their uninfected children (Armistead et al. 1999; Tompkins et al. 1999; Ingram and Hutchinson 2000), varying according to the mother's disease stage and ethnicity and the child's age (Thorne et al. 2000; Schrimshaw and Siegel 2002). The child's age seemed to be the most important factor for the women in my study, but all found the decision to disclose to children extremely difficult to make.

Ten women had told at least one of their children that they were HIV-positive. Some women chose not to hide it so that their children had grown up with it, and others told their children when they were diagnosed. Joy said, "I told the kids straight away. How much they understood I don't know, but I thought this was easier than trying to keep something from them." With repeated bouts of illness, Joy thought that disclosing to her children was the only way to explain everything that was happening:

> I think I had dropped down to 47 kilos and still had this chronic diarrhoea; I mean, I couldn't even do shopping. I would try to do the shopping with the kids and I would get the things to the cash register, that was it and I would poo my pants. I would say, "sorry kids, we are going to have to run". And the anxiety through that was just unbearable. But, the kids were really supportive and they would say, "come on Mum, you've done it again", but no embarrassment.

As well as telling their children, a few women told their children's school principals, usually when either they or their children's father was very unwell. The rationale for this decision was to ensure that others were watching how their children were coping with the news or an ill parent. As well as disclosing to their three children, Samantha and her husband told "their immediate teachers and the principal" when the children's father became "really sick". Samantha justified this decision as the best course of action for her children, because "we thought the kids needed support and so they knew if anything happened within the classroom, why it was actually happening."

Women who did disclose to school principals and teachers reported positive and supportive responses. Samantha's disclosure "went down really well and they were really good." However, there were occasions when peers were less supportive. When Samantha disclosed to the mother of her child's friend, whom she believed would be open-minded to this information, her daughter's friend was subsequently prevented from playing at their house, which Samantha remembered as "hard" for her daughter. Joy reported that her children had experienced a few tussles at school as a result of other children knowing her status. It is not surprising, then, that generally women decided against telling people who were involved in their children's school community in an effort to avoid ramifications for their children.

Partial Disclosure to Children

Most women with young children had not told their children because they judged their children to be too young, but women's choices and approaches to disclosure were varied. Some chose to allow HIV to be freely spoken around children in the belief that it would reduce the shock of sudden disclosure by allowing a gradual awareness. Other women who had decided against full disclosure preferred to explain HIV as "bad blood", "bugs" or a "virus", avoiding the use of the term HIV. This was done to avoid having their child naively repeat "HIV", thereby bringing about unwanted disclosure and potential discrimination. Julia explained, "I was always worried that he'd go to kinder and say 'HIV'. So, I explained it as bug."

A couple of women freely took their treatment in front of children but described it as vitamins or medication for the "bad blood" or unnamed virus. Adele explained that she wanted her daughter to have some knowledge of her status. So, when she asked her why she took pills Adele told her she was "taking vitamins to keep me healthy." Later when her daughter asked why she was not allowed to take the same vitamins as her mother, Adele told her she had "a virus in my body and without the drugs the virus will get out of control and I can get very sick." Adele believed her daughter accepted this amount of information and explained that she was "waiting for her to probe more and to ask more." Whilst she wanted to be "honest", Adele's priority was to protect her child, which for Adele meant limiting what she disclosed about her HIV status to her daughter.

Deciding Not to Tell Children

Most women envisaged a time when they would tell their children, either when their children became sexually active or if they needed to explain illnesses that could occur in the future. However, a few women chose not to tell their children, believing there simply was no need to cause their children any anxiety, particularly if they were well. Monica said about her daughter, "I guess she will fall into that same family category. Like, why tell her, if there's no need?"

Helen's husband was adamant that their daughter never be told that both of her parents were HIV-positive, but Helen thought she would "find out at some point." Helen had also considered that another family member might tell her or that "it will slip out or she'll overhear or something." She then went on to add, "But, I don't know; we might die in a car accident or something, so the need may never be there to even tell her."

Laura explained her daughter's age as one of the main reasons for deciding against disclosing her status when she and her husband were first diagnosed. She understood young children's sense of time to be very different and, because of the rapid progression of her husband's illness and death, Laura "didn't want her thinking that it was going to happen, like, tomorrow for Mum." She did not want her to be "waking up every day thinking, is Mum going to get sick?" Laura went on to say, "I didn't want her to have a childhood that was filled with that sort of anxiety, because I was absolutely positive that she would be paying for it all of her life."

Laura had been diagnosed for 10 years when I met with her and she had still not told her daughter because "it became an irrelevancy in a lot of ways." Laura had stayed well and, because HIV had become a "very small part of my life", Laura had decided "she doesn't need to be concerned with that." Whilst Laura questioned her decision to not tell her daughter, the fear of disclosure negatively impacting on her daughter's life was her justification for keeping this information from her:

> Motherhood brings up those wonderful things about: do you tell your kids? What do you tell your kids? When do you tell your kids? How do you tell your kids? Should you tell your kids? Shouldn't you tell your kids? ... I have come up with all these excuses over the years but the bottom line is I am just too chicken to do it.

Women's decisions about disclosure were very much driven by their desires to protect the people they loved. This was particularly so for women who were mothers, but also applied to family members and friends. Women were aware of the burden that disclosure placed on the recipient and they gave careful consideration to what that information might do to their relationships.

4.2   Public Accounts and Disclosure

Others have written about the decisions made by chronically ill people who decide to publicly declare their illness in an effort to educate the wider public or bring attention to their disease (Hopkins Tanne 2001; Brophy 2003; Sowell et al. 2003). Such accounts are typically quest narratives (Frank 1995), in which "illness becomes a motivator for social action or change" (Thomas-MacLean 2004: 1649). Female celebrities in Australia who have made public their journeys with breast cancer include Olivia Newton-John, Jane McGrath, Kylie Minogue and Belinda Emmett. Susan Sontag (1978) argued that cancer was a highly stigmatised illness but noted in her book, *AIDS and its metaphors* (1990: 104), that "the onus of cancer has been lifted by the emergence of a disease whose charge of stigmatisation, whose capacity to create spoiled identity, is far greater." Lawless et al. (1996a, b: 1371) noted that HIV elicits "judgements of personal responsibility and blame to an extent unseen in other illness." In the past, society categorised HIV-positive women as "innocent" or "blameworthy", depending on how they acquired their HIV infection. Universal blood-handling guidelines have almost eliminated the risk of acquiring HIV through medical procedures or blood products and therefore the category of "innocent" is rarely used now for women. Consequently, most women are considered to blame for their HIV infection, and some women in this study set about publicly challenging that notion.

4.2.1   Public Accounts and the Greater Good

Despite the risk of stigma, some HIV-positive women in Australia have declared their status publicly. They have usually done this in the hope of educating the wider public, reducing transmission rates and reducing stigma for others living with HIV (see also Chaps. 14 and 15 in this volume). Nine women in my study had constructed public accounts of their HIV status that they were prepared to disclose to strangers in the hope that they would educate people about the transmission of HIV as well as help reduce the stereotypes and stigma surrounding HIV/AIDS. Some women were involved in their state-based Positive Speakers' Bureau, whilst others accepted speaking engagements to educate health-care professionals. Eight of these women gave public accounts to media, including television, radio and print interviews.

  . Most women felt they were "making a difference" by disclosing their status publicly. Some women also felt they were "making good out of bad" and that "things happened for a reason." Layla's experience having her first baby made her realize that "a lot of people need a lot of education." When she accepted her first invitation to speak to midwives about her "experience as a positive mother", she described her motivation as "knowing that hopefully the other women would benefit by these people having a better understanding about the needs of positive mothers." Similarly, speaking with young people appealed to some of the women involved in the Speakers' Bureau. Audrey explained the public speaking she did at schools as something she could do "to take the positive out of it and use it to the best of your ability." Denise also envisaged benefiting her own children through the public speaking she did with students: "I thought these young people that we're impacting on are the kids in the generation that my kids are going to grow up with." Denise also explained that she was contributing to the breaking down of stereotypes when she disclosed her drug use in conjunction with her HIV status, because the students said things to her such as, "'Oh, but you don't look like you use drugs and you don't look like someone that's positive'. So, I was challenging that thinking." Other women also thought that, by telling their story, they might help reduce the stigma attached to being an HIV-positive woman and the assumptions people made about them. This was particularly so for women who contracted HIV from their husbands or partners. Joy explained she was simply "a Mum at home looking after my kids, ... and I am not going to be ashamed of that and that is why I will talk and speak publicly and will do whatever I can." Implicit in Joy's account are the categories of guilt and innocence, and, whilst Joy's public narrative might avoid this dichotomy, her private narrative emphasizes her innocence and her justification for refusing to feel shame.

It is important to note that, whilst only a handful of women had constructed a public account for sharing with strangers, all of the women who participated in my study shared their story with at least one stranger: me. Most did so in the hope that it would benefit other HIV-positive women. The advertisement for the study informed potential participants that, "It is also hoped that a booklet discussing pregnancy and motherhood in HIV-positive women will arise from my study. The booklet will be distributed to participants and to organisations that support and care for HIV-positive women." I also asked each woman at the end of her interview why she agreed to participate. Almost all of them responded with altruistic reasons. Miranda's reasoning was typical of many: "Oh, just for other women, really, who are making reproductive choices. Because I know how hard it was. They can make a better choice and it is not so scary."

Goffman (1963: 37) argued that "'speakers' ... provide a living model of fully-normal achievement" and "proving that an individual of this kind can be a good person." Most women in this study had benefited from hearing the narratives of other people living with HIV/AIDS (PLWHA) because it helped to reduce stigma and isolation. Some of these women had reached a stage in their journey as a women living with HIV at which they were able to reflect on the benefits they had gained from hearing these stories and viewed public speaking as an opportunity to benefit others in the same way they had. By participating in public speaking, women were validating their own accounts that emphasized they were just normal women who, by chance, came to be living with this disease and that they were good citizens contributing to the education of others and possible prevention of HIV, as well as the reduction of stigma for PLWHA.

4.2.2   Public Accounts and Children

Of the seven women with children who had constructed public accounts to share with strangers, four had told their children of their status, one had told one child but not her younger child and two women had not told their children, although one of these children knew that her father had died of an AIDS-related illness.

What women were prepared to do with their public accounts was somewhat dependent on whether or not they had disclosed to their children and the age of their child. A few women were prepared to do public speaking and media whilst their children were young and there was little chance of negative consequences or stigma for their child. Once their child started school, they stopped this work in the hope of "protecting" or "shielding" their child. Kate and her husband did media interviews about the birth of their daughter, which included print media with photos and radio interviews. Kate thought her daughter, who was a baby at the time, could "be protected from any hurtful ramifications that could possibly have come up. As she's gotten older we made the conscious decision to shut that stuff down."

Women with older children told of consulting their children about what kind of public work their children were comfortable with. Samantha said she sought her children's "permission" before she did any public speaking. In addition, she and her children had together constructed a public account should anyone question them about Samantha's involvement: "They always say, 'Well, Mum's just a volunteer at the AIDS Council', so if they don't want to say that I'm positive, they just say, 'Mum's a volunteer', which is easy." This allowed for Samantha to pass as a "normal" mother and thereby reduce the risk of enacted stigma. By including their children in the decision about the public accounts women gave, it enabled the women and their children to discuss how they would deal with any questions that might be asked and co-construct public versions that were acceptable to everyone. It also allowed the women to demonstrate to their children that they were sensitive to their children's concerns.

All of the women attempted to protect their children from any potential ramifications related to the public speaking they were involved with. Women who had disclosed to their children made a point of discussing the children's concerns with them. Leanna was involved with the Positive Speakers' Bureau and her son was "always very, very nervous in the beginning with me going to high schools in particular." Leanna promised that she would never speak at his school and never mention his or his father's name to prevent him from being identified. Leanna also spoke of her son's concern about anything that mentioned HIV in their home, such as computer files or pamphlets left around the house, in case a friend might see it. Leanna believed "he was very, very afraid that people would find out and he would be ostracised as a result. I think that was a very real fear for him and it was something that made him feel different to everybody else."

Denise and Laura had teenage daughters to whom they had not disclosed. They both had experienced criticism from others about their decision not to disclose to their children, particularly in relation to the public work they did and the chance that their children might find out through the media. Consistent with women's awareness of the need to protect their children, both women recognised the "emotional load" they would be imposing on them and had therefore decided to avoid giving their children this "burden." Denise's daughter was aware that both her parents had been drug users and spent time in prison because of their addiction. Denise interpreted this information as "enough of an emotional load … without the HIV."[1]

Whilst Laura's daughter did not know about her mother's HIV infection, she did know that her father had died from an AIDS-related illness. Laura believed she was able to pass as an activist who, in her daughter's eyes, was "fighting" against "discrimination that goes on with positive and gay people." Laura attributed her daughter's unquestioning acceptance of any public HIV-related work she had done to this belief. She had spoken publicly about her HIV status to media and had been on television. In an effort to protect her daughter from enacted stigma, Laura said she was "careful about who I speak to and what sort of things I allow to be released." Both Denise and Laura conceded that they would disclose to their children if they were to get sick.

4.3 Managing Unwanted Disclosure and Stigma

Around one in four women had experienced unwanted disclosure. This was either in the form of people they had told telling others, health-care professionals being indiscreet or well-meaning family members insisting on another family member being told even when it was not what the woman herself wanted. A few other women felt they were pressured into disclosing to a parent by another family member who "thought they had a right to know." The consequence to this disclosure was often a very anxious parent who required a great deal of support from his or her daughter. This was often difficult because she was either still grappling with her diagnosis or perhaps lived too far away.

Unwanted disclosure caused additional angst when it directly affected their children. Lily was forced to leave the town in which she and her son were living when an ex-lover told a lot of people, including her neighbors, that she and her son were HIV-positive:

> The discrimination and the abuse we received meant that we were just ostracized from everybody. Nobody talked to us anymore. Zach lost all his playmates and it was just him and me existing, and when we were out we were stared at and talked about and people called out names and abuse. … [My ex-lover] told people that Zach and I had AIDS and that if they touched us they would get it.

---

[1] Denise wrote to me 18 months after we met, saying that her daughter now knew her mother and father were HIV-positive. She found out after she saw a newspaper interview that Denise and her partner had done. Denise believed that her daughter was "more upset about being the only one who didn't know" than about the HIV. Denise also thought that her daughter had "handled it well" and that that could be attributed to her having access to "lots of accurate information" as a result of being around HIV all of her life.

Even women who had not actually experienced unwanted disclosure feared the consequences of it. Monica had not told any of her family about her diagnosis. She did tell her partner who went on to father her child, but after their separation she worried that he would disclose her status against her wishes. She was "concerned" about him because they had "had some really awful times recently", and she was aware that it was "a very good tool for him to use as a mode of threat, which he has done." Adele had not yet disclosed her HIV status to her daughter, but one of her neighbors found out about her status from a previous sexual partner who was contact-traced[2] and subsequently worked out it was Adele. This woman had already disclosed Adele's status without her permission to some of their neighbors, and consequently Adele had "a fear that she would tell somebody that was connected with the school. She is not connected with the school in any way but I have that fear that it would come out at the school." Adele had given considerable thought to how she would handle such a scenario because she believed "a lot of people … would be quite narrow-minded":

> I would try and get somebody else who is experienced and can talk to a group – to stand up in front of a parent meeting – if it came to that, to put my side forward. I couldn't do it because I would get too emotional and I would get too angry. But, I think education would be the answer because I don't want to take Briana out of school. I don't think that would be the way to go, but it would depend on how hard a time she got from the other kids, which would come from the parents because the kids don't know. The teachers and the principal I don't think would be a problem. I get on with them well and I think they are open enough to ideas. It would be parents that are narrow and I guess the only comeback would be that there is nothing wrong with Briana. It's only me.

One act of unwanted disclosure for Adele had resulted in considerable distress for her. Adele's greatest concern was the impact further unwanted disclosure might have on her daughter and consequently she had put a considerable amount of energy into imagining a situation where unwanted disclosure occurred and how she would deal with it when, or if, it did.

However, unwanted disclosure could also inadvertently come from one's children. To prevent ensuing discrimination, many women gave considerable thought to when their child would be able to understand the gravity of the information in relation to how others might react to this news. Goffman (1963: 72) noted that "intimates can come to play a special role in the discreditable person's management of social situations", and women in this study had to consider the role their children would play in managing their spoiled identity. Denise had disclosed her status to her son, but she and her partner were yet to tell their younger daughter. Part of the decision to keep the information from her was the fear that, when she was younger, "she would have gone to school and told the whole assembly":

---

[2] Contact-tracing involves partner notification and is the process of identifying the relevant contacts of a person with an infectious disease (such as HIV) to ensure their awareness of their exposure (Donovan et al. 2006: 2). Although the confidentiality of the infected individual is maintained, sometimes it is possible for the individual who is contact-traced to guess her or his identity.

I wish she could do that, but then what happens when the first time she has someone come and sleep? A couple of years ago my partner said, "oh, what if those parents find out?"I said, "well, is their kid in danger? No". I said, "are we freaks? No". I said, "if they don't like it then they're not, not really her friends". That was what I said on the surface, but there's always that wanting to protect your kids. You don't want them to have to have other kids say mean stuff.

Even adult children did not always understand the risk of disclosure and how their mother expected them to refrain from telling others. Audrey's son told one of his friends about his mother's HIV status without her permission and when this friend revealed that she knew, Audrey was surprised and upset. She told her son "that he didn't have the privilege of telling people my health status; that it was up to me." Her son did not understand her reaction because this friend did not treat her any differently. However, Audrey explained that she felt it was her right to decide who knew and that knowing who knew about her status influenced the kind of conversations she might have. Having others know about their status without their permission or knowledge compromised women's attempts at passing as "normal" and removed their sense of control of managing information about themselves. However, disclosure to a loved one can be burdensome for the person receiving the news and a few women recognized that unwanted disclosure could be avoided by encouraging loved one or friends to confide in one another rather than tell an additional person (see also, Persson and Richards 2008). Laura told the people she disclosed to the names of other people who knew and told them to talk to each other:

When you give that sort of information to someone they have to do something with it because it is really overwhelming… They're going to talk about it to someone, so you need to give them options of people that it doesn't matter if they talk to them and that's what I tried to do.

5   Conclusion

Deciding whether or not to disclose their HIV status to their children is a very difficult and complex decision for mothers living with HIV. Ingram and Hutchinson (1999: 255) have written about the grief and worry that consumes the mental energy of HIV-positive mothers in the United States of America. They found that HIV-positive mothers "grieve multiple day-to-day losses and future losses." Furthermore, these women experience "disenfranchised grief" due to the stigmatised nature of their disease, which often prevents others from knowing what they are going through. Evident in many of the stories women told me is a great deal of pain, loss and grief. Fundamental to these feelings were powerlessness and a sense of losing control of one's life. As Laura explained, "it doesn't feel like you've given it over of your own volition; it feels like it is taken away from you."

The risk of stigma resulted in most women constructing at least two accounts of their HIV status. Generally, women's accounts were private, with different versions constructed for different audiences. Most women with young children had not yet disclosed their status to them, although most envisaged a time when they would.

A few had decided it was too great a burden for their children and considered disclosure only in the context of illness. Those women who did construct public accounts did so in the hope they would educate others and help reduce stigma for other positive women and their families. These women gave careful consideration to their public accounts in a concerted effort to protect their children.

The stigmatized nature of HIV meant that ultimately many women did not tell members of their broader social networks, such as work colleagues and sometime this even extended to friends or family members. The consequence of this nondisclosure was that some women were isolated within their disease which, ultimately, left them unsupported in their anxiety and concerns.

Acknowledgements   Karalyn would like to sincerely acknowledge the women who generously and courageously shared their accounts. She would also like to thank the National Health and Medical Research Council for her Commonwealth AIDS Related Grant (CARG) Ph.D. Scholarship and Dr Jon Willis, Dr Maggie Kirkman and Professor Doreen Rosenthal for their supervision during the study.

References

Alonzo A, Reynolds N (1995) Stigma, HIV and AIDS: an exploration and elaboration of a stigma trajectory. Soc Sci Med 41(3):303–315

Armistead L, Morse E, Forehand R, Morse P, Clark L (1999) African American women and self-disclosure of HIV-infection: rates, predictors and relationship to depressive symptomatology. AIDS Behav 3(3):195–204

Baylies C (2001) Safe motherhood in the time of AIDS: the illusion of reproductive 'choice'. Gend Dev 9(2):40–50

Bennetts A, Shaffer N, Manopaiboon C, Chaiyakul P, Siriwasin W, Mock P et al (1999) Determinants of depression and HIV-related worry among HIV-positive women who have recently given birth, Bangkok, Thailand. Soc Sci Med 49(6):737–749

Berger P, Luckman T (1966) The social construction of reality. Doubleday, Garden City

Brophy J (2003) The Spike Milligan public speaking competition. Psychiatr Bull 27:273

Bruner J (1986) Actual minds, possible worlds. Harvard University Press, Cambridge, MA

Bruner J (1987) Life as narrative. Soc Res 54(1):11–32

Campbell C, Gibbs A (2009) Stigma, gender and HIV: case studies of inter-sectionality. In: Boesten J, Poku N (eds) Gender and AIDS: critical perspectives from the developing world. Palgrave MacMillan, London, pp 29–47

Carovano K (1991) More than mothers and whores: redefining the AIDS prevention needs of women. Int J Health Sci 21(2):131–142

Cazden C (1983) Peekaboo as an instrumental model: discourse development at school and home. In: Bain B (ed) The sociogenesis of language and human conduct: a multi-disciplinary book of readings. Plenum, New York, pp 33–58

Charmaz K (1991) Good days, bad days: the self in chronic illness and time. Rutgers University Press, New Brunswick

Ciambrone D (2001) Illness and other assaults on the self: the relative impact of HIV/AIDS on women's lives. Sociol Health Illn 23(4):517–540

Coll CG, Surrey JL, Weingarten K (eds) (1998) Mothering against the odds: diverse voices of contemporary mothers. Guilford Press, New York

Crossley ML (1998) Women living with a long-term HIV positive diagnosis: problems, concerns and ways of ascribing meaning. Women's Stud Int Forum 21(5):521–533

Davies ML (1997) Shattered assumptions: time and the experience of long–term HIV positivity. Soc Sci Med 44(5):561–571

Donovan B, Bradford D, Cameron S, Conway D, Coughlan E, Doyle L, et al (2006) Australasian contact tracing manual: a practical handbook for health care providers managing people with HIV, viral hepatitis, other sexually transmissible infections (STIs) and HIV–related tuberculosis. www.ashm.org.au. Accessed 30 Sept 2006

Doyal L, Anderson J (2005) 'My fear is to fall in love again ...' How HIV-positive women survive in London. Soc Sci Med 60(8):1729–1738

Draimin BH, Hudis J, Segura J, Shire A (1999) A troubled present, an uncertain future: well adolescents in families with AIDS. J HIV/AIDS Prev Edu Adolesc Child 3(1/2):37–50

Frank A (1995) The wounded storyteller: body, illness, and ethics. The University of Chicago Press, Chicago

Garro LC (1992) Chronic illness and the construction of narratives. In: Good MD, Brodwin PE, Good BJ, Kleinman A (eds) Pain as human experience: an anthropological perspective. University of California Press, Berkeley, pp 100–137

Garro LC (1994) Narrative representations of chronic illness experience – cultural models of illness, mind, and body in stories concerning the temporomandibular joint (TMJ). Soc Sci Med 38(6):775–788

Goffman E (1961) Asylums: essays on the social situation of mental patients and other inmates. Penguin, Harmondsworth

Goffman E (1963) Stigma: notes on the management of a spoiled identity. Penguin, Harmondsworth

Gurevich M, Mathieson CM, Bower J, Dhayanandhan B (2007) Disciplining bodies, desires and subjectivities: sexuality and HIV-positive women. Feminism Psychol 17(1):9–38

Herek G (1999) AIDS and stigma. Am Behav Sci 42:1102–1112

Hopkins Tanne J (2001) Does publicity about celebrity illness improve public health? West J Med 174(2):94–95

Ingram D, Hutchinson S (1999) Defensive mothering in HIV-positive mothers. Qual Health Res 9(2):243–258

Ingram D, Hutchinson S (2000) Double binds and the reproductive and mothering experiences of HIV-positive women. Qual Health Res 10(1):117–132

Kirkman M (1997) Plots and disruptions: narratives, infertility, and women's lives. Unpublished doctoral dissertation. La Trobe University, Melbourne, Australia

Kirkman M (2001) Thinking of something to say: public and private narratives of infertility. Health Care Women Int 22(6):523–535

Lather P, Smithies C (1997) Troubling the angels: women living with HIV/AIDS. Westview Press, Colorado

Lawless S, Crawford J, Kippax S, Sponberg M (1996a) "If it's not on ...": heterosexuality for HIV positive women. Venereology 9(15):15–23

Lawless S, Kippax S, Crawford J (1996b) Dirty, diseased and undeserving: the positioning of HIV-positive women. Soc Sci Med 43(9):1371–1377

Liamputtong P, Haritavorn N, Kiatying-Angsulee N (2012) HIV and AIDS, stigma and AIDS support groups: perspectives from women living with HIV and AIDS in Central Thailand. Soc Sci Med 69:862–868

Marcenko MO, Samost L (1999) Living with HIV/AIDS: the voices of HIV-positive mothers. Soc Work 44:36–45

Mathieson CM, Stam HJ (1995) Renegotiating identity – cancer narratives. Sociol Health Illn 17(3):283–306

McDonald K (2002) I was devastated to think I couldn't have a child: the role of motherhood in the lives of HIV-positive women in Australia. Fertile Imagination Narratives Reprod (Spec Issue) 18(2):123–141

McDonald K (2006a) Do you tell? ... What do you tell? ... When do you tell? ... How do you tell?: HIV positive mothers, disclosure and stigma. HIV Australia 5(4):16–17

McDonald K (2006b) The best experience of my life: HIV positive women on pregnancy and birth in Australia. In: Tankard Reist M (ed) Defiant birth: women who resist medical eugenics. Spinifex Press, North Melbourne, pp 144–158

McDonald K (2006c) Common threads: women's stories of pregnancy, parenting and living with HIV. Australian Research Centre in Sex, Health and Society, La Trobe University and Positive Women Victoria, Melbourne

McDonald K (2008) "What about motherhood?": Women's journeys through HIV and AIDS. Unpublished doctoral dissertation. Unpublished PhD thesis, Australian Research Centre in Sex, Health and Society, La Trobe University, Melbourne, Australia

McDonald K (2011) "The old fashioned way": HIV-positive women's accounts of conception and sex in serodiscordant relationships. Cult Health Sex 13(10):1119–1133

McDonald K (2012) "You don't grow another head": the experience of stigma among HIV-positive women in Australia. HIV Austr 9(4):14–17

McDonald K, Bartos M, de Visser R, Ezzy D, Rosenthal D (1998) Standing on shifting sand: women living with HIV/AIDS in Australia. National Centre in HIV Social Research, La Trobe University, Melbourne

McDonald K, Kirkman M (2011) HIV-positive women in Australia explain their use and non-use of antiretroviral therapy in preventing mother-to-child transmission. AIDS Care 23(5):578–584

Mishler EG (1999) Storylines: craftartists' narratives of identity. Harvard University Press, Cambridge, MA

Moneyham L, Seals B, Demi A, Sowell R, Cohen L, Guillory J (1996) Experiences of disclosure in women infected with HIV. Health Care Women Int 17:209–221

Murphy DA (2008) HIV-positive mothers' disclosure of their serostatus to their young children: a review. Clinical Child Psychol Psychiatry 13:105–122

NCHECR (2006) Australian HIV surveillance report (No. 22 (2)). National Centre in HIV Epidemiology and Clinical Research, The University of New South Wales, Sydney, Australia

Patton C (1993) 'With champagne and roses': women at risk from/in AIDS discourse. In: Squire C (ed) Women and AIDS: psychological perspectives. Sage, London

Persson A, Richards W (2008) From closet to heterotopia: a conceptual exploration of disclosure and 'passing' among heterosexuals living with HIV. Cult Health Sex 10(1):73–86

Riessman CK (1990) Strategic uses of narrative in the presentation of self and illness: a research note. Soc Sci Med 30(11):1195–1200

Sandelowski M, Barroso J (2003) Motherhood in the context of maternal HIV infection. Res Nurs Health 26(6):470–482

Sandelowski M, Lambe C, Barroso J (2004) Stigma in HIV–positive women. J Nurs Scholarsh 36(2):122–128

Scambler G (2009) Health-related stigma. Sociol Health Illn 31(3):441–455

Schrimshaw EW, Siegel K (2002) HIV-infected mothers' disclosure to their uninfected children: rates, reasons, and reactions. J Soc Pers Relat 19(1):19–43

Sherr L (1993) HIV testing in pregnancy. In: Squire C (ed) Women and AIDS: psychological perspectives. Sage, London

Sontag S (1978) Illness as metaphor. Farrar, Strauss & Giroux, New York

Sontag S (1989) AIDS and its metaphors. The Penguin Press, New York

Sontag S (1990) Illness as metaphor and AIDS and its metaphors. Anchor Books, Doubleday, New York

Sowell RL, Seals BF, Phillips KD, Julious CH (2003) Disclosure of HIV infection: how do women decide to tell? Health Educ Res 18(1):32–44

Strauss AL, Glaser BG (1975) Chronic illness and the quality of life. Mosby, St Louis

The Kirby Institute (2012) HIV, viral hepatitis and sexually transmissible infections in Australia Annual Surveillance Report. The Kirby Institute, the University of New South Wales, Sydney, Australia

Thomas-MacLean R (2004) Understanding breast cancer stores via Frank's narrative types. Soc Sci Med 58:1647–1657

Thorne C, Newell ML, Peckham CS (2000) Disclosure of diagnosis and planning for the future in HIV–affected families in Europe. Child Care Health Dev 26(1):29–40

Tompkins T (2007) Disclosure of maternal HIV status to children: to tell or not to tell … That is the question. J Child Fam Stud 16:773–788

Tompkins T, Henker B, Whalen CK, Axelrod J, Comer LK (1999) Motherhood in the context of HIV infection: reading between the numbers. Cultur Divers Ethnic Minor Psychol 5(3):197–208

Williams G (1987) Disablement and the social context of daily activity. Int Disabil Stud 9:97–102

Chapter 9
Dealing with Life: Tactics Employed by Drug-Using Thai Mothers Living with HIV

Niphattra Haritavorn

1 Introduction

Ped, a female injecting drug user, lived in Bangkok: She worked as an outreach worker. One of my friends told me that she used to live with Kum, an injecting drug user who was also working as an outreach worker. Ped gave birth to a boy and then left her son with Kum. During the course of this research, I heard many stories about Ped, most of them negative, about her inability to fulfil her mothering role and to care for her son. One of the staff at the drop-in centre where Kum was working commented on her inability to take care of her son: "Ped left her boy when he was just three months old. She is such a bad mother. Kum loves his son so much and his son also loves him. The boy has never asked about his mother. He sometimes calls Kum's mother '*mae*' (mother) as she is the one raising him. He wouldn't even recognise his real mom." Ped left her family after they discovered that she was a drug addict: It is now many years since she has seen them. Ped told me that her mother discriminated against people using drugs: "My mother said she would rather have a daughter working as a prostitute than a drug addict daughter like me. I haven't been home for many years because she would hit me if she found out I was still using drugs." After moving out of the family home, Ped lived with Kum, who provided her with drugs. Talking about her time with him, she said: "I just used drugs. I did not have to worry about anything because Kum was a drug dealer at that time." Ped's life changed dramatically after she found out about her unplanned pregnancy and HIV status, "It was unintended and unplanned. My periods stopped after I started using drugs. I first thought that maybe drugs caused me to be sterile, but in fact they didn't. My boyfriend noticed my body changing and asked me to go to hospital. I was so shocked to know that I was seven months pregnant. Worse still, they told me that I was HIV-positive. It was a double shock and I didn't dare to tell the nurse and doctor I was a drug addict. If the nurse knew, she would suggest terminating my baby." During the pregnancy, Ped tried to stop using drugs for the sake of her child, but she couldn't. "When I first knew I was pregnant, I stop injecting drugs for a few months, but later on I start injecting drug again. All my friends are drug users, and we all talked about drugs. I couldn't stop taking drug that long. My boy was very thin and small. I cried a lot

N. Haritavorn (✉)
Faculty of Public Health, Thammasat University, Piychart Building 10th Floor,
Klong Luang, Rangsit, Pathumthani 12121, Thailand
e-mail: niphattraha@yahoo.com

P. Liamputtong (ed.), *Women, Motherhood and Living with HIV/AIDS:*
A Cross-Cultural Perspective, DOI 10.1007/978-94-007-5887-2_9,
© Springer Science+Business Media Dordrecht 2013

when I first saw him. He had craving symptoms just like me. He was not like other children. He cried a lot." Ped raised her son for three months before asking Kum's parents to adopt him. She recalled the time when she gave her son away: "I held him in my arms then handed him to Kum's mother. I was sad but I couldn't say anything. He will have a happier life with Kum's mother. I don't want to raise him in the drug community … he might grow up to be a drug addict like me and Kum." Ped's story is like other women I interviewed, the compelling story this woman told me revolved around the role of motherhood.

Ped's story is the typical lived story of Thai women using drugs who are faced with decision-making regarding their mothering role and the well-being of their children. The image of parents' drug use as a form of moral decay is nearly always one that is totally negative and unacceptable in most, if not all, societies worldwide (Keller et al. 2002; Klee 1998). Such images lead to judgements that are based on simple associa-tion, for example, assumptions that drugs and femininity are in essence incompatible (Banwell and Bammer 2006; Friedman and Alicea 2001). Because the role of mother-hood is strongly linked to social norms, cultures and practises (Woodward 2003), it has a significant impact on the female addict's sense of self (Rosenbaum 1988; Taylor 1993), with many women who use drugs finding themselves unable to fulfil the mother role. Using drugs distances women from socially ascribed feminine practises (Campbell 2000). Mothers who use drugs face more discriminatory action. While mothers who use drugs are frequently viewed by society as selfish, uncaring women who sacrifice their children's well-being in the pursuit of their own personal pleasure, the reality is that some women use drugs as a means of coping with the difficulties associated with childrearing (Klee 1998; Rosenbaum 1988).

The majority of women are expected to be first and foremost women – to give priority to the well-being of their children above all else (Bradley 2007). Imbued with this notion, society in general finds female drug users' modes of caring for their children unacceptable: Pregnant women using drugs are targeted by policy-makers as symbolic distortions of maternity and femininity (Campbell 2000). According to Boyd (2004), maternal cocaine use was initiated in the 1980s based upon the assumption that a mother using drugs was unfit for the mothering role and that her drug use endangered the development of the foetus. In response, the state constructed strategies to mandate the mother's taking of drugs. Policies ranging from child removal to incarceration are used as forms of punishment for pregnant drug users (Campbell 2000). In some instances, the state uses its power to control or punish the women's behavior by threatening to remove their children unless they enter treat-ment programs (Boyd 2004; Paone and Alperen 1998; Taylor 1993). These penalties see pregnant drug users targeted through social policy which leads women injecting drugs to believe that their bodies (and minds) are unfit for reproduction and, that in the interests of all concerned, abortion should be considered (Ettorre 2004).

Such strategies portray drug-using mothers as a collectivist rather than an individualist problem (Campbell 2000; Kandall 1996). Strategies in the form of segregation, controlling and rebellion underpin the particular forms of social distinction and discrimination that impact upon mothers who use drugs in Thailand. These strategies, however, are a symbolic dramatization of drug-using women's experiences of stigmatization. Gender meaning and imagery, particularly that relevant to the role of mother, become crucial points of the tactics employed by drug-using mothers. Research suggests that women's representation as "good mothers" is expressed in the form of tactics employed to lessen the impact of their drug life-style and HIV/AIDS upon their children. In this chapter, I explore the ways in which Thai women's injecting practises revolve around the role of mother and the tactics they employ to cope with gender expectations of being a mother, tactics that revolve around social expectations of "good" mothers. Being a mother who use drugs and living with HIV challenge the hegemonic notion of motherhood. Living with HIV exacerbates the life of drug-using mother as AIDS is interpreted to their understanding as well as public recognition as pollution.

2 Conceptual Framework: Gender Habitus and Drugs

The concept of habitus helps us understand the gender constructions which govern men's and women's behavioural patterns and actions in each society, particularly the social construction of motherhood. Bourdieu (1977:72) refers to habitus as the "objective structure of subjective experiences", that is, "habitus" as the objective structure or "the structured structures predisposed to function as structuring structures, that is, as principles of the generation and structuring of practices and representation." Habitus objective structure acts as a formalised code for regulating behavior, which takes various forms including laws, cultures, norms, roles, religions and beliefs. Through social interaction, the individual living within a particular habitus internalizes these objective structures by extension forming their embedded dispositions (Swartz 1997). The practices of members of the same groups, class or experiences create degrees of group conformity, implying that there is a chance of sharing the same habitus (Earle and Letherby 2003). This has implications for the sharing habitus of men and women.

In principle, habitus represents gendered norms and expectations. The gender habitus has traditionally exercised control over the lives of men and women to ensure cohesion and conformity to gender expectations and norms (Bourdieu 2001). The habitus of males and females differ based on their individual socialization and opportunity structures (Dumais 2002). One important role of women, or what society expects from them, is the duty of reproduction and childrearing (Earle and Letherby 2003; Woodward 2003). What concerns society in general is the impact of unhealthy maternal habits upon children, such as mothers taking drugs or drinking alcohol (Cobrinik et al. 1959; Zelson 1973).

Like gender, drug use is socially constructed based upon expectations and practises. It takes place in a specific, cultural context and is shaped by the structuring structures that inform consumption and experience (Cohen 2006; Lam 2008; McDonald 1994). There are, however, implicit tensions between a drug-using habitus and a female gender habitus in particular to motherhood. Substance-abusing mothers who attribute a polluting and destructive capacity to their children in the process violate the perceived traditional norms of parental care (Kettinger et al. 2000; Street et al. 2008). The duty of the pregnant woman is to protect her developing fetus rather than harm it through drug use; thus, unarguably pregnancy and drug use are incompatible (Rosenbaum 1988). Murphy and Rosenbaum (1998:1) delineate the degree to which the pregnant drug user breaks the gender habitus:

> A pregnant woman is supposed to take care of herself to protect her forming fetus. Women who purposely poison their wombs by using drugs are seen as failing in their reproductive role, and they must take their place among the most stigmatized groups in modern society.

The deterioration of the role of drug-using mothers is critical in the Thai context given that traditionally motherhood is the core of family foundation. In Thai society, a mother is referred to as *mae*, as Mulder (2000:70) describes:

> As a source of goodness, mother symbolizes virtue and selflessness. She is the pivot of one's moral obligations that revolve around the family. Her purity symbolizes the wholeness of the home. It is thus not too far-fetched to conclude that mother easily becomes the foremost reference point of one's conscience, that conscience is consciousness of her, and that she is the primary superego representative of most Thais.

Understanding the lives of Thai mothers injecting drugs and living with HIV requires interpretation of the meanings of mother. In Thailand, the imposition of the motherhood and reproductive roles on a woman often means she is excluded from male space (Whittaker 2002). Muecke (1984:462) notes on the role of Thai mother as 'while women could live without husbands, they could not live without children'. As in many societies, motherhood is the pivotal role for Thai women (Keyes 1984; Mulder 2000; Liamputtong 2007). More importantly, it represents the creation of a socially informed gendered role. Liamputtong states that the role of the Thai mother is inextricably linked to the Thai moral framework, that is, the good and responsible mother as she (2007:178) notes that "Women must ensure that their newborn infants and young children are free of 'risk', which posts danger on their lives or has ill consequences. As good responsible mothers, women make sure that their children are healthy and well."

Notably, gender habitus is considered to fundamentally direct how Thai men and women feel, act or think. Mother's reproduction is seen as being based on the nature of women. Both strategy and agent learn to correspond to the formative conditions of habitus (Hillier and Rooksby 2005; Krais 2006). Mother using drugs employs several tactics associated with prescribed role as mother in gender habitus. Taking drugs impinges upon women's status. That is, it also has direct implications for the status of mother using drugs in Thai society. Furthermore, taking drugs and living with HIV/AIDS threatened the status of women, especially as a mother. Mothers taking drug and living with HIV/AIDS are perceived to mark harm in the well-being of their children.

3   The Study

Drug users are a hidden population or hard-to-reach group (Lee 1994; Page and Singer 2010). Hence, research requires specific methods of data collection, in particular, the ethnographic method. Significantly, the ethnographer has to try to capture the grassroots' point of view through living or spending time among them so that he/she can both understand and determine the meaning of their behavior accurately. Page and Singer (2010:17) maintain that "the prime directive in the ethnographic study of drug use is to achieve an understanding of how and why the behaviours of interest take place in a given natural habitat and what forms these behaviours take." The ethnographic form of research has been used as a key means of studying illicit drug-taking as it provides the researcher with "hands-on" insight into the drug context and drug behaviour (Taylor 1993; Bourgois 1995; Bungay et al. 2010; Page and Singer 2010). The focus of this study is to explore the tactics that drug-using Thai mothers employ and to observe and record their lived experiences.

In order to understand the lived reality of female injecting drug users, I used several forms of qualitative research: ethnography, in-depth interviews, participant observation and focus group discussions. Each of the two focus groups comprised five key informants. I conducted in-depth interviews with 25 female injecting drug users living with HIV/AIDS in Bangkok and its suburbs in 2008. All of the interviews were analyzed using thematic analysis method and transcribed verbatim for coding. Permission for the study was obtained from the Thammasat Ethical Review Committee.

According to the data collected, the women interviewed ranged in age from 20 to 47 years. Twenty were Buddhist and the remaining five were Muslim. They reported a wide range of illicit drug consumption including heroin, methadone and amphetamine, among which heroin was the drug of first choice. All were injecting drug users. Ten had graduated from primary school, 12 from junior high school and the rest were in vocational school. Five of the women are now working as outreach workers with various Thai NGOs. The remainder are unemployed. Fifteen live with either their parents or in-laws, while the rest live with partners who also use drugs. Their average income is between 3,000 and 6,000 baht (US$100–150) per month. Most have government health insurance: The five among them who were outreach workers have social security insurance. All of the women are now on antiretroviral treatment.

4   Tactics of Mother Using Drugs

Women using drugs internalize the value of a mother, that is, what mothers are supposed to be. As Woodward (2003:18) notes: "Motherhood is recognizable and identifiable through the discursive and symbolic regimes which produce meanings about the experience, and through which we make sense of our identities." Motherhood is represented within cultural values and meanings expressed in the caring of children. In their attempts to fulfil social expectations of "good" mothers, women using drugs have to employ tactics that are compatible with certain tasks and responsibilities. The mother hegemonic notion predominantly influences the lives of the women using drugs who participated in this study. Many drug-using parents, aware of the possible danger to their children, find themselves confronting personal dilemmas in their attempts to combine their drug use with their parental responsibilities. Mothers, expressing concern about how their children would grow up in an environment where drugs are visible, attempt to lessen the impact of their drug use on their children by refusing to take on the mothering role. The desire to prevent their children from becoming enmeshed in lifestyles similar to their own is another reason why women send their children away to live either with their parents or in-laws. These are the tactics that women using drugs employ. Notably, living with HIV/AIDS becomes the exacerbating factor that cause suffering for women.

Mothers who inject drugs learn how to balance their drug use and normality by establishing specific tactics. Based on Certeau's (1988) definition, "tactics" are the ways in which the marginalised attempt to cope with – or subvert – strategic forces. Those employing tactics are subject to the power of authorities or external forces: In response, they devise their own ways of dealing with/lessening any impacts (Certeau 1988). Mothers who use drugs and living with HIV/AIDS create "tactics" that will allow them to maintain both their drug lifestyle and their mothering role, tactics such as not administering drugs in front of their children. Tactics women injecting drug use to cope with motherhood is linked with social conceptions of gender and drug habitus, particularly this tactic formation is serving to facilitate both habitus and also HIV/AIDS.

5 Taking Antiretroviral: A Means of HIV Protection

Women who use drugs are exposed to, and infected by, HIV through unprotected sex and needle sharing. Most of the women who use drugs I interviewed found out their HIV status when they became pregnant. They received HIV testing at the hospital and the result turned out to be positive. Children are one reason that they decided to continue living. Rak and Yui recalled the time they knew about her HIV status:

> I didn't know whether I was infected with HIV until I was pregnant. My boyfriend knew all the time that he was HIV-positive, but he rarely used condoms when he had sex with me. He was such a selfish person. (Rak, 31 years old)

> When I first knew my result, I thought of committing suicide, but when I thought of my child, I couldn't. It is all my fault not her fault. I feel sorry for her to have a mother like me, a drug user and also HIV-positive. Thus, I try the best as I can to provide the good environment for her. (Yui, 37 years old)

Women injecting drug users represent one of the most vulnerable groups currently requiring access to antiretroviral (ARV) treatment to prevent mother-to-child transmission. Taking antiretroviral required discipline as injecting drug users are viewed as non-compliant, untreatable and undisciplined (Carrieri et al. 1999; Aceijas et al. 2006; Kiatying-Angsulee et al. 2006). This type of attitude can easily be exploited to exclude injecting drug users from both antiretroviral treatment and methadone programs. Some health workers remain opposed to treating HIV-positive drug users because of prevailing judgemental attitudes about drug users. Similarly, this has led implicitly to how mother injecting drugs are treated. Nuu (35 years old) told me about her antiretroviral experiences that

> A nurse told me that I was HIV-positive. She suggested me to take ARV medicine as it would prevent my child from being infected with HIV. She warns me seriously that I have to be punctual about taking medication. If I wasn't take medicine on time, there is a chance that my child will get infected with HIV. It was difficult for me because at that time I was still using drugs. What people injecting drugs think most is heroin rather than ARV. But, I have tried to take medicine every time. I did set up the alarming on my mobile phone to remind me that it's medication time.

Although taking ARV is not compatible to their lifestyle, women in this study try to adhere to the medication regime for the sake of their children. Hence, several ways are formed to achieve this objective. Unprotected sex is not only directly involved in risk of HIV transmission but also unplanned pregnancy. Upon discover the result of their HIV status, women face the dilemma of whether to give birth or to abort them.

6   Ceasing or Terminating: Dilemma of Mother Using Drugs and Living with HIV

Generally speaking, the women interviewed did not take the absence of menstruation as an indication of pregnancy; rather, they attributed it to their drug-taking. Hence, most women's pregnancies were unplanned. Nok (27 years old) said about her first pregnancy:

> Since I used drugs, my period stopped. At first I thought I was getting fat, but my husband told me to go and see the doctor. I was so shocked when the doctor told me I was six months pregnant. I told the doctor that I was not ready to have a child and I may have to abort it.

Confirmation of pregnancy causes a dilemma. The woman has to make a decision regarding her public and private lives. Women envision their future lives without drugs. They now have a chance of normalcy: They can either quit using drugs and take her place in the public sphere or continue to consume drugs in private. Most of the women, after learning of their pregnancy, attempt to control their drug behavior in the hope that one day they can stop using permanently. Ying (35 years old) described how hard she tried to control her drug behavior:

> After knowing my pregnancy, I wanted to quit using drugs. Pregnancy became the light in my life. I did lessen my drug use. I was proud of that. But, in the seventh month, I saw my boyfriend using drugs. I could not resist it. Finally, I relapsed and started using drugs again.

Pregnancy determines the point at which a woman can enter public space and access the necessary health services. But, the negative attitude of hospital staff towards pregnant addicts may result in failure to provide adequate care (Rosenbaum 1988). Interaction worsens when the health professionals become aware of the mother's addiction. Some women choose to abort as the health professionals suggest, the reason being that they feel unable to perform the mothering role. Lek (33 years old) told me about her abortion that

> I aborted my baby as health professionals suggested. I was HIV-positive and drug-using mother. There are many concerns about the well-being of my baby. The nurse said there is a chance that my baby will not be infected if I adhere to ARV, but because I am using drugs, she was afraid that I may not be able to take medicine punctually.

For women living with HIV, their infection influences their decision to terminate the pregnancy (Pivnick et al. 1991). Abortion is easy to accept when they know that they are HIV-positive. Most of the women I interviewed for this study knew their HIV status and of the uncertainty it brought to their lives and to their children's futures. But, being asked to abort implies social judgement, the perception that they are unable to perform the mothering role.

> I didn't know that I was pregnant when I was first tested for HIV/AIDS. The HIV test result was positive. Everyone told me to get an abortion because I was handicapped (can't walk), am HIV-positive and a drug user. They thought, with all that, how can I raise the child? My husband was in prison. Finally, I decided to keep the child. (Jeab, a 23-year-old female)

> But, when my daughter was two years old, I asked my boyfriend's relatives to adopt her. Because of my HIV-positive status and economic constraints, I figured it would better for her if I sent her away. If I die either by overdose of AIDS, no one would take care of my girl. So, it would better to send her off to my in-law. Since then, I have never seen her again. (Took, a 40 year old female)

Infant born to an addict mother experiences low birth weight and withdrawal symptoms or cardiac defects and other illnesses (Blinick 1971; Glass 1974; Källén and Otterblad Olausson 2003). Some of the women did not know that their heroin addiction could be passed on to the foetus. However, even if they had known, they felt unable to control their drug use during their pregnancies.

> I did not know that my heroin addiction would pass on to my son. I knew it might cause some effect, but I did not expect a severe outcome. I was frightened when I saw him crying all the time. I did not know what to do and the nurse told me that my boy was crying because he was craving drugs just like me. (Nom, 28 years old)

Although a few women claimed that they were afraid of being mothers, most tried to perform the mother role after the birth by incorporating mother responsibility into drug discourse. They genuinely suffered when they saw their babies' craving symptoms. Women with young children have little option but to accommodate them within the drug community because many have no one to look after them.

7   Telling a Lie: Concealing Their Lifestyle

Parents who are dependent upon drugs are easily stereotyped by society. The drug-using mother is subject to conflict and dilemma as she attempts to combine her drug use with her parental responsibilities. They genuinely do not want their children to experience their drug lifestyle. When children become accustomed to those around them taking drugs, they naturally start to question their mother's behavior, especially their injecting of drugs. A typical question asked by children is as follows: "Why do you have to inject yourself? Why are you always sleepy?" Faced with these questions about their behaviour, the women have little option but to lie. They commonly answer: "I was sick and the doctor prescribed me with injecting drugs. Or, I took some allergy medicine which makes me feel sleepy." Lying assuages their feelings of guilt; as well, they are aware of their children's inability to maintain secrecy.

Socialization raises concern in drug-using parents. Mothers fear that their children may learn the truth from neighbors or friends. More importantly, they fear that their children may be stigmatized as children of drug-addicted mothers living with HIV/AIDS. People living with HIV/AIDS are still stigmatized in Thai society (Chan et al. 2008; Li et al. 2009; Liamputtong et al. 2009). At the same time, they do not underestimate their children's ability to recognize illicit behavior. Below are two women's accounts of how they conceal their drug use and HIV status from their children:

> Whenever my daughter saw me holding the brown paper bag, she rushed to grab the glass and spoon from me. She prepared the equipment for injection even though she was only three years old. What she did scare me. I was afraid that if she stayed with me, she would grow up like me, a drug user. (Mok, a 26 year old female)

> My son did not know that I was a drug user living with HIV/AIDS. When my son saw me injecting heroin in the bathroom, he asked what I was doing and why did I hurt myself. I lied to him that I was sick and the doctor prescribed me with injections. I knew he suspected what I was doing. He may know I use drug but did not know I was HIV-positive. Having mother using drugs is worst yet, how could I tell them I am HIV-positive. (Yui, a 31-year-old female)

To avoid discrimination being directed towards their children, mothers employ tactics not to protect themselves but to protect their children. As I have mentioned above, lying is one tactic they use to minimize their own emotional pain and stigmatization upon their children. When a child socializes his/her mother's drug behavior and HIV/AIDS, that is, discusses it in the school grounds, for example, the mother seeks ways of safeguarding her child. For this reason, women employ the above concealment tactics. Due to the stigma and discrimination surrounding women using drugs, mothers feel compelled to keep their drug behavior secret. When mother face the burden of taking care of children, they ask the help of their relatives. Leaving their children ensures that women maintain social expectations as they could provide a healthy environment for them.

8   Leaving My Boys/Girls

It is the role of the parent, especially the mother, to protect the psychological well-being of the child; as well, as much as possible she must provide a healthy environment for the child to grow up in. The state does not typically concern itself solely with women's mental states and standards of childrearing: Care extends to the physical environment and social context (Klee 1998). Hence, the mother living with HIV feels that living with them may transfer the pollution to their children as Mod, a 35-year-old woman, said about her HIV status that: "Even though I knew that HIV is not easy to transmit, I tried not to share food with my boy. I am afraid he might infect HIV. Every day, I was worried about the future of my boy. If I died of AIDS, what would he do? Finally, I ask my parents to adopt him." For the women using drugs, AIDS is equated to death and risk.

Thai women who use drugs are reluctant to assume the mothering role: They find it painful to watch their offspring growing up in a drug-taking environment. Hence, many opt to relinquish care of their children to the hands of their relatives. The responsibility often has to be shared with the elderly, for example, the mother's parents or in-laws. Family support for child rearing is still common practise in Thailand (Liamputtong et al. 2004; Soonthorndhada 1992).

The Thai family structure takes the form of extended family. In Bangkok, due to economic constraints, women in general tend to live with either their parents or in-laws; thus, they typically turn to them for help with childcare. In cases of drug-using mothers, sometimes they voluntarily surrender their children to relatives in the belief that removing them from the drug environment will ensure a better life.

> My in-laws took care of my son. I rarely visited them because my in-laws did not want me to be there. They were afraid that my addiction would pass to my son and I also did not want them to lose face. I think he may be embarrassed to have a mother who is a drug addict. (Lek, a 35-year-old female)

Jing, a 31-year-old woman whose child was being raised by her relative, recounted the following:

> I slept in a small house with my boyfriend. My aunt adopted my son. He was lucky living with them so I had nothing to worry about, but she did say to my son that if he was not well-behaved, she would ask me to take him back. I think it is because she was afraid that he would be "bad" like me when he grew up.

Some families use "motherhood" as a form of punishment for their drug-taking daughters/sisters. Although some mothers try to maintain contact with their children, access is often refused by caretakers, who fear that the child will be discriminated against by friends or neighbors should he/she be connected to a drug-using mother. Thus, caretakers exercise a particular level of control over the involvement of the mother, who must abide by the conditions and rules set by former, most of which relate to the mother's drug consumption. If the mother can control her drug use, or cease using, she may be able to perform the function of mother.

> My sister adopted my daughter when she was young. They, my family, thought that I was not able to raise her and I did not deserve to be a mother because of my drug use. My daughter called me "aunt" and called my sister "mom." My sister asked her to do so. Sometimes she would call me "mom" when I behaved well, especially when I stopped using drugs. You know, I was so happy when I heard her call me "mom" even though I haven't raised or supported her. (Ying, a 30-year-old female)

But, other motives drive women who use drugs to ask their relatives or in-laws to take care of their children: Many simply want (or have) to continue their drug lifestyle. Too, a 35-year-old woman said: "My in-laws are caring for my son. I rarely see him. But, I call them once a month checking that he is fine." For women, leaving their children is a means of protection of being caring mothers. Leaving their children with others distances them from their mothers: Many of the latter have not seen their children for years. However, the mothers are convinced that their children are better off being raised outside of a drug environment.

9 I Can Be a Mother Using Drugs and Living with HIV

In Rosenbaum's (1988) study, in the heroin world, a mother using heroin who can take care of children is respected as they could combine motherhood and heroin consumption. Some homeless women have no choice but to raise their children themselves. Although women using drugs and living with HIV/AIDS in my study appear to reject the mothering role by giving their children to others, some opt to try to balance this role with their drug lifestyle and HIV/AIDS. In the process, they try to keep their children away from drugs as much as possible. But, the reality is that it is an almost impossible task for them due to limited income and childcare needs. In such cases, women often work as drug dealers to gain more income for their children.

In this way, children inadvertently become part of the drug social network. Some of the women admitted that they have carried their children in their arms when selling drugs. In this way, they use their children as a form of self-protection from harassment. They carry their children everywhere they go: when buying drugs or visiting the drug seller's house. Ta, a 27-year-old mother, told me that

[w]hen my son was young, I carried him everywhere – and to the drug seller's house. I did not think that he would remember what I did or where I went since he was only 2 years old. But, he did remember. When he was 4 years old, we sat on a bus and passed Klong Toey (a drug community in central Bangkok). He pointed out the place where I was arrested.

Raising their children in a drug community is difficult for women. They feel tremendous guilt because they are unable to provide a healthy environment for their children, a regret invoked by their excessive drug use. The action of separation can have a profound impact upon the amount of drugs they consume as they have no maternal responsibilities to observe. When they are accused by others of being drug-using mothers, they find solace in using more drugs. Having others raise their children relieves them of the risk of their children observing their drug practise. Usually, children will acknowledge their mother's behavior when they reach primary school age. Nok (a 27-year-old female) said:

It was difficult to tell him I am a drug addict, but my son accidentally found out by himself. He has never asked me and I have never said anything. I thought he knew from school that using drugs was a bad habit. That was why he has never told his friends about this.

Since all of women are prescribed with antiretroviral drugs which require women to adhere to medicine strictly, this raises the curiosity of their children as to what kind of illness their mother is suffering from. Also because of taking ARV and methadone, the women have to go to hospital quite often. They have to take their children to either hospital or methadone clinic with them.

Raising their children by themselves, women feel burdened because unlike other mothers, they are less active in caring for their children. The Thai medical and social welfare system has ignored the difficulties women using drugs confront. In fact, the violence drug-using women confront in everyday life is not only violence inflicted upon the physical body: It is also gender habitus related.

10   Conclusion

Living in a drug community and having HIV, women are faced with the dual dilemma of either ceasing their drug use for the sake of their children or pursuing their drug consumption. Living with HIV exacerbates the situation of drug-using mothers. Public opinion requires a "good" mother to devote her life to her children and behave in an exemplary fashion. Using drugs is not an option. There is no opportunity in Thai discourse for mothers who use drugs and living with HIV/AIDS to combine their mothering role with their drug-taking. Having internalized the prescribed role of mother, of whom they should be, women have constructed the tactics to balance the life in public and private space. The women in my study attempt to employ several tactics to fulfil the social expectations of motherhood. They have agency to manage their life as mother using drugs and living with HIV/AIDS. This account of the tactics women use is articulated in response to motherhood in Thai social context. The tactics Thai women injecting drug use implicitly represent Thai gender habitus. Rather, the construction of mother using drug context is generated within an interplay of gender and drug habitus. The women internalize social and cultural roles of motherhood which they saw as unfit to their lifestyle. Thai women using drugs have suffered the most from gender prescribed roles, thereby, they opt to form several tactics to lessen the impact upon themselves and the well-being of their children. Here, I will suggest that there is the need for broadscale care and prevention on women using drugs. Harm reduction, today, have ignored women using drugs. The emotional burden of caring for children and the subjective experiences of mothers who use drugs have yet to be recognised by Thai Ministry of Public Health and local NGOs.

References

Aceijas C, Oppenheimer E, Stimson G, Ashcroft R, Matic S, Hickman M, The Reference Group on HIV/AIDS Prevention and Care among IDU in Developing and Transitional Countries (2006) Antiretroviral treatment for injecting drug users in developing and transitional countries 1 year before the end of the 'treating 3 million by 2005. Making it happen. The WHO strategy' ('3by5'). Addiction 101(9):1246–1253

Banwell C, Bammer G (2006) Maternal habits: narratives of mothering, social position and drug use. Int J Drug Policy 17(6):504–513

Blinick G (1971) Fertility of narcotics addicts and effects of addiction on the offspring. Soc Biol 18:34–39

Bourdieu P (1977) Outline of a theory of practice. Cambridge University Press, Cambridge

Bourdieu P (2001) Masculine domination. Polity Press, Cambridge

Bourgois P (1995) In search of respect: selling crack in El Barrio. Cambridge University Press, Cambridge

Boyd S (2004) From witches to crack moms. Carolina Academic Press, Durham

Bradley H (2007) Gender. Polity Press, Cambridge

Bungay V, Johnson J, Varcoe C, Boyd S (2010) Women's Health and use of crack cocaine in context: structural and 'everyday' violence. Int J Drug Policy 21(4):321–329

Campbell N (2000) Using women gender, drug policy, and social justice. Routledge, New York

Carrieri MP, Moatti JP, Vlahov D, Obadia Y, Reynaud-Maurupt C, Chesney M, The MANIF 2000 Study Group (1999) Access to antiretroviral treatment among French HIV infected injection drug users: the influence of continued drug use. J Epidemiol Commun Health 53(1):4–8

Certeau MD (1988) The practice of everyday life. University of California Press, Berkeley

Chan K, Stoové M, Sringernyuang L, Reidpath D (2008) Stigmatization of AIDS patients: Disentangling Thai nursing students' attitudes towards HIV/AIDS, drug use, and commercial sex. AIDS Behav 12(1):146–157

Cobrinik RW, Hood RT Jr, Chusid E, Slobody LB (1959) The effect of maternal narcotic addiction on the newborn infant. Pediatrics 24(2):288–304

Cohen A (2006) Youth culture and identity: consumerism, drugs and gangs in urban Chiang Mai, northern Thailand. Unpublished material, Department of Anthropology, Macquarie University, Sydney

Dumais S (2002) Cultural capital, gender, and school success: the role of habitus. Sociol Educ 75(1):44–68

Earle S, Letherby G (2003) Introducing gender, identity and reproduction. In: Earle S, Letherby G (eds) Gender, identity and reproduction: social perspectives. Palgrave Macmillan, Hampshire, pp 1–12

Ettorre E (2004) Revisioning women and drug use: gender sensitivity, embodiment and reducing harm. Int J Drug Policy 15(5–6):327–335

Friedman J, Alicea M (2001) Surviving heroin: interviews with women in methadone clinics. University Press of Florida, Gainesville

Glass L (1974) Narcotic withdrawal in the newborn infant. J Natl Med Assoc 66(2):117–120

Hillier J, Rooksby E (2005) Habitus: a sense of place. Ashgate, Hants

Källén BAJ, Otterblad Olausson P (2003) Maternal drug use in early pregnancy and infant cardiovascular defect. Reprod Toxicol 17(3):255–261

Kandall S (1996) Substance and shadow: women and addiction in the United States. Harvard University Press, Cambridge, MA

Keller T, Catalano R, Haggerty K, Fleming C (2002) Parent figure transitions and delinquency and drug use among early adolescent children of substance abusers. Am J Drug Alcohol Abuse 28(3):399–427

Kettinger L, Nair P, Schuler M (2000) Exposure to environmental risk factors and parenting attitudes among substance-abusing women. Am J Drug Alcohol Abuse 26(1):1–11

Keyes CF (1984) Mother or mistress but never a monk: Buddhist notions of female gender in rural Thailand. Am Ethnol 11(2):223–241

Kiatying-Angsulee N, Sringernyuang L. Haritavorn N (2006) Beyond the targets: assessment of public and private ARV treatment programs. Thailand country working paper. HAI, Amsterdam

Klee H (1998) Drug-using parents: analysing the stereotypes. Int J Drug Policy 9(6):437–448

Krais B (2006) Gender, sociological theory and Bourdieu's sociology of practice. Theory Cult Soc 23(6):119–134

Lam NT (2008) Drugs, sex and AIDS: sexual relationships among injecting drug users and their sexual partners in Vietnam. Cult Heal Sex 10(suppl 1):S123–S137

Lee R (1994) Dangerous fieldwork. Sage, London

Li L, Lee S-J, Thammawijaya P, Jiraphongsa C, Rotheram-Borus MJ (2009) Stigma, social support, and depression among people living with HIV in Thailand. AIDS Care 21(8):1007–1013

Liamputtong P (2007) The journey of becoming a mother among women in northern Thailand. Lexington Books, Lanham

Liamputtong P, Yimyam S, Parisunyakul S, Baosoung C, Sansiriphun N (2004) When I become a mother!: discourses of motherhood among Thai women in northern Thailand. Women's Stud Int Forum 27(5–6):589–601

Liamputtong P, Haritavorn N, Kiatying-Angsulee N (2009) HIV and AIDS, stigma and AIDS support groups: perspectives from women living with HIV and AIDS in central Thailand. Soc Sci Med 69(6):862–868 (Special issue: Women, mothers and HIV care in resource poor settings)

McDonald M (1994) A social anthropological view of gender, drink and drugs. In: McDonald M (ed) Gender, drink and drugs. Berg, Oxford, pp 1–32

Muecke MA (1984) Make money not babies: changing status markers of northern Thai women. Asian Surv 24(4):459–470

Mulder N (2000) Inside Thai society: religion, everyday life, change. Silkworm Books, Chiang Mai

Murphy S, Rosenbaum M (1998) Pregnant Women on Drugs: Combating Stereotypes and Stigma. New Brunswick: Rutgers University Press

Page J, Singer M (2010) Comprehending drug use: ethnographic research at the social margins. Rutgers University Press, New Brunswick

Paone D, Alperen J (1998) Pregnancy policing: policy of harm. Int J Drug Policy 9(2):101–108

Pivnick A, Jacobson A, Eric K, Mulvihill M, Hsu A, Drucker E (1991) Reproductive decisions among HIV-infected, drug-using women: the importance of mother-child coresidence. Med Anthropol Q 5(2):153–169

Rosenbaum M (1988) Women on heroin. Rutgers University Press, New Brunswick

Soonthorndhada A (1992) Domestic role behavior, expectations and applications: past to present. Institute for Population and Social Research, Salaya

Street K, Whitlingum G, Gibson P, Cairns P, Ellis M (2008) Is adequate parenting compatible with maternal drug use? A 5-year follow-up. Child Care Health Dev 34(2):204–206

Swartz D (1997) Culture & power: the sociology of Pierre Bourdieu. University of Chicago Press, Chicago

Taylor A (1993) Women who use drugs: an ethnography of a female injecting community. Clarendon, Oxford

Whittaker A (2002) Water serpents and staying by the fires: markers of maturity in a northeast Thai village. In: Manderson L, Liamputtong P (eds) Coming of age in Southeast Asia. Curzon Press, Surrey, pp 17–41

Woodward K (2003) Representation of motherhood. In: Earle S, Letherby G (eds) Gender, identity and reproduction: social perspectives. Palgrave Macmillan, Hampshire, pp 18–32

Zelson C (1973) Infant of the addicted mother. N Engl J Med 288(26):1393–1395

Chapter 10
Senegalese Women Living with HIV Versus the 2009 WHO Recommendations for PMTCT: Meanings for Resistance Regarding Infant Feeding

Alice Desclaux

1 Introduction

> Since access to medicines is now permitted by the Global Fund, (…) it is necessary to convince, to somehow educate these women to let them know that their lives will be better, their infants will be healthy and they won't leave orphans behind. (Carla Bruni-Sarkozy, Global Ambassador to the Global Fund to Fight AIDS, Tuberculosis and Malaria for the protection of mothers and children against AIDS, December 1, 2009)[1]

The history of the prevention of HIV transmission through breastfeeding in sub-Saharan Africa can be narrated by distinguishing three phases in international policies: ignorance of a public health issue before 1998, prevention based on behavioral change until late 2009, and prophylactic use of antiretrovirals since 2010. In summarizing the strategy held by United Nations agencies and GFATM (Global Fund to Fight AIDS, Tuberculosis and Malaria), Carla Bruni-Sarkozy asserts that a global understanding of PMTCT (Prevention of Mother-to-Child Transmission of HIV) is now a matter of access to pharmaceuticals and women's information. Do women in sub-Saharan African countries agree with this statement? What do they think about the latest World Health Organization's recommendations that opened the "antiretroviral era" in the field of breastfeeding and HIV

---

[1] "Ces femmes ont accès aux traitements qui vont permettre à leur enfant de naitre en bonne santé, complètement en bonne santé, et de continuer elles-mêmes à se soigner par la suite (…). Puisque maintenant l'accès aux médicaments est permis par le Fonds Mondial, (…) il faut absolument convaincre, éduquer en quelque sorte ces femmes pour qu'elles sachent que leur vie sera meilleure, que leurs enfants seront en bonne santé et qu'elles ne laisseront pas des orphelins." Carla Bruni-Sarkozy, Global Ambassador to the Global Fund to Fight AIDS, Tuberculosis and Malaria, for the protection of mothers and children against AIDS. TV5 Monde, http://www.youtube.com/watch?v=gdgzIFkT5B4

A. Desclaux (✉)
IRD, UMI TRANSVIHMI (IRD, Université de Montpellier 1, Université Cheikh Anta Diop de Dakar, Université de Yaoundé), BP 1386, CRCF, Hôpital de Fann, Dakar, Senegal
e-mail: alice.desclaux@ird.fr

P. Liamputtong (ed.), *Women, Motherhood and Living with HIV/AIDS: A Cross-Cultural Perspective*, DOI 10.1007/978-94-007-5887-2_10,
© Springer Science+Business Media Dordrecht 2013

(WHO 2009a, b)? How do they interpret this policy at the local level and would they comply with "education for prevention" requested by international experts?

The aim of this chapter is to present and analyze HIV-positive women's perceptions of—and reactions to—the latest WHO recommendations in a West African country, Senegal, where unexpected resistance and a protest movement arose. Then, I will attempt to shed light on underlying rationales on the part of international organizations, national public health institutions, and HIV-positive women as well as the role claimed by women in prevention. This will lead us to specify the continuities and shifts concerning spaces for women's decision-making after a change in preventive policies from a behavioral-based model to a pharmaceutical-based model. This analysis is focused on understanding the expected social roles in these policy models and their potential consequences on women's ability to protect their children in West Africa.

2   Theoretical Framework and Historical Perspectives

2.1   African HIV-Positive Women: Therapeutic Citizens or Good Patients?

The HIV/AIDS epidemic has been described globally as bringing a "revolution" to the patient-healer relationship and the distribution of health expertise (Epstein 1996; Barbot 2002). At first, the involvement of community-based organizations in the care of persons living with HIV when biomedical institutions were unable to provide treatment opened a field of intervention alongside biomedical care. It was later encouraged by transnational organizations and international agencies through, for instance, the promotion of the 1994 GIPA principles.[2] Field activities progressively included support and self-support, psychosocial and economic help, counseling related to testing or adherence to treatment, and defense against stigma and advocacy for persons "infected or affected by HIV." In Africa, community-based organizations played a major role in organizing care and support (see TASO in Uganda), in obtaining access to treatment (see Treatment Action Campaign in South Africa), and in setting ethics for care and research (see Coalition Respect in West and Central African countries) (Eboko et al. 2011). This movement has been heterogeneous and

---

[2] The GIPA Principle was formalized at the 1994 Paris AIDS Summit when 42 countries agreed to "support a greater involvement of people living with HIV at all levels and to stimulate the creation of supportive political, legal, and social environments." The Greater Involvement of People Living with HIV and AIDS (GIPA) Declaration was signed in 1994. UNAIDS prefers the umbrella term "people living with HIV." For historical reasons, this policy brief continues to use the acronym GIPA. UNAIDS (2007). The Greater Involvement of People Living with HIV and AIDS. Policy Brief, 4p. March 2007 http://www.unaids.org/en/resources/presscentre/featurestories/2007/march/20070330gipapolicybrief/

emphasized either advocacy and the defense of rights or care and support delivery, according to organizations and country contexts.

Since its rise during the late 1980s, the HIV patients' movement has been strong and well acknowledged in developed countries. This led to a shift regarding the relevant theoretical models for the role of the patient, who appeared as a "reformer," while "community participation" became a necessary component in public health programs. In Africa, Nguyen considered the emergence of "therapeutical citizenship," adapting the concept of "biological citizenship" to social mobilizations and HIV experience in Côte d'Ivoire (Nguyen 2005). This model acknowledges the shift from an individualistic difficult experience of HIV infection shaped by suffering to a collective "positive" experience emphasizing advocacy. However, ongoing discussion examines the extent to which this model can be applied to the majority of persons living with HIV in West African countries, or whether it only concerns a minority with privileged access to education and personal autonomy that enabled them to join organizations and participate as active members.

Women's involvement as patients and as PLHIV-association members has only recently been analyzed at the local level in West Africa; a global social-science analysis is still missing (Desclaux et al. 2011). Women are usually considered as "natural caregivers" in families, especially for children, and are responsible for family compliance to biomedical prescriptions. Recent analyses in Cameroon, a Francophone Central African country, have shown that health professionals consider women living with HIV as "good patients," compliant and able to communicate about their bodies and ailments, focused on their infants' care rather than their own interests, and tenacious and altruistic enough to overcome social difficulties in order to get treatment for members of the family unit (Djetcha 2011). This image of "good wives and good mothers," who are active though victims of HIV transmission, is reinforced by the high number of women involved in community care and support activities, much higher than the number of men—considered by health professionals as less compliant, vindictive, and selfish, also shown in Burkina Faso (Bila 2011).

Beyond gender stereotypes, these perceptions fit with the model of care and patient role that puts forward compliance to medical prescriptions following patients' "therapeutic education" about biomedical knowledge. According to this model, women would apply health professionals' prescriptions and adapt their social context to the requirements of pharmaceutical treatment, without any critical opinion or expertise: their role as patients would be defined by obedience and hope (Blystad and Moland 2009). Are Senegalese women living with HIV "therapeutic citizens" or "compliant patients needing to be educated and convinced?" The social effects of and reactions to the WHO 2009 recommendations regarding infant feeding and HIV provide an opportunity to document this issue; this will aid in understanding the experience of HIV-positive women living in West Africa.

Before considering recent women's reactions, it is necessary to present the history of international recommendations regarding infant feeding and HIV and the role they assign women in addition to women's attitudes and interpretations until 2009.

2.2   A Quick Analytical History of Prevention of HIV Transmission Through Breastfeeding

The first phase in international policies—ignorance of a public health issue—lasted 13 years: though HIV transmission through breastfeeding was discovered in 1985, it was only in 1998 that United Nations agencies published the first international recommendations for prevention.[3] These recommendations opened the second phase—prevention based on behavioral change—and proposed a variety of feeding options (formula feeding, reducing the duration of breastfeeding, resorting to a wet nurse, pasteurization of breast milk, use of animal milk, and so on). Mothers were supposed to apply the option that presented the lowest risk in each individual case and contextual setting. In 2001, these recommendations were simplified: formula feeding and exclusive breastfeeding with early and rapid weaning (between 4 and 6 months) were the only "informed choice" options for mothers; in other words, women living in developed countries would use formula to avoid any HIV risk, and women living in resource-poor countries would select an option by "weighing risks" in their own setting. They would then "stick to their choice" and faithfully practise risk reduction in addition to applying behavioral control of breastfeeding through methods such as exclusiveness of breast milk use, care for nipples and infant mouth candidiasis, and care for infant nutrition and development. In 2003, the options were prioritized, and the required conditions for formula feeding were more narrowly defined.[4]

In 2004, the extension of antiretroviral coverage in low-resource countries led to considering the situation of women who need treatment for their own health and launching studies on the efficacy of antiretrovirals as a prophylaxis to make breast-feeding "safe." As study results were gradually published showing the reduction in HIV-transmission rates, more and more health-care providers experimented with "protected breastfeeding,"[5] a French-language idiom for prophylactic use of antiret-rovirals taken by the mother or by the infant during the period of breastfeeding. For health professionals, this strategy represented progress insofar as it avoids the financial costs related to formula (with pharmaceutical-related costs assigned to others), management difficulties, and the risk of stigma associated with breast milk substitutes. In November 2009, the third phase in preventive policies officially began when WHO published recommendations based on the use of antiretroviral treatment combined with a feeding option—exclusive breastfeeding for 6 months, followed by mixed breastfeeding until "12 months," or formula feeding (WHO 2009a). The choice between these feeding options would be made at the national or

---

[3] For an analytical presentation of the successive versions of these recommendations, see Desclaux and Alfieri (2009).

[4] Formula feeding should only be chosen if it is "AFASS," meaning accessible, feasible, acceptable, sustainable, and safe from the mother's point of view; if it is not, maternal breastfeeding should be "chosen."

[5] Allaitement protégé.

regional level, rather than the individual level as done previously. The national PMTCT program would then supply formula—or not—according to national decisions. African countries opted for exclusive breastfeeding as the only strategy, sometimes with a transition period when women who had already started formula feeding their infant at the date of publication of the recommendations would continue to be supplied until weaning. By contrast, developed countries maintained infant feeding with formula for all HIV-positive women. This new strategy is part of a global "vision" that aims to eliminate mother-to-child HIV transmission in 2015 (WHO 2010a). See also Chap. 12 in this volume.

2.3   Behavioral Strategy and Women's Choice Regarding Infant Feeding

For 11 years (between 1998 and 2009), the preventive strategy was behavioral, based on women's individual choice, a rather unusual concept in the field of public health in low-income countries. One may question the relevance of interpreting this attribution of the decision to women as part of the "HIV culture" emphasizing patient responsibility and community participation in health matters.

At the field level, women were informed during a "breastfeeding counseling session" conducted during pregnancy. They were then supposed to discuss options with a counselor and choose the one that best corresponded to their individual and contextual situation to reduce or eliminate HIV-related risks, while also avoiding other infectious and nutritional risks inherent to breastfeeding alternatives. Why suggest that women choose when health workers might have prescribed an option after considering individual situations? The rhetoric of women's "informed choice" was fairly explicit in successive versions of recommendations and "guidelines" that direct their implementation, though most recent recommendations set up criteria that reinforced the guidance role of health workers. Health professionals provide various explanations for keeping choice in the international recommendations before 2009, which have been discussed elsewhere (Desclaux et al. 2005). The choice would be the following: a woman's right, outlined in the first recommendations in 1998, that should not be refuted to avoid questioning a gender-sensitive approach; a condition holding women to one feeding option for the entire required duration; a way to articulate and adapt the "global to the local" (in other words, strategies defined on an international level for individual situations that are too diverse to be reduced to a single national standard); and a relationship model between patient and health-care services in the context of HIV that fits in with counseling as applied to testing, which assumes a voluntary approach or informed consent. Other interpretive paths can be presumed to explain the divergence between attribution of the decision to women in the South and prescription of a single preventive strategy (formula feeding) in the North. Delegating choice to women in the South reflects the inability of the health-care systems to propose measures that are effective enough and available to all. It could also be interpreted as "cultural shaping" for prevention, involving operations (individual decision, anticipation, and "rational balancing" of risks) that fit into a Western model of risk management prevailing in public health and inspiring United Nations officials (Peretti-Watel and Moatti 2009).

On the contrary, in the field of infant feeding and nutrition (not considering HIV), women's choice is seldom at stake since all medical discourses converge to encourage breastfeeding. Besides being based on a scientifically attested and ideologically influenced rationale, the content of these local discourses is shaped by UNICEF/ WHO programs such as "Baby Friendly Hospitals." They drive an a priori opposition to formula feeding whatever the mother's situation, inherited from the 1980s when medical discourses were fighting the influence of multinational companies that had extensively provided formula in Africa during the 1970s, leading to an increased prevalence of diarrhea and malnutrition among infants (Van Esterik 1989). Though the extension of poverty in West Africa over the last 30 years eliminates the possibility for accessing formula for the majority of women, health professionals still seem to consider that women must be educated to the benefits of breastfeeding to avoid formula, and the notion of women's choice is not relevant in biomedical recommendations regarding overall infant feeding. In the field of mother-and-child health—and particularly regarding infant feeding—mothers are not seen as legitimate "reformers," and health professionals' authoritative knowledge shapes power relationships in a very different way than in the field of HIV: here, mothers take on the role of patient rather than community participant.

3   The Study

This analysis regarding women's attitudes towards WHO recommendations on breastfeeding and HIV is based on investigations about the experience of people on antiretrovirals for several years in Senegal.[6] The enquiries about infant feeding and women's roles were added to the overall study as part of a personal long-standing anthropological interest for infant feeding and HIV matters in West Africa initiated before PMTCT programs considered this issue (Desclaux and Taverne 2000; Desclaux and Alfieri 2009). Data collection was primarily based on observation and individual and collective interviews with resource persons, members of the Aboya association (PLHIV association) and women who benefited from the association in Dakar and its suburbs. This was part of an ethnographic approach based on field immersion for 3 years in a multidisciplinary research center on HIV in Dakar.

---

[6] ANRS Project 1215 'Evaluation de l'impact bio-clinique et social, individuel et collectif, du traitement ARV chez des patients VIH-1 pris en charge depuis 10 ans dans le cadre de l'ISAARV (Initiative Sénégalaise d'Accès aux traitements ARV)', coordinated by B. Taverne and I. Ndoye.

Senegal is a West African country of 13 million inhabitants with a Human Development Index of 0.411 (ranked 144th out of 177), a life expectancy at birth of 56.2 years, and a 3.5 mean number of years of education (UNDP 2010). Some 33.5 % of the population lives below the poverty line of 1.25 USD a day (2000–2008). The estimated HIV prevalence rate in the general adult population is 0.9. The epidemic is considered to be concentrated, i.e., mainly affecting vulnerable groups who have much higher prevalence rates. The number of HIV-positive pregnant women in 2009 is estimated between 2,000 and 5,900 (for about 400,000 pregnant women), and between 16 and 45 % among them had access to antiretroviral treatment for PMTCT, which mean they accessed prevention of HIV transmission partially or totally through breastfeeding (UNICEF 2010).

4   Main Issues: Women's Interpretation in Context

4.1   A Collective Protest Movement in Dakar

On April 21, 2010, at the Fann Clinical Research Center, doctors involved in the Prevention of Mother-to-Child Transmission (PMTCT) program, researchers and representatives from the Ministry of Health have gathered to examine the implications of new WHO recommendations for PMTCT, how they should be applied in Senegal, and directions for subsequent research. Twenty women, members of the Aboya association, enter the already-crowded space and sit on the floor in front of the screen. They speak Wolof in a space where French is the usual language; two have come with their children. First off, they came to protest, as indicated by the red handkerchiefs tied around their wrists, against the interrupted provision of formula[7] that had no longer been available in health-care services for several months. For the association president, this unexplained interruption prepared the groundwork for the implementation of new recommendations, and the Aboya members wanted to express their desire to maintain their "freedom to choose" between two preventive infant feeding options. According to them, their ability to protect their children from HIV transmission depends on this choice.

At the time of the Aboya protest, women's associations from other West African countries had not voiced criticisms. Activists in the international fight against AIDS had remained silent, which is usually the case for infant feeding strategies, seen as a matter of scientific evidence and expert opinion unchallenged by users groups. At the global level, new recommendations had not changed the situation in developed countries where women would go on using formula with antiretrovirals, which limited the reasons for mobilization. In Africa, since their publication, public critics of WHO recommendations were only heard at the local level, for instance, in the South

---

[7] This term is used by United Nations agencies with "formula feeding." In this article, we will use the terms used "in the field" among health-care teams.

African media.[8] Aboya members did not claim to be supported by AIDS experts at the local level. Do local dimensions explain such a protest by Senegalese women?

4.2   Senegal's 2010 National Free-Formula Policy in Context

The goal of the protest was unexpected because the "new recommendations," which endorse treatment of mothers for their own well-being (and not only to protect their children) and advocate reassurances that breastfeeding is safe with antiretrovirals, are considered an advance at the international level (Morris 2010). When adopting WHO recommendations at the national level, public health experts adapted them to the local norms and sanitary context as specified in WHO documents and chose exclusive breastfeeding (Ministère de la santé et de la prévention médicale du Sénégal 2011). "Protected breastfeeding" was considered more accessible and more acceptable than previous options in a country where 98 % of all children are breast-fed, and 42 % are still breastfed between 20 and 23 months (WHO 2010b). Practicing prolonged breastfeeding like HIV-negative women do would then reduce the risk of stigma for HIV-positive mothers, in a country where stigma is still a leading concern among persons living with HIV, even when healthy on antiretrovirals.

Like WHO and UNICEF, international funding agencies such as GFATM believed that providing breast milk substitutes was no longer cost effective in 2010 and no longer saw it as their responsibility. Yet, since these products have not received the same attention at the global level as other means of prevention such as condoms or antiretroviral drugs, there is no system for efficient production, supply, and distribution of breast milk substitutes "for medical use" that national programs could implement. In addition, costs were not negotiated, and it became more expensive than HAART (Desclaux 2004). Moreover, the WHO strategic plan for PMTCT does not propose strengthening health-care systems in this domain (WHO 2010). Without support from international donors for this measure, Senegal's national program was unable to continue providing formula, since breaks in stock were recorded when funding was still available. It then fell on women who wished to apply this option to supply themselves with breast milk substitutes at the high market price. Although international experts maintain that 2009 recommendations allow any woman to exercise her "right to choose" (if she can get formula and if her situation fulfills the required criteria), this "choice" is henceforth limited by the economic inaccessibility of formula in Senegal and more generally in sub-Saharan Africa. New strategic directions for international agencies and organizations led to imposing

---

[8] In South Africa, the Daily Dispatch published a paper entitled "State plan to halt free baby milk" (Dec 7, 2010, by Ntando Makhubu) that quoted a former provincial health MEC, Dr Trudy Thomas: "'To remove formula is extremely irresponsible, extremely un-medical and extremely uninformed' because many more babies would die of HIV and malnutrition."

modes of prevention on Senegalese women that are identical to those for sites and countries in Africa that are less advanced in PMTCT.[9]

4.3 The End of a Senegalese Achievement?

Let us revisit the Senegalese situation in 2010. The interviews show that by "freedom of choice," the members and beneficiaries of the Aboya association mainly request that they could continue to resort to formula feeding. Previously, provision of substitutes by the health-care system was one of the guiding principles of the national PMTCT program implemented in 2005 (Ministère de la Santé et de la Prévention Médicale 2005). Until 2009, the majority of Senegalese HIV-positive women opted for this feeding method.[10] Since the pilot phase (2000–2004), health-care services, and associations in Dakar and its suburbs demonstrated their capacity to ensure this infant feeding method, even in difficult socioeconomic conditions. The support provided by community participation through associations and non-governmental organizations include follow-up care for women undergoing PMTCT, individual or collective counseling sessions, home visits, nutritional care and supplementation for mothers and infants, social help to tackle the issue of disclosure to partners, and economic support at the family level, according to each woman's needs. Decentralization of the PMTCT program supported this model and promoted a community approach involving numerous association actors in monitoring formula feeding. Many actors believe that the practise of formula feeding with no adverse health impact is a success of the psychosocial support provided in Senegal. This is consistent with results of public health studies in other contexts that showed that social support is the most important factor for compliance to any innovative infant feeding pattern—whether exclusive breastfeeding or formula feeding (Msellati and Van de Perre 2008). Senegal was accredited with achieving safe PMTCT including formula feeding and exclusive breastfeeding, particularly in Dakar's suburbs where the association Synergie pour l'Enfance became a West African expert for the care of HIV-positive children.

Moreover, selection of formula feeding by the PMTCT program had an important advantage compared to breastfeeding besides reduction of HIV-transmission risk: when an infant is formula fed, an early diagnosis at 6 weeks is possible, which means that the infant may get antiretroviral treatment if he/she is HIV positive. If HIV negative, since he/she is no longer exposed to HIV through breastfeeding, he/she can receive follow-up like any "vulnerable" child. When infants are breastfed,

---

[9] Analysis of the epidemiological impact of this measure regarding the goal of eliminating mother-to-child HIV transmission in 2015 will be conducted.

[10] No national survey exists on feeding modalities for infants exposed to HIV; various sectoral studies, notably MD dissertations, report percentages ranging between 86 and 94 % of women opting for formula feeding.

even if the risk of transmission is very low, its continuation delays diagnosis until the date of weaning plus 6 weeks. Senegal had been a leader in setting up early HIV diagnosis and conditions for implementation in low-resource and decentralized sites such as DBS[11] that enables HIV testing on infants living far from large cities. Since the 2009 recommendations, the meaning of such early diagnosis is questioned as test results at 6 weeks that were "definitive for MTCT" have become transitional.

The combination of these achievements—women's choice, formula feeding with support, early child HIV diagnosis and care—led to better results in Senegal than in other West African countries since the evaluation of the program's pilot phase (2000–2004) reported a mother-to-child HIV-transmission rate of 4 %.[12] Since the strategy proposed by WHO in 2009 is supposed to reduce the risk of HIV transmission from mother to child to under 2 % for formula feeding and under 5 % for breastfeeding, local pediatricians did not perceive it as progress compared to previously obtained results.

In 2010, stockouts lasting several months were followed by a complete break in supply of breast milk substitutes from health-care services. This situation led to complaints from Aboya members and PLHIV-association leaders. Health-care services managers in charge of PMTCT also complained, confronted by managing complex and difficult situations for some women during a transition they were unprepared to handle. Though this break was not exactly linked to the change in strategy, it was interpreted as such, and field actors had a rough experience, which might have undermined their confidence in health administrators' commitment to PMTCT at the field level.

4.4   Women's Perceptions of HIV Risk

However, Aboya members' critics go much further than discussing the transmission rates reported with "protected breastfeeding"; for them, despite the reduction of risk, no mother would consciously take any risks for HIV transmission. In Dakar, as in other sites we surveyed in West Africa, women who breastfed report their constant worry about "transmitting HIV to their child" (Desclaux and Alfieri 2008). This grammatical construction using the active voice, which echoes the phrasing used by most of the interviewed women, not only reflects the lexical insensitivity that many authors have attached to "mother-to-child transmission programs" that designate the mother as the source of contamination. It also attests to the burden of guilt carried by breastfeeding mothers, which most of them can only let go of after 18 months, when their child's HIV status is disclosed—at least when it is negative. When asked about which preventive option they would choose in conditions of sufficient resources,

---

[11] Dried Blood Spots: this technique enables easy management of taking and transporting blood samples to laboratories.

[12] More recent national data are not available, which constitutes a major barrier to discussing strategic directions for Senegal's PMTCT program.

women from the Aboya association almost all identify formula feeding. As in other survey sites, concerns about HIV surpass the advantages of maternal breastfeeding that they mention though. The psychological impact of an HIV transmission on the mother and the mother-child relationship following the "choice" to breastfeed has not been documented yet, but our interviews attest to how worrisome risk is for a mother, no matter what its probability is. Also, the transmission rates related to the various infant feeding options, with or without antiretrovirals, do not constitute concrete reference points that clarify "choice" for mothers. Other psychological dimensions arise that prevent women from accepting options which do not totally eliminate risk.

4.5 A Different Interpretation of Pharmaceutical-Based Prevention and Formula

Another issue is related to confidence concerning the use of antiretrovirals for prevention. Because they support persons in their association who undergo PMTCT or antiretroviral treatment or because they themselves are taking antiretrovirals, the Aboya members fear that treatment observance by mother and child cannot be ensured, although it is essential in the context of the new recommendations for obtaining "protected breastfeeding." The examples they cite show that during the postpartum period, women are in a fairly precarious psychological and relational situation that is not conducive to taking a treatment that is hard to hide from a suspicious family circle. It is also usually an uneasy period for disclosing HIV status to partners, which is sometimes necessary before dispensing treatment to the infant (Desclaux and Alfieri 2010). On the other hand, weaning before 1 year, which is requested of the majority of HIV-positive women following 2009 recommendations, does not seem to be more socially acceptable than formula feeding. The alleged advantage regarding stigma avoidance might be minimal.

Besides these limitations of pharmaceutical-based prevention, some women seem to overestimate the advantages of formula. Several association members who personally experienced having had a child, who is untouched by HIV infection, believe it was "thanks to the formula," which means they do not consider pre- and intrapartum transmission risk. Finally, they are particularly sensitive to the dilemmas of women who, after resorting to formula feeding for one child, cannot use it for the next one, thus causing further risk. Also, they see the new recommendations as abandoning a strategy that eliminates transmission risk in all cases for a strategy that only reduces it in an uncertain way.

In interviews, Aboya members bring up other advantages to formula feeding that they were able to evaluate after 10 years of practise in the national program: the possibility of leaving their children in the care of another person to go to a doctor's appointment or to work, thus securing income-generating activities that forbid keeping a child "on her back" to breastfeed him or her. In this domain, the preventive strategy has allowed some women to discover that beyond its importance for HIV, formula feeding could facilitate managing social obligations. Although the discourses seek to remain within the boundaries of a rationale justified by HIV prevention, they show that women now know that formula can be a way to increase their autonomy just as in developed countries. They appreciated the escape from upholding the image of the "eternal African woman," constantly carrying a child on "her back" if not at "her breast." This demand from Senegalese women reflects the situation of many African women living in urban areas where health conditions may allow them to practise formula feeding while avoiding the dangers of infection and malnutrition. Through medicalization during the era of AIDS exceptionalism, they could experience the advantages of formula, owing to associations, that other women could not discover due to poverty.

4.6   From Complaint to Mobilization

The imposition of the new strategy is also perceived by associative members as regressive and denigrating their competence in a domain where association actors had gained experience and assurances of their effectiveness. The associations' memory—particularly Aboya's—is marked by case histories of mothers who either could or could not protect their children. This concrete and human dimension of a collective experience when many women were alternatively or simultaneously beneficiaries (i.e., receiving psychosocial support, care, material help, and family mediation), active members in PLHIV associations, care providers, and mothers has greater weight in constructing their representations of preventive measures than the epidemiological arguments of experts, whether quantitative or abstract, defined in a locus far from Senegal. Divergences clearly appear in interpretations of the new preventive measures. When international agencies consider a simplified strategy validated through the efficacy of antiretroviral drugs, Senegalese women consider the complexification of individual histories of prevention because the duration of risk experience is extended for mothers.[13] They foresee that the variety of women's individual cases will have to be managed without freedom of choice, in frequently difficult family and social contexts and with uncertainty about the efficacy of preventive measures. Meanwhile, some high-level staff members from the national AIDS committee interpret women's reaction as immobilism towards innovation, with one declaring during a meeting on PMTCT recommendations: "Everybody is reluctant to change. It was the same problem at the beginning of the PMTCT program when we changed to formula feeding."[14]

Requests about the new recommendations were first expressed by an association of women living with HIV who demand to be understood as such. During the aforementioned meeting, the Aboya president complained, "I have not seen women

---

[13] The period of time when risk remains, like the mother's uncertainty about her child's serological status, can now be close to 2 years between prenatal counseling and child HIV diagnosis.

[14] A high-level staff member in the Ministry of Health, during a workshop for revision of PMTCT national guidelines, Feb. 2010.

living with HIV in the group of experts.[15] You continue to see us as 'beneficiaries' and call on us when everything has already been decided." In Senegal, where for nearly 15 years sociological analyses have been describing the participation of associations in the fight against AIDS as "decreed" by the national committee (Delaunay et al. 1998; Mbodj 2007), community claims were exceptionally related to public health policy. Here, women "beneficiaries," uninfluenced by international associations, join their leaders in asking for participation in decisions and recognition as "experts." An objection, expressed in terms of a claim by "beneficiaries," has been transformed into a request, expressed as affirming expertise, relative to the "right to choose" the way to feed her child. The launch of this mobilization, which was followed by other declarations in the following weeks, seemed all the more remarkable since the experiences of women treated in the PMTCT programs have been characterized in other African countries by their social vulnerability (Blystad and Moland 2009).

5 Conclusion

The adoption of WHO recommendations and prevention of HIV transmission through breastfeeding does not seem to be only a matter of antiretrovirals and women's education. Women have opinions, and in Senegal, they are critical about these recommendations in light of their previous achievements in PMTCT.

Regarding prevention of HIV transmission through breastfeeding, women had managed, at least in the Dakar region and with the support of health teams and associations within the national PMTCT program, to construct an experience based on the same strategy as in developed countries. The mobilization of Senegalese women brings attention to the issue of acceptability of a decline in the efficacy of services offered by the health-care system.[16] Neither generalization to remote areas of Senegal of the positive results in PMTCT achieved in Dakar under the previous strategy nor achieving the previous level of efficacy with WHO 2009 recommendations is guaranteed. Analysis of the rationales and relationships of power and the scientific and political legitimacy at work in the decision-making process on a national vs. an international level, which led to an interruption in funding of breast milk substitutes in the Senegalese PMTCT program, still needs to be conducted with a focus on economic aspects, on the one hand, and on power and legitimacy relationships between institutions, on the other hand.

---

[15] This group of experts was created by the Ministry, and it is responsible for defining ways to adapt the new WHO recommendations in Senegal.

[16] Based on the new recommendations, interruption in the supply of breast milk substitutes would likely cause an HIV-transmission rate that is 3 points higher than expected if the use of breast milk substitutes had been maintained.

Returning to the "regular" recommendations that only promote exclusive breast-feeding for all women, in the name of "normalization" or "end of HIV/AIDS-related exceptionalism," not only causes a reduction—whether perceived or objective—in the preventive efficacy of PMTCT in Senegal, it also causes a disappearance of the decision-making space that was once open to HIV-positive women. The launch of collective mobilization of Senegalese women to keep this "freedom to choose" reminds us that for this measure to be applied, access to formula must be ensured by the health-care system, as is the case for a drug or therapeutic nutritional product; if these conditions are not met, the concept of "individual choice," still advanced by international institutions, becomes insignificant under economic constraints.

Mobilization of Dakar's associations also shows that, while other aspects of the PMTCT systems could have a major impact in terms of transmission risk, breast-feeding remains the predominant concern, like a "symbolic sponge" soaking up the stakes and fears. Its social signification also holds, as in other contexts analyzed by Badinter (2010); the rise in power of discourses and measures that exclusively promote breastfeeding seem to go along with a step backwards in the recognition of women's rights. This may be the case in Dakar, where women have begun to collectively demand an "effective choice" rather than an individual choice that has become virtual.

As beneficiaries, mothers, and providers, Senegalese women are in a position to present their acquired skills as expertise. These women voice their perceptions about risk and priorities for prevention, which are radically different from those proposed to them by WHO. Are they aligning themselves with situations in regions of the poorest African countries and reintegrating the role of "patients" as mothers observing prescriptions from caregivers or are they continuing to apply expertise from community actors and asserting a freedom of choice as mothers that allows them to protect their children? These are the terms through which women from Senegalese associations perceive their roles and the changes that are reserved for them through the new strategies. When shifting to pharmaceutical-based prevention, these strategies favor, as attested when antiretrovirals became available for HIV treatment, a shift back to the vertical relationship between health professionals managing technical knowledge and mothers who bear the patient role. However, women, now engaged in associative groups and collective expertise, request community participation, since the social support and global care which they manage are acknowledged as an essential component of prevention.

Although WHO presents its partnerships and synergies with "bilateral donors, nongovernmental organizations (NGOs), foundations, the private sector, people living with HIV, faith-based organizations, multilateral agencies, and national governments" as an important element in advances in PMTCT (WHO 2010a, b: 20), women's demands in favor of the ability to choose introduce a dissonance in the "strategic vision." This is probably because advances in reducing HIV transmission through breastfeeding presented in the new strategies do not come along with any advances in recognizing women's expertise (not to say that they promote going backwards in this domain).

References

Badinter E (2010) Le conflit. La femme et la mère. Flammarion, Paris

Barbot J (2002) Les malades en mouvement. La médecine et la science à l'épreuve du sida. Balland, Paris

Bila B (2011) Différences de recours au traitement des personnes vivant avec le VIH et valeurs liées au genre au Burkina Faso. In: Desclaux A, Msellati P, Sow K (eds) Les femmes à l'épreuve du VIH dans les pays du Sud. Genre et accès universel à la prise en charge. ANRS, collection Sciences sociales et sida, Paris, pp 31–42

Blystad A, Moland KM (2009) Technologies of hope? Motherhood, HIV and infant feeding in eastern Africa. Anthropol Med 16(2):105–118

Delaunay K, Blibolo AD, Cissé-Wone K (1998) Des ONG et des associations: Concurrences et dépendances sur un "marché du sida" émergent. Cas ivoirien et sénégalais. In: Deler JP, Fauré YA, Piveteau A, Roca PJ (eds) ONG et développement: Société, économie, politique. Karthala, Paris, pp 115–141

Desclaux A (2004) Transmission par l'allaitement: la prévention par les substituts du lait maternel négligée. Transcriptases ANRS Informations, Numéro spécial Bangkok, automne, 33–35

Desclaux A, Alfieri C (2008) Allaitement, VIH et prévention au Burkina Faso. Les déterminants sociaux ont-ils changé ? Science et Technique, Série Sciences de la santé, Special issue n°1, 117–126

Desclaux A, Alfieri C (2009) Counseling and choosing between infant-feeding options: overall limits and local interpretations by health care providers and women living with HIV in resource-poor countries (Burkina Faso, Cambodia, Cameroon). Soc Sci Med 69(6):821–829

Desclaux A, Alfieri C (2010) Facing competing cultures of breastfeeding: the experience of HIV-positive women in Burkina Faso. In: Liamputtong P (ed) Infant feeding practices: across-cultural perspective. Springer, New York, pp 195–210

Desclaux A, Taverne B (eds) (2000) Allaitement et VIH en Afrique de l'ouest: De l'anthropologie à la santé publique. Karthala, Paris

Desclaux A, Crochet S, Querre M, Alfieri C (2005) Le "choix informé" des femmes séropositives qui doivent alimenter leur enfant: Interprétations locales, limites et nouvelles questions. In: Desgrées du Lou A, Ferry B (eds) Sexualité et procréation confrontées au Sida dans les pays du Sud. CEPED, Paris, pp 245–262

Desclaux A, Msellati P, Sow K (eds) (2011) Les femmes à l'épreuve du VIH dans les pays du Sud. Genre et accès universel à la prise en charge. ANRS, Paris

Djetcha S (2011) Le traitement antirétroviral, support de relations pour les femmes, objet de dissimulation pour les hommes au Cameroun. In: Desclaux A, Msellati P, Sow K (eds) Les femmes à l'épreuve du VIH dans les pays du Sud. Genre et accès universel à la prise en charge. ANRS, collection Sciences sociales et sida, Paris, pp 43–53

Eboko F, Bourdier F, Broqua C (2011) Les suds face au sida. Quand la société civile se mobilise. Editions IRD, Marseille

Epstein S (1996) Impure science: AIDS, activism and the politics of knowledge. University of California Press, Berkeley/Los Angeles

Mbodj FL (2007) Les associations de personnes vivant avec le VIH au Sénégal: Genèse d'une participation décrétée. In: Diop MC, Benoist J (eds) L'Afrique des associations. Entre culture et développement. CREPOS-Karthala, Paris, pp 215–229

Ministère de la Santé et de la Prévention Médicale (2005) Politique nationale de prévention de la transmission mère-enfant du VIH au Sénégal. Division de lutte contre le sida et les IST, March 2005, Dakar.

Ministère de la santé et de la prévention médicale du Sénégal (2011) Directives nationales sur la prévention de la transmission Mère-Enfant du VIH au Sénégal, Dakar

Morris K (2010) New WHO guidelines on antiretrovirals welcomed worldwide. Lancet Infect Dis 10(1):11–12

Msellati P, Van de Perre P (2008) Maternal HIV infection and infant feeding: support is the key. AIDS 22:2391–2392

Nguyen VK (2005) Antiretroviral globalism, biopolitics, and therapeutic citizenship. In: Ong A, Collier SJ (eds) Global assemblages: technology, politics and ethics as anthropological problems. Blackwell, Malden, pp 124–144

Peretti-Watel P, Moatti JP (2009) Le principe de prévention. Le culte de la santé et ses dérives. Seuil, Paris

UNDP (2010) The real wealth of nations: pathways to human development. Human Development Report 2010. UNDP, New York

UNICEF (2010) Children and AIDS: Fifth stocktaking report. Washington: UNICEF/NYHQ2006-1376. http://www.childinfo.org/hiv_aids.html. Accessed 12 July 2010

Van Esterik P (1989) Beyond the breast-bottle controversy. Rutgers University Press, New Brunswick

WHO (2009a) HIV and infant feeding. Revised principles and recommendations. Rapid advice. Geneva: WHO. http://whqlibdoc.who.int/publications/2009/9789241598873_eng.pdf. Accessed 12 July 2010

WHO (2009b) Use of antiretroviral drugs for treating pregnant women and preventing HIV infection in infants. Rapid advice. Geneva: WHO. http://www.who.int/hiv/pub/mtct/rapid_advice_mtct.pdf. Accessed 12 July 2010

WHO (2010a) PMTCT strategic vision 2010–2015. Preventing mother-to-child transmission of HIV to reach the UNGASS and millennium development goals. Moving towards the elimination of paediatric HIV. Geneva: WHO. http://www.who.int/hiv/pub/mtct/strategic_vision.pdf. Accessed 12 July 2010

WHO (2010b) Indicators for assessing infant and young child feeding practices. http://www.who.int/child_adolescent_health/documents/9789241599757/en/index.html. Accessed 28 July 2010

Chapter 11
Improving Access to Mother-to-Child Transmission (PMTCT) Programs in Africa: An Ongoing Process

Philippe Msellati

1 Introduction

Until now, prevention of mother-to-child transmission of HIV (PMTCT) is the most effective intervention for combating new HIV infections. For more than 12 years, pediatric AIDS has been virtually eradicated from Northern developed countries (McKenna and Xiaohong 2007; Yéni 2010). According to the most recent UNAIDS report (2010), in developing countries the evolution of PMTCT is very different from country to country. In Africa, in the last 5 years, real progress has been observed in Southern Africa, where four countries (Botswana, Namibia, Swaziland, and South Africa) and in some countries of Eastern Africa reached the coverage of 90% of HIV-infected pregnant women with prophylaxis or treatment. In Central and West Africa, progression exists but is slower, as less than 30% of HIV-infected pregnant women have received any treatment or prophylaxis for PMTCT in 2009.

UNAIDS has called for a virtual elimination of mother-to-child transmission (MTCT) of HIV by 2015. This objective could only be realized if there is a significant increase in actions to prevent transmission to children in countries where programs are not optimal. However, pediatric AIDS has long been in Africa as they are already 2.3 million children living with HIV, which represent around 90% of HIV-infected children in the world. They are around 1.3 million children in need of antiretroviral treatment, and even if it is a dramatic improvement, coverage is still below 30% of the need. But, with antiretroviral treatments, these children have a real future as teenagers and young adults. This is another topic which will not really be addressed in this chapter, but must be underscored.

P. Msellati (✉)
Hôpital Central de Yaoundé, MD, PhD, UMI233 IRD/UCAD/Université de Montpellier 1/Université Yaoundé 1, Centre de coordination et de recherches du site ANRS Cameroun, BP 16854, Yaoundé, Cameroon
e-mail: philippe.msellati@ird.fr

P. Liamputtong (ed.), *Women, Motherhood and Living with HIV/AIDS: A Cross-Cultural Perspective*, DOI 10.1007/978-94-007-5887-2_11, © Springer Science+Business Media Dordrecht 2013

This chapter is based on the combination of a literature review, an analysis of databases, and empirical evidence collected during 15 years of PMTCT implementation, childcare research, and treatment programs in Central, East, and West Africa. In a previous paper, I discussed how to improve mothers' access to PMTCT programs in West Africa (see Msellati 2009). This question is still important even if the PMTCT field is the subject of many publications with a very rapid updating. For example, recommendations for PMTCT were modified three times between 2006 and 2010. It is a field where things move fast in technical matters but much more slowly, as usual, for behavioral changes.

One way to progress in the scaling up of PMTCT is to analyze why in some countries, implementation has been possible and in others these programs do not work properly. It seems important to analyze the process of PMTCT programs at several levels (site, regional, and national) and step-by-step through literature, databases, and qualitative studies. It should be the better way to understand the successes and failures of the programs and how to "scale up" PMTCT programs, where there are gaps or obstacles and how to try to go through these obstacles. It includes analyses of the health system, health workers' expectations and limitations, mothers' expectations, and relationship between mothers and the care system.

2   PMTCT: Theoretical Understanding

As UNAIDS and WHO describe it (2003), PMTCT is based on four components and strategic approaches: (1) primary prevention of HIV infection in young women in childbearing age, (2) prevention of unwanted pregnancies in HIV-infected women, (3) prevention of mother-to-child transmission of HIV, and (4) appropriate treatment care and support for HIV-infected women and their children and families.

About the first component, as most pediatric HIV infections are acquired from the HIV-infected mothers, the most effective means of preventing pediatric infection is the prevention of HIV infection in women of childbearing age. There are many interventions in the field of education campaigns. But, as the prevalence among young women and young men in Africa shows, they work poorly as there are three to five times more 15–19-year-old HIV-infected girls than young men. Young women could be often involved in sexual relations with older men ("sugar daddies") for many reasons (such as need of money or protection, social promotion, and sexual abuse), and these older men have a higher probability of being infected than teenager boys.

Some poverty and development experimental researches show possibilities of efficient interventions among young women at secondary schools. These interventions, as Dupas describes (2009), based on targeted information about "sugar daddies" and specific risk in relation with them, had a real efficacy in terms of sexual behavior change, measured by pregnancy incidence. Another work, also in

Kenya, presented by Duflo et al. (2009), showed that offering free school uniforms to girls had an impact on school attendance and also on unwanted pregnancies (and therefore on risk of exposure to HIV and other STDs).

The second component of PMTCT is prevention of unwanted pregnancies in HIV-infected women. It has not been promoted as far as other components but adequate family planning services are an essential component of PMTCT. According to Delvaux and Nöstlinger (2007) and Curtis and colleagues (2009), the safety of contraception methods, including hormonal and intrauterine methods, is quite well established. The integration between the two health programs (reproductive health/family planning and PMTCT) should be implemented as a cost-effective strategy to reduce mother-to-child transmission of HIV, as Johnson and colleagues (2009) advocate for. In East Africa, several teams (Elul et al. 2009; Keogh et al. 2009) have shown that fertility desires are different among HIV-infected women and that preventing unwanted pregnancies among them should be addressed as a priority by family planning and PMTCT programs. This prevention component could decrease the number of HIV-exposed children by 40%.

The third component is the most addressed in the literature. PMTCT is a package of interventions such as voluntary counseling and testing for pregnant women, ARV prophylaxis for pregnant women and children, infant feeding counseling, and postnatal follow-up until diagnosis of HIV infection in exposed children. The majority of papers published in the last 5 years have highlighted failures of programs either from a quantitative point of view (Noba et al. 2001; Penda and Msellati 2010; Toro et al. 2010) or from a qualitative one (Painter et al. 2004; Levy 2009; Larsson et al. 2010) more than on technical aspects of PMTCT in itself. But some papers, particularly in recent years, show improvements and successes of these PMTCT programs and give some keys for scaling up access (Chandisarewa et al. 2007; Doherty et al. 2009; Lim et al. 2010; Muchedzi et al. 2010). With the improvement of antiretroviral drugs access, this component is highly related with the fourth component.

When we consider broad figures, from United Nations Agencies (UNAIDS 2010), worldwide, 53% (40–79%) pregnant HIV-infected women in low- and middle-income countries received antiretroviral medication to prevent the mother-to-child transmission of HIV in 2009. But this percentage recovers quite different things as the effectiveness of antiretroviral drugs in preventing mother-to-child transmission of HIV varies with the type of regimen used and the duration over which it is given. Combination regimens of antiretroviral drugs are more efficacious than monotherapies, as Leroy showed in 2005 (Leroy et al. 2005). In the countries that provided disaggregated data for their prevention of mother-to-child regimens, around 30% of HIV-infected pregnant women received single-dose nevirapine, while 54% received a combination regimen. About 15% of all HIV-infected mothers received ongoing antiretroviral therapy for their own health.

In new guidelines, WHO recommends (2009) that all pregnant women, as other adults, should receive highly active antiretroviral treatment when they are eligible for treatment with a higher threshold than previously, around 350 CD4, for their own health. Over that limit, HIV-infected pregnant women should receive a combination of antiretroviral drugs rather than nevirapine alone during pregnancy and delivery. For women living in developing countries and unable to provide a safe alternative infant feeding to breastfeeding, they should breastfeed and receive a prophylaxis during the duration of breastfeeding and a week after the end of breastfeeding.

3   Indicators of Effectiveness of PMTCT Programs

As Stringer and colleagues (2008) point out, some indicators of PMTCT effectiveness have been elaborated, to measure *in fine* the proportion of HIV-infected mothers/exposed infants that receive the intervention and the proportion of HIV-infected children at 15 months of life among all HIV-exposed children. HIV-free survival at 15 months or 2 years of age among children of HIV-infected pregnant women should be the best indicator for the success of PMTCT programs. But this indicator is seldom available as most health structures are not used to following mothers and children for a long period of time. Thus, the attrition is very important and the proportion of HIV-exposed or HIV-infected children still followed at 15 months of age is very low.

4   Antenatal Care Offer and Coverage

Coverage for PMTCT is in strong relation with coverage of antenatal care, and as Druce and Nolan (2007) argue, there have been a lot of mis-opportunities to link the two activities. When there is a low attendance to antenatal care, there is definitely a low coverage of counseling and testing for HIV among pregnant women (see also Chap. 19 in this volume). Some countries have quite an excellent coverage of antenatal care, and as a consequence, it is easier to implement a PMTCT program. Others have a good geographical coverage of PMTCT but the antenatal care is not good, and therefore, the performances of PMTCT program are poor. This is what Penda and Msellati have showed in their recent study in Cameroon (2010).

5   HIV Counseling and Testing in Pregnant Women

For Rwanda, Lim and colleagues (2010) reported that there can be improvements in PMTCT as far as there is a comprehensive learning from the field and meetings where improvements are identified, discussed, and experimented. Step-by-step, with an active biweekly supervision, it was possible to improve PMTCT care in 17 health centers. In 15 health centers, 95% of HIV-infected pregnant women received PMTCT services. Even antenatal care attendance improved as well as the proportion of women delivering in participating health centers (56–72%). Coverage of cotrimoxazole prophylaxis was 98% in exposed children.

One study described by Labhard and colleagues (2009) show that in rural Cameroon, PMTCT programs have to be adapted in rural areas, especially in settings where they are only nurses to lead the clinics. Training and providing equipment are major components. Authors also underscore the need to avoid any shortage of tests and drugs.

In Zimbabwe, Shetty and colleagues (2008) pointed out that it was possible to develop a PMTCT program in urban areas with peer counselors. In Malawi, Levy (2009) examined women's decisions about HIV testing and PMTCT. Women accept HIV testing for expected benefits on their own health and their infant's health (see also Chap. 4 in this volume). But they are often disappointed because of health system weakness, absence of good referral for their own health, and absence of integration of care. According to Painter and colleagues (2004) in Côte d'Ivoire, and Anand and colleagues (2009) in Kenya, site factors as health workers' attitudes could be more important than women factors in acceptance of HIV test.

In 2007, WHO provided guidelines for provider-initiated HIV testing and counseling (PITC) which is also called "opt-out" approach of HIV testing (WHO 2007). Until that time, in antenatal care units, health workers had to propose explicitly the HIV test and to ask the women if they wanted to be tested or not. With these guidelines, after a pretest counseling on HIV, women are not asked any more if they want the HIV test, they have to explicitly refuse it. In terms of acceptance of the test, it makes a dramatic difference and a real increase. Certainly, from a public health point of view, it is good as it improves rates of HIV acceptance. Chandisarewa and colleagues (2007) reported improvement in acceptance and return for results. But attrition of the number of women is still important even in this study. HIV testing is only the entry point for a long process through pregnancy, delivery, and infancy that makes PMTCT work. What if women did not understand they had an HIV test? And what happens if this test was positive? How would they manage such "bad news" during pregnancy?

As Kakimoto pointed out (2008), we need a cautious evaluation of consequences of HIV testing at a large scale. Similarly, in some places in Africa, results of HIV testing are immediately given back to the women at the end of the antenatal session. It is not always easy for pregnant women to learn in such a rapid process they are HIV-infected, as a vast majority of them are surprised by this result, as Painter and colleagues (2007) showed in Abidjan. This method, while it improves the proportion of pregnant women learning about their HIV status, could have a limited impact if the stress produced by this news overwhelms the capacities of HIV-infected women to manage the PMTCT process.

In Mulago Hospital, in Uganda, Namukwaya and colleagues (2011) reported a dramatic difference between highly active antiretroviral therapy (HAART) and other regimens on rate of HIV infection in children, from 1.7% with HAART to over 30% in mothers who did not take any drug. The paper also shows the same cascade in this population where acceptance of HIV test among pregnant women is

99.7% and return for treatment or prophylaxis in HIV-infected women is 96.5%. They are around 60% that deliver in the same sites, and only 30% of children were early tested. We can always improve HIV testing (by new techniques or improvement in counseling), but we will still not understand why women do not come back for delivery and postnatal follow-up.

6 PMTCT Intervention and Access to Care for HIV-Infected Pregnant Women

From 1999 and the results of a randomized trial reported by Guay and colleagues (1999), the use of nevirapine for PMTCT has been recommended for a decade. The intervention is easy to implement and allows around 50% of reduction of HIV transmission from mother to child with a very low cost. However, quick emergence of resistance to nevirapine, which was also one of the most used drugs for treatment, hampered this intervention, as Arrivé and colleagues (2007) described it. As resistance occurs, it is necessary to use other drugs than nevirapine, both in mothers, as Lockman and colleagues (2010) have proved, and infected children who were exposed to nevirapine during pregnancy, as Palumbo and colleagues (2010) have proved. However, it remains as a possible intervention when nothing else is possible in remote rural places. But, as Stringer and colleagues (2010) showed in different African countries, even for such a simple intervention, in a large population of exposed children, they were only 51% who have actually a good coverage of nevirapine.

Since the last decade, there are PMTCT programs that include access to care for women and families. Some initiatives, as FSTI (Fonds de Solidarité Thérapeutique Internationale) or MTCT-Plus, have implemented HIV/AIDS care and treatment to families identified through PMTCT programs (Noba et al. 2001; Abrams et al. 2007). As reported by Toro (2010), these programs improve dramatically the proportion of retention of women in PMTCT and the mortality of HIV-infected women. Muchedzi and colleagues (2010) studied obstacles and challenges that pregnant women have to overcome to access HAART. And Stinson and colleagues (2010) noticed in South Africa that even when HAART and PMTCT programs are present, services fail to initiate a high proportion of eligible pregnant women on HAART.

7 PMTCT and Men

For at least one decade, there is an advocacy for the involvement of male partners of pregnant women in PMTCT. But, in most of the African countries, this involvement remains marginal and less than 10% of partners come for HIV testing through these PMTCT programs. We have to admit that antenatal care units are seldom men friendly and that it is certainly something that has to be improved. Aluisio and colleagues (2011) showed in Nairobi that a much higher attendance of men than usual (31%) is associated with a reduction in HIV infection and mortality in HIV-exposed children. Katz and colleagues (2009) in Kenya also presented ways to involve men and to increase HIV testing among them. In Côte d'Ivoire, in a prospective qualitative study, Tijou and colleagues (2009) described decision-making process about PMTCT and breastfeeding among couples. PMTCT actions should be an interaction between three actors (health workers, women, and their partners). In Uganda, Larsson and colleagues (2010) identified, through a qualitative study among fathers of HIV-exposed infants, many reasons that men argue for not having a test. They worry about relations in the couple after testing and prefer to have the opportunity to test themselves on their own, without "control" of their partner. In Uganda, as in other places, a misbelief has never been really addressed. When a woman is tested for HIV and share this result with her partner, quite often the partner consider that his HIV status is the same as the status of his partner. Therefore, it is useless to do the test! This should be specifically addressed in information campaigns.

8   Breastfeeding Under HAART and New Recommendations

Following the results of several clinical trials, WHO changed recommendations on breastfeeding HIV-exposed children (Kilewo et al. 2009; The Kesho Bora Study Group 2011). Clinical trials showed that HAART given to the mother until 6 months of breastfeeding was safe and prevented most of postnatal HIV infections. Curiously, in its recommendations, WHO extrapolated, without data, the protection duration of HAART until 1 year of age and proposed exclusive breastfeeding until 6 months and then mixed feeding. This recommendation of HAART during breastfeeding, either in mothers or in children, will certainly decrease dramatically postnatal transmission of HIV. But firstly, we do not know if it is feasible and if women are able to understand and follow all changes of feeding recommendations. Secondly, it is even more difficult for women who choose infant feeding alternatives to express their choices and to obtain infant formula. That reinforces health inequalities in a field where health authorities tried to reach equity. Thirdly, if a mother breastfeeds her HIV-exposed child until 1 year, it will be useless to test the infant before 1 year (as exposed), and the HIV-infected children will not be diagnosed in time and remain untreated. Even with HAART during breastfeeding, there will still be failures, and some children will be HIV-infected. These children will probably be resistant to several antiretroviral drugs such as nevirapine used in prophylaxis regimen in exposed children during breastfeeding. These rare HIV-infected children will be "scapegoats" of PMTCT programs.

9 Infant Testing and Large Access Testing in Children

Greater efforts are needed to scale up early testing of HIV-exposed infants, reduce the rate of loss to follow up among them, and further integrate HIV care with services for child health. As a clinical trial conducted by Violari and colleagues (2008) has shown, it is important to treat all HIV-infected children as soon as the diagnosis is carried out. And this diagnosis should be done as early as possible from 6 weeks of age. Unfortunately, until 12–15 months of life, we cannot use antibodies as a diagnosis tool, just as a first sorting tool to identify HIV-exposed children. Then, we need to use much more sophisticated techniques, such as real-time polymerase chain reaction tests, which are often available only in capital cities in Africa. For several years now, new techniques were developed as dried blood spots (DBS) for HIV (as it is used for decades for metabolic diseases in West countries in neonates). These DBS can be easily collected and transported from remote places to reference laboratories as it allows 1 month to 6 weeks to use them. It is only if this is developed everywhere in PMTCT sites in Africa that we can expect to have a real scale-up of early testing in exposed children and treatment in HIV-infected children. We can also expect to lower attrition in mothers if programs are able to give the diagnosis of exposed children early in life. In high prevalence settings, as emphasized by Rollins et al. (2009) and Kellerman and Essajee (2010), universal testing of children should be promoted, including immunization programs. Health workers should systematically propose the HIV test to ill children services, children in tuberculosis departments, malnourished children services, and also siblings of HIV-exposed children.

10 Conclusion

In conclusion, we can say that there has been a huge work on PMTCT during the last decade. The drug regimens for treatment and prophylaxis are effective, and there are regular improvements. There have also been improvements in programs and scaling up in Southern and East Africa. The effectiveness of PMTCT is not always good, and the eradication of mother-to-child transmission of HIV, as an objective, will be difficult to achieve by 2015. But we learn and progress day by day. There has been a very interesting and enlightening experience in South Africa that Doherty and colleagues (2009) developed. After a situation assessment, they improved training and supervision on a day-to-day basis in a district hospital. Improvements in coverage were really important in CD4 testing as well as in nevirapine intake and early diagnosis. This quality improvement intervention as a process and a way to identify, analyze, and resolve bottlenecks in PMTCT should be used everywhere when PMTCT indicators are not good. It is probably one of the best ways to try to achieve an eradication of mother-to-child transmission of HIV in Africa.

References

Abrams EJ, Myer L, Rosenfield A, El Sadr WM (2007) Prevention of mother to child transmission services as a gateway to family based human immunodeficiency virus care and treatment in resource limited settings: rationale and international experiences. Am J Obstet Gynecol 197:S101–S106

Aluisio A, Richardson BA, Bosire R, John-Stewart G, Mbori-Ngacha D, Farquhar C (2011) Male antenatal attendance and HIV testing are associated with decreased infant HIV infection and increased HIV-free survival. J Acquir Immune Defic Syndr 56:76–82

Anand A, Shiraishi RW, Sheikh AA, Marum LH, Bolu O, Mutsotso W et al (2009) Site factors may be more important than participant factors in explaining HIV test acceptance in the prevention of mother-to-child HIV transmission programme in Kenya, 2005. Trop Med Int Health 14:1215–1219

Arrivé E, Newell ML, Ekouevi DK, Chaix ML, Thiebaut R, Masquelier B et al (2007) Prevalence of resistance to nevirapine in mothers and children after single-dose exposure to prevent vertical transmission of HIV-1: a meta-analysis. Int J Epidemiol 36:1009–1021

Chandisarewa W, Stranix-Chibanda L, Chirapa E, Miller A, Simoyi M, Mahomva A et al (2007) Routine offer of antenatal HIV testing ("opt-out" approach) to prevent mother-to-child transmission of HIV in urban Zimbabwe. Bull World Health Organ 85:843–850

Curtis KM, Nanda K, Kapp N (2009) Safety of hormonal and intrauterine methods of contraception for women with HIV/AIDS: a systematic review. AIDS 23(suppl 1):S55–S67

Delvaux T, Nöstlinger C (2007) Reproductive choice for women and men living with HIV: contraception, abortion and fertility. Reprod Health Matters 15(suppl 29):46–66

Doherty T, Chopra M, Nsibande D, Mngoma D (2009) Improving the coverage of the PMTCT programme through a participatory quality improvement intervention in South Africa. BMC Public Health 9:406. doi:10.1186/1471-2458-9-406

Druce N, Nolan A (2007) Seizing the big missed opportunity: linking HIV and maternity care services in Sub-Saharan Africa. Reprod Health Matters 15:190–201

Duflo E, Dupas P, Kremer M (2009) Education and fertility: experimental evidence from Kenya. Massachusetts Institute of Technology. Working Paper

Dupas P (2009) Do teenagers respond to HIV risk information? Evidence from a field experiment in Kenya. PWP-CCPR-2009-066. California Center for Population Research: Online Working Paper Series

Elul B, Delvaux T, Munyana E, Lahuerta M, Horowitz D, Ndagije F et al (2009) Pregnancy desires, and contraceptive knowledge and use among prevention of mother-to-child transmission clients in Rwanda. AIDS 23(suppl 1):S19–S26

Guay LA, Musoke P, Fleming T, Bagenda D, Allen M, Nakabilto C et al (1999) Intrapartum and neonatal single-dose nevirapine compared with zidovudine for prevention of mother to child transmission of HIV-1 in Kampala, Uganda: HIVNET 012 randomised trial. Lancet 354:795–802

Johnson KB, Akwara P, Rutstein SO, Bernstein S (2009) Fertility preferences and the need for contraception among women living with HIV: the basis for a joint action agenda. AIDS 23(suppl 1):S7–S17

Kakimoto K (2008) Response to opt-out approach to prevent mother-to-child transmission of HIV. Bull World Health Organ 86:D

Katz DA, Kiarie JN, John-Stewart GC, Richardson BA, John FN, Farquhar C (2009) Male perspectives on incorporating men into antenatal HIV counseling and testing. PLoS ONE 4:e7602. doi:10.1371/journal.pone.0007602

Kellerman S, Essajee S (2010) HIV testing for children in resource-limited settings: what are we waiting for? PLoS Med 7. doi:10.1371/journal.pmed.1000285

Keogh SC, Urassa M, Kumogola Y, Mngara J, Zaba B (2009) Reproductive behaviour and HIV status of antenatal clients in northern Tanzania: opportunities for family planning and preventing mother-to-child transmission integration. AIDS 23(suppl 1):S27–S35

Kilewo C, Karlsson K, Ngarina M, Massawe A, Lyamuya E, Swai A et al (2009) Prevention of mother-to-child transmission of HIV-1 through breastfeeding by treating mothers with triple antiretroviral therapy in Dar es Salaam, Tanzania: The Mitra Plus study. J Acquir Immune Defic Syndr 52:406–416

Labhardt ND, Manga E, Ndam M, Balo JR, Bischoff A, Stoll B (2009) Early assessment of the implementation of a national programme for the prevention of mother-to-child transmission of HIV in Cameroon and the effects of staff training: a survey in 70 rural health care facilities. Trop Med Int Health 14:288–293

Larsson EC, Thorson A, Nsabagasani X, Namusoko S, Popenoe R, Ekström AM (2010) Mistrust in marriage – reasons why men do not accept couple HIV testing during antenatal care: a qualitative study in Eastern Uganda. BMC Public Health 10:769. http://www.biomedcentral.com/1471-2458/10/769

Leroy V, Sakarovitch C, Cortina-Borja M, McIntyre J, Coovadia H, Dabis D et al (2005) Is there a difference in the efficacy of peripartum antiretroviral regimens in reducing mother-to-child transmission of HIV in Africa? AIDS 19:1865–1875

Levy JM (2009) Women's expectations of treatment and care after an antenatal HIV diagnosis in Lilongwe, Malawi. Reprod Health Matters 17:152–161

Lim Y, Kim JY, Rich M, Stulac S, Niyonzima JB, Smith Fawzi MC et al (2010) Improving prevention of mother-to-child transmission of HIV care and related services in Eastern Rwanda. PLoS Med 7. doi:10.1371/journal.pmed.1000302

Lockman S, Hughes MD, McIntyre J, Zheng Y, Chipato T, Conradie F et al (2010) Antiretroviral therapies in women after single-dose Nevirapine exposure. N Engl J Med 363:1499–1509

McKenna MT, Xiaohong H (2007) Recent trends in the incidence and morbidity that are associated with perinatal human immunodeficiency virus infection in the United States. Am J Obstet Gynecol 197:S10–S16

Msellati P (2009) Improving mothers' access to PMTCT programs in West Africa: a public health perspective. Soc Sci Med 69:807–812

Muchedzi A, Chandisarewa W, Keatinge J, Stranix-Chibanda L, Woelk G, Mbizvo E et al (2010) Factors associated with access to HIV care and treatment in a prevention of mother to child transmission programme in urban Zimbabwe. J Int AIDS Soc 13:38. doi:10.1186/1758-2652-13-38

Namukwaya Z, Mudiope P, Kekitiinwa A, Musoke P, Matovu J, Kayma S et al (2011) The impact of maternal highly active antiretroviral therapy and short-course combination antiretrovirals for prevention of mother-to-child transmission on early infant infection rates at the Mulago national referral hospital in Kampala, Uganda, January 2007 to May 2009. J Acquir Immune Defic Syndr 56:69–75

Noba V, Sidibe K, Kaba K, Malkin JE (2001)Voluntary screening and prevention of mother-to-child transmission of HIV among pregnant women in Côte d'Ivoire: a public health program of the International Therapeutic Solidarity Fund. Paper presented at the 8th American conference on retrovirus and opportunistic infections, Chicago, USA, 4–8 February

Painter TM, Diaby KL, Matia DM, Lin LS, Sibailly TS, Kouassi MK et al (2004) Women's reasons for not participating in follow up visits before starting short course antiretroviral prophylaxis for prevention of mother to child transmission of HIV: qualitative interview study. BMJ 329:543–548

Painter TM, Diaby KL, Matia DM, Lin LS, Sibailly TS, Kouassi MK et al (2007) Faithfulness to partners: a means to prevent HIV infection, a source of HIV infection risks, or both? A qualitative study of women's experiences in Abidjan, Côte d'Ivoire. Afr J AIDS Res 6:25–31

Palumbo P, Lindsey JC, Hughes MD, Cotton MF, Bobat R, Meyers T et al (2010) Antiretroviral treatment for children with peripartum nevirapine exposure. N Engl J Med 363:1510–1520

Penda I, Msellati P (2010) Bottle neck of HIV PMTCT programmes in Cameroon. Analysis of 2008 data from "littoral" region. Paper presented at the XVIII International AIDS conference, Vienna, Austria, 18–23 July 2010. Abstract CDE1196

Rollins N, Mzolo S, Moodley T, Esterhuizen T, van Rooyen H (2009) Universal HIV testing of infants at immunization clinics: an acceptable and feasible approach for early infant diagnosis in high HIV prevalence settings. AIDS 23:1851–1857

Shetty KA, Marangwanda C, Stranix-Chibanda L, Chandisarewa W, Chirapa E, Mahomva A et al (2008) The feasibility of preventing mother-to-child transmission of HIVusing peer counselors in Zimbabwe. AIDS Res Ther 2008(5):17

Stinson K, Boulle A, Coetzee D, Abrams EJ, Myer L (2010) Initiation of highly active antiretroviral therapy among pregnant women in Cape Town, South Africa. Trop Med Int Health 15: 825–832

Stringer EM, Chi BH, Chintu N, Creek TL, Ekouevi DK, Coetze D et al (2008) Monitoring effectiveness of programmes to prevent mother-to-child HIV transmission in lower-income countries. Bull World Health Organ 86:57–62

Stringer EM, Ekouevi DK, Coetzee D, Tih PM, Creek TL, Stinson K et al (2010) Coverage of nevirapine-based services to prevent mother-to-child HIV transmission in 4 African countries. J Am Med Assoc 304:293–302

The Kesho Bora Study Group (2011) Triple antiretroviral compared with zidovudine and single-dose nevirapine prophylaxis during pregnancy and breastfeeding for prevention of mother-to-child transmission of HIV-1 (Kesho Bora study): a randomised controlled trial. Lancet Infect Dis 11:171–180

Tijou Traore A, Querre M, Brou H, Leroy V, Desclaux A, Desgrées-du-Loû A (2009) Couples, PMTCT programs and infant feeding decision-making in Ivory Coast. Soc Sci Med 69: 830–837

Toro PL, Katyal M, Carter RJ, Myer L, El Sadr WM, Nash D et al (2010) Initiation of antiretroviral therapy among pregnant women in resource-limited countries: CD4+ cell count response and program retention. AIDS 24:515–524

UNAIDS (2010) Global report: UNAIDS report on the global AIDS epidemic 2010. Geneva, Joint United Nations Programme on HIV/AIDS. UNAIDS/10.11E | JC1958E, Geneva

Violari A, Cotton MF, Gibb DM, Babiker AG, Steyn J, Madhi SA et al (2008) Early antiretroviral therapy and mortality among HIV-infected infants. N Engl J Med 359:2233–2244

World Health Organization (2003) Strategic approaches to the prevention of HIV infection in infants. Report of a WHO meeting, Morges, Switzerland, 20–22 March 2002. World Health Organization, Geneva. http://www.who.int/hiv/mtct/StrategicApproaches.pdf. Accessed 23 May 2011

World Health Organization (2007) Guidance on provider-initiated HIV testing and counselling in health facilities. World Health Organization, Geneva. http://whqlibdoc.who.int/publications/2007/9789241595568_eng.pdf. Accessed 23 May 2011

World Health Organization (2009) HIV and infant feeding. Revised Principles and Recommendations. Rapid Advice. World Health Organization, Geneva

Yéni P (2010) Prise en charge médicale des personnes infectées par le VIH. Rapport 2010. Recommandations du groupe d'experts. Direction Générale de la Santé. Agence Nationale de Recherches sur le SIDA et les hépatites virales, Paris

Part III
Women, Mothers and Care

Chapter 12
Psychological Distress Among HIV-Positive Pregnant and Postpartum Women in Thailand

Ratchneewan Ross

1 Introduction

Over 67 million people live in Thailand (Central Intelligence Agency [CIA] 2010). By the end of 2009, it was estimated that 530,000 Thais were HIV-positive, most of whom (98.1%) were 15 years of age or older (Joint United Nations Programme on HIV/AIDS [UNAIDS] 2010). The 2009 HIV infection rate for Thailand was reported at 1.3% and one-third of these were female (UNAIDS). HIV infection rates among pregnant Thai women were found to be particularly alarming, ranging from 1 to 3% of the total population across different regions of Thailand in 2008 and 2009 (National AIDS Prevention and Alleviation Committee [NAPAC] 2010).

In Thailand, most HIV transmission has been found to be through heterosexual activity and related to husband/partner's earlier or present promiscuity (NAPAC 2010). When infected with the virus, Thai women can feel stigmatized and depressed. Ingram and Hutchinson (1999: 122) note that "our society expects women to be mothers, yet at the same time, it negatively judges HIV-positive women who choose to become pregnant or refuse to abort an existing pregnancy. These double messages engendered strong emotions among the women."

It is vital for health-care professionals to understand HIV-positive pregnant and postpartum Thai women in relation to their lived experiences, psychological disturbances, and also how they cope with HIV through their religious beliefs and practises. This knowledge will lead to more effective health care, education, research, and policies to address the psychological needs of Thai mothers with HIV (see also Chap. 15 in this volume).

R. Ross (✉)
College of Nursing, Kent State University, Kent, OH, USA 44242
e-mail: rross1@kent.edu

P. Liamputtong (ed.), *Women, Motherhood and Living with HIV/AIDS:*
A Cross-Cultural Perspective, DOI 10.1007/978-94-007-5887-2_12,
© Springer Science+Business Media Dordrecht 2013

In this chapter, I will include topics concerning HIV-positive pregnant and postpartum Thai women in relation to their lived experiences, psychological disturbances (depressive symptoms), physical symptoms, a Buddhist way to cope with HIV infection, telephone support, and recommendations for health-care professionals. The chapter is based on findings from different studies conducted in Thailand. Throughout the chapter, I will refer to them accordingly.

2 Psychological Distress Among Thai Mothers with HIV Infection

Like HIV-positive women in other countries, women in Thailand often feel shocked, depressed, and stigmatized—in many cases, suffering from suicidal ideation and/or attempts (Jirapaet 2001; Ross et al. 2007a; see also Chap. 15 in this volume). A hermeneutic phenomenological study examined the lived experience of 10 pregnant women in Thailand after the acknowledgment of their HIV status (Ross et al. 2007a). Using Van Manen's analysis technique, results showed that "the struggle" was the core theme of the participants' experience, unfolding into four subthemes: struggling alone, sharing one's struggling, struggling for the baby, and struggling through ups and downs. Upon learning of their HIV diagnosis, the women usually felt shocked and ashamed, even though most of them knew that their spouse or partner had spread the virus to them. Their fear of stigmatization and rejection from family and friends increased their feeling of struggling all alone. At least half of the participants admitted that they were depressed and had suicidal ideas. However, these ideas were kept at bay due to their consciousness of responsibility to their fetus. Later, most of the participants began to share their struggle with others by disclosing their HIV status to family, friends, or others in a support group (see also Chap. 15). Most of them found that these actions were helpful and enabled them to be more mindful and to think more about their unborn infant. Some of them began to acknowledge more their baby's existence and thus felt more that they were struggling for their baby. A few participants started talking to their unborn child, saying it had given them hope and a positive outlook, although at times, they felt concerned about mother-to-child transmission. One participant stated:

> I keep talking with my baby about whatever I do, like, …Baby, Mom is going to go to the prenatal clinic today so that people at the hospital can check on us. Dad is not here because he has to work. The three of us will …fight…the disease together. We will never be alone… (Ross et al. 2007a: 738)

The participants admitted that, in their struggles, they unavoidably passed through ups and downs. Inadequate support and low income tended to add to their vulnerability, while good support from family and support groups were likely to revive their energy.

In a cross-sectional correlational study conducted by Ross et al. (2012a) in Thailand, 63% of the 207 pregnant and postpartum female participants revealed their HIV status to someone—mostly to their spouse, mother, and sister. While about three-quarters (78%) of these were happy with their HIV disclosure, one-seventh (12.9%) were not. The rest (9.1%) were not sure whether or not they were happy with their disclosure. In this study, when using logistic regression, predictors of HIV disclosure included age, employment status, and family support. Older mothers were almost five times more likely to disclose their HIV status than younger mothers. Unemployed mothers were roughly twice as less likely than their employed counterparts to reveal their status. Women with more family support were more likely to disclose their HIV status than those with lower support.

Research of depression/depressive symptoms among HIV-positive mothers is crucial for health-care providers. It has been reported that depressive symptoms of HIV-positive individuals were correlated with nonadherence to antiretroviral therapy, faster progression to AIDS, and poor quality of life (Antelman et al. 2007; Adewuya et al. 2008; Campos et al. 2008). Ross et al. (2009) examined depressive symptoms and their predictors among 127 HIV-positive pregnant Thai women to find ways that could help health-care professionals decrease depressive symptoms for the general population of HIV-positive mothers in Thailand. In their correlational, cross-sectional study, the Center for Epidemiological Studies Depression Scale (CES-D; Radloff 1977) was used to measure depressive symptoms ($\alpha=.91$). Self-esteem, emotional support, and physical symptoms were included as predictors of depressive symptoms. Self-esteem was measured by the Rosenberg Self-Esteem Scale (R-SE; Rosenberg 1989) and showed a Cronbach alpha of .81. Emotional support was measured by the Multidimensional Scale of Perceived Social Support (MSPSS; Zimet et al. 1988, 1990) with a Cronbach alpha of .88. The CES-D, R-SE, and MSPSS scales were translated into Thai with back translation. Physical symptoms were captured by a two-item questionnaire created by Ross and team and had a Cronbach alpha of .80.

Results from this study showed that, based on Radloff's CES-D (1977) cutoff scores (≥16), about three-quarters (78%) of the women reported depression to some degree. A little over half (55.1%) of the participants' scores fell in the range of 23–60, indicating possible clinical depression. Using simultaneous multiple regression, significant predictors of depressive symptoms included all three interested predictors of self-esteem as well as emotional support and physical symptoms: Women who reported less emotional support, lower self-esteem, and more physical symptoms experienced more depressive symptoms than other participants. In addition, family financial status significantly predicted depressive symptoms: Women with financial hardship reported more depressive symptoms than those with no financial difficulty. Among these four variables—self-esteem, emotional support, physical symptoms, and financial status—self-esteem was the strongest predictor, with its unique contribution of 16.5% for depressive symptoms. The model as a whole yielded 41.2% of the explained variance in depressive symptoms (Ross et al. 2009).

Ross et al. (2011) also examined depressive symptoms among 85 HIV-positive postpartum Thai women (6 weeks after delivery) in another correlational, cross-sectional study. As with their previous study, interested predictors of depressive symptoms in this study included self-esteem, emotional support, and physical symptoms, plus infant health status, using the same scales to measure the first three variables. Cronbach alphas were reported at .92 for CES-D, .87 for self-esteem, .72 for emotional support, and .82 for physical symptoms. Infant health status was measured by a single-item questionnaire developed by the researchers: "How is your infant's health status in general?" There were two possible answers: "Not in good health" (*score* = 0) or "In good health" (*score* = 1) (Ross et al. 2011: 38).

In this study, Ross et al. (2011) found that the prevalence of depression among HIV-positive postpartum mothers was comparable to that of their pregnant counterparts at 74.1% when the CES-D cutoff score of ≥16 was used, and almost half (45.6%) of the participants indicated clinical depression when the cutoff score of ≥23 was applied. Simultaneous multiple regression was used and showed that self-esteem and infant health status were significant predictors of depressive symptoms in this group, but not emotional support and physical symptoms. An additional significant predictor was education. Women with higher self-esteem, a positive perception of their infant's health status, and a higher educational background were less depressed than participants with lower levels in the same three areas. Like the previous study among HIV-positive pregnant Thai women, self-esteem was found here to be the strongest predictor of depressive symptoms with its unique variance of 19.3%. Overall, the three predictors (self-esteem, infant health status, and education) significantly accounted for 29.5% of depressive symptoms among HIV-positive postpartum women.

Ross et al. (2011) compared and noted three interesting points related to their two studies of depressive symptoms among HIV-positive Thai mothers (Ross et al. 2009, 2011). First, they pointed out that emotional support from family and friends was not a significant predictor of depressive symptoms among postpartum women with HIV, but it was a significant predictor among pregnant women with HIV. The researchers argued that tangible support may be a more helpful type of support than emotional support for postpartum mothers because these new mothers are more likely to need tangible assistance, for example, with household chores and baby care. They posited that such support could lessen their feelings of being burdened, thus decreasing their stress and depressive symptoms.

Secondly, Ross et al. (2009, 2011) found that the most frequently reported physical symptom among both pregnant and postpartum HIV-positive mothers was fatigue. Of the 43 pregnant women who reported some physical symptoms, 27 (63%) stated that they experienced fatigue. Of the 29 postpartum mothers who reported physical symptoms, 18 (62.1%) reported that they experienced fatigue. Rates of fatigue between these two groups of Thai mothers with HIV were high and comparable.

Thirdly, a mother's physical health was a significant predictor of depressive symptoms in pregnant mothers but not in postpartum mothers. Ross et al. (2011b: 41) noted that "these conflicting findings may be explained in part by the fact that the life context of HIV-positive postpartum mothers is different from that of their HIV-negative counterparts. Given that mothers with an HIV have concerns about the possibility of mother-to-child transmission, their own physical symptoms may be put on the back burner."

Ross et al. (2012b) examined the effects of telephone support by a registered nurse (RN) on depressive symptoms among HIV-positive pregnant women in Thailand. Emotional and informational support was provided over the phone by an RN during an 8-week period. This mixed-methods study showed that telephone support minimized depressive symptoms in the intervention group over time using two-way repeated measures of analysis of variance to analyze the data.

Results from in-depth interviews in Ross et al.'s study (2012b) elucidate how telephone support can be effective. HIV-positive pregnant participants stated that the support helped them to put things into perspective and also helped them to feel that someone was always there for them. Participants additionally stated that practical guidance from the nurse helped them to worry less, thus decreasing their depression. An example of practical guidance by the RN was given by a 19-year-old HIV-positive pregnant Thai participant: She shared with the research team that she had two major physical concerns/incidents which truly worried her. The first involved a day when she went shopping for hours. That night she experienced swollen legs, worrying that something might have been wrong with her legs. She decided to call the RN and was instructed to raise her legs overnight. After following the RN's instructions, she was relieved in the morning to find that her legs were back to normal. The other incident took place when her physician informed her that she was infected with German measles. Although the physician had told her that she was not infected with German measles, the young mother did not feel at peace until she was reassured by the RN, who confirmed that her lab result was indeed negative for German measles. With the RN's support, the participant stated that she felt better physically and psychologically.

3   Finding Peace: Thai Mothers' Buddhist Way to Live with HIV Infection

This section will cover how some HIV-positive, Buddhist Thai mothers have coped spiritually with their infection. In Thailand, the majority (94.6%) of the population is Theravada Buddhist (Klunklin and Greenwood 2005; CIA 2010). A hermeneutic phenomenological study examined the Buddhist beliefs and practises of seven HIV-positive postpartum Thai women (Ross et al. 2007b). In this study, Ross et al. (2007b) interviewed seven postpartum women in Thailand in terms of how they coped with their HIV infection through their Buddhist beliefs and practises. All seven had received the virus from their partners who had frequented sex workers. Using van Manen's (1990) data analysis technique, *Finding*

Peace was found to be the central theme of the participants' experiences along with three subthemes: *finding peace through belief in karma, finding peace through belief in Buddhist's Five Precepts, and finding peace through belief in Buddhist's Four Noble Truths.*

The postpartum women in the study stated that their belief in *karma* enabled them to accept their infection and take care of themselves spiritually (see also Balthip et al. 2012; Chap. 15 in this volume). They believed that, in their past life, they must have done something wrong so that their karma came back to them negatively in their present life. One participant said:

> I must have done something very bad in my past life, so in this life I got this disease to pay off my sin. That's good in a way to be sick in this life. I just have to move on and hope for the better life for my next birth. Whenever I think about this whole bad karma, it helps me accept the truth and feel *sa-ngob jai* (peaceful). (Ross et al. 2007b: 231)

The participants also tried to do good deeds in their current life, believing that such good deeds would help them get on better with their infection and be better off in their next life. Examples of good deeds as practised by the participants included liberating animals (a Buddhist's custom is to free, e.g., birds and turtles), giving alms to Buddhist monks, and donating money to the less fortunate (Ross et al. 2007b).

To help their peace of mind, Buddhist's Five Precepts (corresponding with half of the Ten Commandments in Christianity) were followed by the postpartum mothers in the study. These precepts prohibit killing, stealing, lying, illegitimate sexual behaviors, and illicit drug use or intoxicating drinks. The Four Noble Truths were also pursued by all participants. These truths include the concepts that "(a) life is suffering, (b) the cause of suffering is *tanha* (personal desire), (c) overcoming *tanha* is attainable, and (d) a path to the cessation of suffering exists" (Ross et al. 2007b: 231). According to the Buddha, suffering inevitably occurs at four moments in life: birth, sickness, aging, and death. A birth yields labor pain and birth trauma. Sickness causes pain and discomfort. Aging is a path to sickness and death. Death occurs after dying and causes its survivors suffering.

However, suffering from these four moments is avoidable in Buddhism through termination of one's personal desire (*tanha*) and through self-awareness by perceiving oneself as an imaginary entity, or as being selfless and mindful of suffering (Flanagan 2005). In this way, one can be free from suffering. In Buddhism, neither one's body, one's mind, nor one's spirit is real. Thus, when one is selfless, thinks about oneself as being unreal, and is mindful of one's suffering, one can limit self-interest and, in theory (or theologically), be emancipated from suffering. For health-care professionals wishing to empathize with their Buddhist patients, the concepts being discussed here will be highly useful to understand in terms of their practice.

Meditation, praying, and also the *Middle Way* were practiced by most of the HIV-positive Thai mothers in this study in order to help them feel peaceful and mitigate their suffering. The *Middle Way* in Buddhism is "the path between the two extremes of self-indulgence and self-mortification. [Simply put] according to the Buddha, too

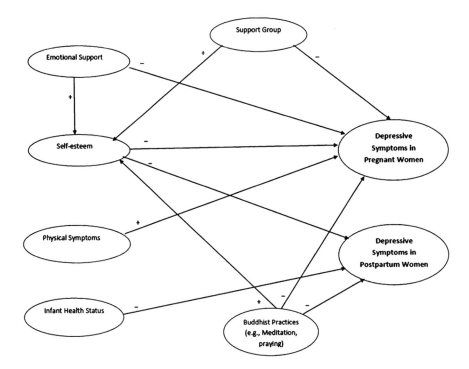

Fig. 12.1 A summary model of depressive symptoms among HIV-positive pregnant and postpartum women in Thailand

much or too little of any emotion, thought, or activity is not wholesome..." (Ross et al. 2007b: 233). One participant stated about the *Middle Way*:

> I don't feel too bad about the disease and the whole thing now. The Buddha taught us that the *Middle Way* is the best way for us to journey along. If we are too passionate or have too strong emotions and feelings toward things and situations, we are not going to live our lives *yang sa-ngop jai* (peacefully). (Ross et al. 2007b: 233)

The qualitative results from the above studies related to religious beliefs and practises are supported by a correlational, cross-sectional quantitative study where the data were drawn from the parent study (Ross et al. 2009) in that almost all of 127 HIV-positive, pregnant, Thai women believed in Karma to some degree, ranging from believing a little to strongly believing in karma (Brazofsky and Ross 2009). When Buddhist practises were examined in relation to depressive symptoms using Pearson product–moment correlations, meditation ($r=-.188$, $p<.05$), doing good deeds ($r=-.205$, $p<.05$), and watching TV or listening to the radio about religious teachings and stories ($r=-.220$, $p<.05$) were found to be reversely associated with depressive symptoms: The more the HIV-positive Thai women engaged in such religious activities, the fewer depressive symptoms they reported. Figure 12.1 summarizes a model of depressive symptoms and their predictors among HIV-positive pregnant and postpartum women in Thailand.

4   Conclusion and Implications

Psychological distress is found to be common among HIV-positive pregnant and postpartum mothers in Thailand. Thai mothers with an HIV infection tend to experience stigmatization, depressive symptoms, and suicidal ideation. Depressive symptoms have been found to be linked with a lower quality of life and faster progression to AIDS. Through qualitative and quantitative studies in Thailand, factors related to depressive symptoms among HIV-positive pregnant women have been found to include self-esteem, emotional support, physical symptoms, and Buddhist practises (meditation, doing good deeds, and listening to or watching religious stories). Factors associated with depressive symptoms among HIV-positive postpartum women include self-esteem, a negative perception of infant's health status, and religious practises.

Due to high rates of depression among HIV-positive pregnant and postpartum women, health-care providers in Thailand should develop a policy and procedures to support routine screenings for depressive symptoms in these populations. Depressive symptoms can first be assessed using a questionnaire, such as the CES-D scale. When a CES-D score of 23 or higher is shown, the patient should be transferred to appropriate practitioners so that a clinical diagnosis can be confirmed and treatment of depression can be administered appropriately. Health-care professionals can also encourage certain religious practises as being beneficial to HIV-positive, pregnant and postpartum, Thai women living in a Buddhist culture, since these practises have been found to be associated with fewer depressive symptoms in both groups.

Increasing self-esteem among the target population will also be beneficial. Action research in Thailand among 10 HIV-positive pregnant Buddhist women revealed that strategies that increased self-esteem among them included counseling, education about HIV infection and the prevention of its transmission, support groups, emotional support, hope, religious practises (e.g., praying, meditation, going to the temple), reading, exercising, and doing errand work (Sawatphanit et al. 2004).

Evidence also shows that self-esteem, as a learned phenomenon, can be strengthened through an individual's perception of social inclusion (Leary et al. 2004). Therefore, programs that increase a sense of belonging can escalate an HIV-positive mother's self esteem. Such programs may include support groups, exercise clubs, and other like venues. Health-care professionals should encourage HIV-positive pregnant and postpartum Thai women to join a group of their own personal interest.

Emotional support should also be made available to HIV-positive pregnant Thai women whenever possible. This can be done through counseling within the women's families so that family members might better express their love and care for these Thai women. Again, emotional support through support groups among Thai mothers with HIV has been found to be beneficial (Liamputtong et al. 2009; see also Chap. 15). For HIV-positive postpartum Thai mothers, tangible support should also be encouraged along with emotional support. Newborn care and house chore assistance could help provide these postpartum mothers with sorely needed, even if brief, a respite from such work stress.

When an HIV-positive perinatal Thai woman voices her concern about her own or her infant's physical symptoms, health-care professionals should seriously respond to the concern. A real cause of such symptoms should be further investigated and treated accordingly. These actions will likely help the woman to have more peace of mind, thereby decreasing her depressive symptoms, and increasing her health overall.

As mentioned earlier, telephone support by an RN was found to be helpful in lessening depressive symptoms among HIV-positive pregnant women in Thailand (Ross et al. 2012b). Thus, emotional and informational telephone support could be expanded to more effectively care for HIV-positive perinatal Thai women. It should be helpful as well if similar telephone support models are developed for and tested among HIV-positive pregnant and postpartum women in other cultures.

Health-care students should also be informed about the psychological distress of HIV-positive pregnant and postpartum Thai women. The helpful strategies mentioned above can be shared with students so that they will be equipped with this knowledge for their future practises.

Finally, further research should be conducted to examine predictors of depressive symptoms among HIV-positive pregnant and postpartum Thai women longitudinally so that definite causation of these predictors can be made. Important predictors that should be included in future research are stigma, self-esteem, different types of social support, support groups, physical symptoms, infant health status, and religious practises. Future research which includes some of these predictors as interventions will be helpful. In addition, research of the emotional and informational benefits of telephone support among HIV-positive pregnant and postpartum Thai women should be explored in a large sample in Thailand as well as other cultures so that the results can be more generalizable. These recommended studies will add new knowledge to the field and advance our practise so that HIV-positive pregnant and postpartum women in Thailand will receive optimal health care through which their psychological needs can be met and their quality of life maximized.

References

Adewuya A, Afolabi M, Ola B, Ogundele O, Ajibare A et al. (2008) Relationship between depression and quality of life in persons with HIV infection in Nigeria. Int J Psychiatry Med 38(1):43–51

Antelman G, Kaaya S, Wei R, Mbwambo J, Msamanga GI, Fawzi WWBS et al. (2007) Depressive symptoms increase risk of HIV disease progression and mortality among women in Tanzania. J Acquir Immune Defic Syndr 44(4):470–477

Balthip Q, Boddy J, Siriwatanamethanon J (2012) Achieving harmony: moving from experiencing social disgust to living with harmony in people with HIV/AIDS in the Thai context (Chapter 21). In: Liamputtong P (ed) Stigma, discrimination and HIV/AIDS: a cross-cultural perspective. Springer, Dordrecht

Brazofsky SE, Ross R (2009) Religious activities, belief in karma, depression and CD4 levels among HIV-positive, Buddhist, Thai pregnant women. Paper presented at the Robinson Memorial Hospital Research Day: Women's Health Issue, Ravenna, OH, 8 May 2009

Campos LN, Guimaraes MD, Remien RH (2008) Anxiety and depressive symptoms as risk factors for non-adherence to antiretroviral therapy in Brazil. AIDS Behav [E-pub ahead of print]

Central Intelligence Agency (2010) The world factbook. https://www.cia.gov/library/publications/the-world-factbook/geos/th.html. Accessed 1 Mar 2011

Flanagan A (2005) Buddhism. Retrieved from http://buddhism.about.com/cs/ethics/a/BasicsKama.htm

Ingram D, Hutchinson SA (1999) Defensive mothering in HIV-positive mothers. Qual Health Res 9(2):243–258

Jirapaet V (2001) Factors affecting maternal role attainment among low-income Thai, HIV-positive mothers. J Transcult Nurs 12:25–33

Joint United Nations Programme on HIV/AIDS (2010) Global report: UNAIDS report on the global AIDS epidemic/2010. http://www.unaids.org/globalreport/Global_report.htm. Accessed 1 Mar 2011

Klunklin A, Greenwood J (2005) The status of women and the spread of HIV/AIDS in Thailand. Health Care Women Int 26:46–61

Leary MR, Schreindorfer LS, Haupt AL (2004) The role of low self esteem in emotional and behavioral problems: why is low self-esteem dysfunctional? In: Kowalski RM, Leary MR (eds) The interface of social and clinical psychology. Psychology Press, New York, pp 116–128

Liamputtong P, Haritavorn N, Kiatying-Angsulee N (2009) HIV and AIDS, stigma and AIDS support groups: perspectives from women living with HIV and AIDS in central Thailand. Soc Sci Med Spec Issue Women Mothers HIV Care Resour Poor Settings 69(6):862–868

National AIDS Prevention and Alleviation Committee (2010) UNGASS country progress report: Thailand. http://data.unaids.org/pub/Report/2010/thailand_2010_country_progress_report_en.pdf. Accessed 1 Mar 2011

Radloff LS (1977) The CES-D scale: a self-report depression scale for research in the general population. Appl Psychol Meas 1:385–401

Rosenberg M (1989) Society and the adolescent self-image. Wesleyan University Press, Middletown

Ross R, Sawatphanit W, Draucker C, Suwansujarid T (2007a) The lived experiences of HIV-positive, pregnant women in Thailand. Health Care Women Int 28(8):731–744

Ross R, Sawatphanit W, Suwansujarid T (2007b) Finding peace (*Kwam Sa-ngob Jai*): a Buddhist way to live with HIV. J Holist Nurs 25:228–235

Ross R, Sawatphanit W, Zeller R (2009) Depressive symptoms among HIV-positive pregnant women in Thailand. J Nurs Scholarsh 41(4):344–350

Ross R, Sawatphanit W, Mizuno M, Takeo K (2011) Depressive symptoms among HIV-positive postpartum women in Thailand. Arch Psychiatr Nurs 25(1):36–42

Ross R, Stidham AW, Drew D (2012a) HIV disclosure by perinatal women in Thailand. Arch Psychiatr Nurs 26(3):232–239

Ross R, Sawatphanit W, Suwansujarid T, Stidham AW, Drew D, Creswell JW (2012b) The effect of telephone support on depressive symptoms among HIV-positive pregnant women in Thailand: an embedded mixed-methods study. J Assoc Nurses AIDS Care. doi:10.1016/j.jana.2012.08.005 [E-pub ahead of print]

Sawatphanit W, Ross R, Suwansujarid T (2004) Development of self-esteem among HIV positive pregnant women in Thailand: action research. J Sci Technol Humanit 2(2):55–69

van Manen M (1990) Researching lived experience: human science for an action sensitive pedagogy. State University of New York Press, Albany

Zimet GD, Dahlem NW, Zimet SG, Farley GK (1988) The multidimensional scale of perceived social support. J Pers Assess 52(1):30–41

Zimet GD, Powell SS, Farley GK, Werkman S, Berkoff KA (1990) Psychometric characteristics of the multidimensional scale of perceived social support. J Pers Assess 55(3&4):610–617

Chapter 13
HIV Is My "Best" Problem: Living with Racism, HIV and Interpersonal Violence

Josephine Mazonde and Wilfreda (Billie) Thurston

1 Introduction

We began our study with the belief that understanding women's experiences of HIV/AIDs and gender-based violence could only be accomplished within a socio-ecological framework that acknowledged structural forces that shape women's lives (Thurston and Vissandjée 2005; Navarro et al. 2006). In this context, the environment includes economic, social, institutional and cultural elements that affect an individual and in turn will affect the community's well-being (Green et al. 1996; Thurston and Vissandjée 2005). We used critical feminist perspectives and critical theory in general, standpoint epistemologies and gender and power perspectives (Wingood and DiClemente 1997; Smith 1999; Gupta 2000; see also Chap. 1 in this volume) to further shape our project.

These theoretical foundations help in understanding the societal basis of HIV/AIDS and IPV as global concerns. The way women are exposed to these two issues does not occur randomly but rather follows the already established social forces of power inequality, gender role inequality and cultural expectations that shape how women are treated by their male counterparts. From the perspective of feminist

J. Mazonde (✉)
249 Citadel PT NW, Calgary, AB T3G 5L2, Canada
e-mail: nnani28@hotmail.com

W. Thurston
Department of Community Health Sciences, Faculty of Medicine,
University of Calgary Institute for Gender Research,
3330 Hospital Drive NW, Calgary, AB T2N 4N1, Canada

Department of Ecosystems and Public Health, Faculty of Veterinary Medicine,
University of Calgary Institute for Gender Research,
3330 Hospital Drive NW, Calgary, AB T2N 4N1, Canada
e-mail: thurston@ucalgary.ca

P. Liamputtong (ed.), *Women, Motherhood and Living with HIV/AIDS:*
A Cross-Cultural Perspective, DOI 10.1007/978-94-007-5887-2_13,
© Springer Science+Business Media Dordrecht 2013

standpoint epistemology, it is necessary to provide women with an environment without pressures from men because men have traditionally determined what women's needs are and how they are interpreted. Smith (1999) states that women-to-women talk might be more productive in understanding women's personal experiences.

We also brought our personal histories to the project. As a young woman, mother, nurse, midwife, educator and researcher, Josephine Mazonde lived in the developing world during the inception of HIV in the early 1980s. Like many people, she had a choice whether or not to turn a blind eye to what the world was facing – this mysterious disease no one understood at the time. But, she did not turn her back to it, and as a young nurse working in rural areas of Botswana, she started with very basic strategies of prevention. When visiting traditional doctors and churches, she targeted the young people with prevention education, drawing in parents, until the whole community saw the need for collaborative action. The struggle against HIV continued in all areas of the country and there came a time when the government, chiefs and other leaders realized the need to aggressively attack the "monster." Josephine extended her work on a voluntary basis, working nights, weekends and holidays, reaching out to schools, churches, prisons, district multidisciplinary committees and later at a national level through Knowledge, Innovation and Training Shall Overcome AIDS (KITSO).

Before becoming an academic researcher, Wilfreda Thurston was involved in starting a sexual assault centre and later a shelter for women fleeing domestic violence. She was director of the shelter before going back to complete a doctorate in health promotion for women. In studying women's health, she made the connection between HIV and violence against women, recalling how little had been known about this in the shelter. Her research has continued to examine how the health system does or does not act to prevent violence against women. She has also focused on gender as a determinant of women's health and the promotion of Aboriginal women's health.

Despite our backgrounds, neither of us was entirely prepared for the stories about the depth of strength required to survive the intersections of HIV/AIDS and IPV in a wealthy western city.

2 Background

2.1 Women and HIV/AIDS

The prevalence of HIV in Canada increased from 52,000 in 2002 to 58,000 in 2007; more women are being diagnosed with HIV and AIDS and they now represent about 20% of all Canadians infected with HIV. Generally, groups that are at high risk include men who have sex with other men, intravenous drug users, Aboriginal people and people from countries where HIV is endemic (Public Health Agency of Canada 2006).

The medical approach to HIV/AIDS management has instigated strategies that serve medical personnel well but pay minimal attention to social, economic and political conditions. This approach currently excludes information about how those infected and affected understand their experiences around HIV and AIDS. People living with HIV/AIDS have diverse experiences based on factors such as gender, ethnicity, socioeconomic status and government policies, as well as the attitudes of individual care providers. This diversity of experience results in the isolation of certain groups of people, including women, especially women from minority populations; intravenous drug users; and sex trade workers. The result is perpetual stigma and marginalization of such groups and fear of being identified with the condition (Committee on HIV Prevention Strategies 2001; Krishnatray et al. 2006).

Research has shown that women's bodies, specifically the receptive mucosal membrane in the genital tract, make it easier for women than men to contract HIV (Kathewera-Banda et al. 2005). Moreover, studies have also shown a difference in vulnerability across a woman's reproductive life. Quinn and Overbaugh (2005) point out that adolescent girls are more vulnerable than mature women, either because their immature genital tract exposes them to irritations and tears or because of their behavioral high-risk activities. Biological changes, such as high levels of progesterone in pregnancy and those created with the use of hormonal contraceptives, also affect risk. Progesterone is seen to enhance susceptibility to HIV, interfering with the immune response to infection. Another vulnerability is linked to gender norms and beliefs around sex, sexuality, sexual risk-taking and fidelity (Quinn and Overbaugh 2005).

How people define a disease will influence its management. The original perception of how HIV/AIDS spread and its medical description directed an approach to management that followed the medical model of diagnosis and treatment. This approach conflicts with some cultures, gender roles and political support. Kleinman et al. (2006: 144) suggest the "cultural construction of clinical reality" which encompasses the interplay of biological, psychological and sociocultural aspects of illness as a more culturally inclusive model of managing illnesses. Brach and Fraser (2000) refer to this kind of approach as based in cultural competency, which they consider a factor that would reduce racial and ethnic health disparities. They suggest that this approach goes beyond knowledge of cultural diversity to the acquisition by care providers of skills in dealing with culturally diverse populations.

A culturally competent approach would recognize gender and the fact that women's vulnerability to HIV/AIDS is rooted in almost every aspect of life across the range of health determinants, from their biological make-up to economic, social and political conditions (Kathewera-Banda et al. 2005). Low education among women continues to fuel their vulnerability to HIV; education would improve their access to information, the labour force and increased self-esteem that would help them rise above the poverty line. Also, a gap in knowledge perpetuating the ignorance and stigma around HIV/AIDS is created by the lack of inclusive care services where HIV/AIDS is an integral part of every service provided to women.

The community expects certain roles of women, especially the caregiver role (Lewis 2006; UNAIDS 2006). Women diagnosed with HIV/AIDS face different challenges than men. For most, they do not only have to take care of themselves but also provide care and attention to others who need and expect it. Further, they often do not have others to take care of them, which add more burdens to their physical, social, emotional and economic situations. The pressures from their multiple roles isolate women from social activities and adversely affect their self-care. Stress further weakens their immune systems and adds to quick diagnoses and stigma. Women are also exposed to further risk of infection by forced sex from their partners as well as other forms of abuse, hence the greater incidence of HIV/AIDS among women than men for a long period of time. Moreover, violence or the fear of violence has been identified as interfering with women seeking HIV/AIDS information, voluntary testing and counselling (Goldstein and Manlowe 1997), further compounding the spread of HIV. Moreno (2007), in her study with Latina women, outlined how HIV and IPV share risk factors that impact both HIV prevention and management. She related IPV and HIV to childhood trauma, such as sexual, physical and verbal abuse. This in turn affects women's ways of dealing with relational issues as it affects their trust, lowers their sense of self-worth and also results in self-blame.

Women's combined experiences of abuse and surviving HIV may impact their parenting skills and activities because of the physical, emotional and psychological trauma they experience. Ultimately, the children may also display signs of distress that then exacerbate the woman's stress, resulting in cycle of trauma for everyone (Jaffe et al. 1990; Levendosky and Graham-Bermann 2000). Mothers experiencing both HIV and IPV, however, continue to express a need to live *for* their children; the distresses of HIV and IPV become secondary to this goal (Wilson 2007).

2.2   Interpersonal and Domestic Violence

The World Health Organization and other international agencies have recognized violence against women as a global human rights issue (UNAIDS 2004). IPV also affects men, but the rates differ greatly (Trainor 2002). According to Piot (1999), IPV causes more deaths than other recognized epidemics such as malaria, cancer, road traffic incidents and war. Piot further states that in the United States, a woman is assaulted by her spouse at least every 15 s, and in India about 45% of men abuse their female partners. In other parts of the world, women are used sexually for ritual cleansing. Sexual abuse of women is also seen as a weapon of war and as a sign of masculinity for men (Dunckle et al. 2004).

IPV is related to sexual and power imbalances between women and men. Johnson and Ferraro (2000) describe contexts of violence, issues of power used by men to control women and the social effects of violence against women. They suggest that IPV revolves around political, social, economic, cultural and gender issues. The social aspects of IPV have many implications in women's lives, relating to economics, politics, health, justice, education, employment and human rights. Considering that 25–54% of adult females will experience IPV in their lifetime (Bonomi et al. 2006), IPV presents a challenge to women's health and well-being. Bonomi and colleagues contend that IPV exposes women to physical, mental and psychosocial issues relative to the intensity and duration of the abuse. They further state that lack of data on long-term effects of IPV has inversely affected screening and intervention measures by care providers.

With reference to human rights, Wagman (2008) suggests that IPV not only undermines women's rights to fundamental freedom but also increases their risk to HIV and other sexually transmitted infections (STIs) and reduces quality of life. Research conducted in South Africa revealed that experience of violence and controlling behavior from male partners was strongly related to the increased risk of HIV infection among women (Dunckle et al. 2004). According to Human Rights Watch, rape and sexual assault within marriage is not uncommon and husbands may physically force wives to have sex against their will even where there is a possibility of HIV infection (Schleifer 2004). The threat of violence often results in women deferring decisions about sexual practises to their male partners, such as the use of male or female condoms which the men often reject. For women who experience IPV, low self-esteem, substance abuse and low power to initiate condom use lead to unprotected sex and are factors that make them vulnerable to HIV infection (Beadnell et al. 2000). A study conducted in South Africa among pregnant women revealed the link between IPV and increased risk factors for HIV, including having multiple sex partners, alcohol use and engaging in unprotected sex (Dunckle et al. 2003).

While IPV can result in HIV infection, research has also revealed that IPV can be a consequence of HIV (Medley et al. 2004). For example, in studies of American women's experiences of HIV disclosure, Gielen et al. (1997, 2000) variously found that 18% of women living with HIV reported disclosure-related violence, 4% reported physical abuse after disclosure and 45% reported emotional, physical or sexual abuse following their diagnosis.

3   Janey's Story

Our first hint that getting at the intersections in experiences of HIV/AIDS and IPV in women's lives would be a challenge was the difficulty in recruiting participants to our study. Through our many recruitment efforts, we encountered Janey (a pseudonym) who agreed to participate and met with Josephine several times to tell her story. Janey was between 30 and 35, unemployed, involved in the sex trade, had about a high school education, used street drugs and did not have a permanent address. She was proud of her Aboriginal[1] identity. She is identified as a lesbian. She had been HIV positive for about 10 years when telling her story and had experienced IPV.

Janey was a talented writer who used her writing as a way of letting her voice be heard by the world. Most of her writing showed signs of rage towards the unfair treatment and injustice inflicted by colonizers, who took advantage of Aboriginal

---

[1] Aboriginal is used to include First Nations, Inuit and Métis ancestry in Canada.

peoples, abused the women and children and took a precious resource, the land. She was very aware of systemic discrimination against Aboriginal people and believed her experiences with abuse, drug use and the sex trade were all rooted in her childhood experiences, mostly in boarding schools and group homes. Research in Canada supports her beliefs. Kirmayer et al. (2009: 27), for instance, indicated that the damage done to Aboriginal peoples by the residential school system that operated up to the 1960s has been extensive, as is the "ongoing effects of a chaotic and constricted present and murky future." A national Truth and Reconciliation Commission was established in Canada after the June 2008 apology from the Prime Minister in the House of Commons to former students, their families and communities (Truth and Reconciliation Commission of Canada 2011).

To work towards being drug-free, Janey had gone to a detoxification centre in the city. She reported doing very well and was very proud of herself. She wanted to pursue her desire to get clean and empower other women and children in regard to drug use and HIV. However, while she talked freely about her drug use and HIV, she did not want to address IPV in any detail. Each time the topic of abuse was brought up, she would react with extreme anger. At one point, she said she did not want to talk about it because of the pain it brought to her. We can see from this that failure to address the violence has continued to disrupt Janey's life; while it festers under the surface, service workers and others may not understand her outbursts or may see her relapses as personal weakness while she is actually carrying great personal pain as well as the pain of oppression and harm done to her people.

Janey mistrusted the system that she believed was oppressive, and this led her to not use the government-run programmes, either health care or the legal system. She said that care providers were more interested in the disease (i.e. her HIV status) than in her as a person. She was very selective about the services she used because she wanted care providers who would look at her and see a total human being, needing company and acceptance, instead of just focusing on the disease and seeing her only as a subject of care services. This desire matches what the system refers to as client- or patient-centred care and it has long been recognized that such care is a paradigm shift that has been difficult to achieve (Bensing et al. 2000).

Janey connected HIV to gender-based violence, her childhood experiences of abuse as well as partner violence. The trauma she experienced as a child and adolescent led to suicidal and other behaviors, such as drug use and involvement in the sex trade that are considered high risk for HIV infection. The abuse by others also led to self-abuse, which included causing physical harm to herself by going for days without food and water, taking only drugs and alcohol, as well as provoking other people with the intention of getting hurt. Janey got into drugs and the sex trade as a teenager, and this exposed her to IPV and HIV. She came to believe that she deserved the abuse and her description of how she contracted HIV suggested a form of self-negligence rooted in the cycle of abuse:

> …after a certain period of time I decided I didn't care anymore. It all added up everything from my life and from being out in the streets with different partners. It all added up and I finally just, ah, I went out and I delivered [used] the used needles with some people that

were HIV positive just because I couldn't kill myself, which I did commit suicide in all different ways and it never worked. I always ended up in the hospital or being saved somehow.

Hopelessness led to engaging in behaviors exposing her to HIV and more IPV.

3.1   Cycle of Abuse

The experience of surviving HIV/AIDS and IPV negatively impacted Janey's life and created a cycle that was difficult to escape. Her drug use and involvement in the sex trade exposed her to HIV reinfection with a different strain of HIV and to other STIs, such as hepatitis C. It also exposed her to additional physical, sexual and psychological abuse by others and led to self-destruction and a desire to die and, hence, attempts at suicide:

It [abuse] affected me and I decided I didn't want to feel anything because I wanted too much as a kid. So I started doing the drugs and the alcohol and I got into the needles and when I figured out a way and I couldn't commit suicide through everything else…you know, you're doing crazy things like ripping, taking the drugs from a drug dealer and thinking you know they will come back and shoot you or, you know, get somebody to beat, to beat you or kill you. Whatever, right. I did everything I could to try and get somebody to be, to kill me or I took pills or, you know, drank and did pills or hung, I tried to hang myself, everything. I tried everything.

The childhood trauma that she experienced contributed to her use of drugs and alcohol and work in the sex trade. She used alcohol and drugs to numb herself from the pain she experienced during her childhood. She acted with the intention to aggravate anger in other people, such as drug dealers, with the aim of getting hurt or killed. The suicide rate among Aboriginal teens is three to six times that of non-Aboriginal teens (Kirmayer et al. 2009). The rates vary, however, by community depending on how much community has been able to restore self-governance and cultural identity (Chandler and Lalonde 2009).

Janey indicated that her self-abuse started very early in life. She wanted both to avoid feeling the pain of abuse experienced as a child and adolescent and also to gain attention that seemed not to come:

…but when I was a kid I did different things. I, you know, I'd take Gravol or, you know, go sniff inhalants or solvents. I just did a lot of other things to, to try avoid feeling what I was feeling so I'd, I'd slash my wrists, my wrists for I don't know for how many years while I was in the, ah, in the group homes, the government homes.

In summing up the impact of the abuse in her life, Janey said that everything left her feeling like a "piece of shit." Her childhood trauma was part of a cycle of abuse by others as well as self-abuse. It was part of the legacy of residential schools in Canada that created a generation that had not witnessed parenting or the kindness and love of parents and extended family. When they came to have children, they were often at a loss as to how to care for them and the pain of the parents was inflicted on the children (Tsosie 2010).

The physical, emotional, spiritual and sexual abuse experienced by Janey included a rape that resulted in a teenage pregnancy. This was part of the painful truth of IPV that Janey was hesitant to discuss. Later, Janey had another child from a consensual relationship. Because of her other social problems, however, her children were with their grandmother and Janey had little contact with them. She expressed a longing for a better relationship, especially as the children grew into teenagers, but she recognized that her ability to parent was severely compromised by the HIV and her social status.

3.2 HIV: A Reason to Live

An HIV diagnosis can motivate some women to take charge and to reshape their lives (Barroso and Sandelowski 2004; see also Chaps. 12, 14 and 15 in this volume), and this is what Janey recounted. Almost immediately after she was diagnosed with HIV, she decided she wanted to live. She referred to this as a "blessing from above":

> …when I first converted [sero-positive] I thought, I thought that was basically the end of my life. I spent my whole life trying to commit suicide but then when I found out I was HIV positive, I figured out I wanted to live and that's what kind of turned my head; actually it's a gift from the skies and I don't know if you've ever heard anybody say that before.

The diagnosis not only restored her will to live, it also created a desire to find out who she really was and why things happened the way they did. This influenced the strategies she employed in her process of survival. She decided to work with a spiritual leader, and she preferred to work with her traditional healer to using the mainstream services. In fact this was not the first time we had heard that an HIV diagnosis had changed a life for the better (Wilson 2007).

Janey talked about wanting to live and to achieve a better quality of life by getting clean from drugs, having improved relationships with her children and empowering herself, other women and youth in relation to HIV and drugs. She never, however, talked about empowering herself or others regarding childhood abuse, IPV or sex trade work. As mentioned above, the experience of violence was not de-stigmatized enough for Janey and the residual pain from the experiences of violence and the oppression of her people was not healed. Although Janey reported doing well while working with her traditional healer, she went back to drug use and sex work. During some interviews, she seemed to be in a state of hopelessness and to feel defeated. She fought back, however, and decided to book into an addictions rehabilitation centre:

> …to me it…was my wake-up call and start, you know, trying to live life and do something with myself and I did that for, for a little while. I saw a traditional healer and did a 180 degree turn around and took care of myself and got healthy and got help that I needed for my drug and alcohol issues and went to counselling and did everything for myself and I was doing pretty good.

While there was support for getting off drugs and for adhering to medications for the HIV, Janey again did not receive care for her history of abuse. Care providers (nurses, doctors and social workers) who interacted with her during her visits for health services, like HIV/AIDS care, did not speak to IPV. As a result, Janey did not get the impression that addressing IPV was important to her success. She also described the care providers as being cold and too clinical. When asked, "How is the help you received or are still receiving regarding HIV and abuse (IPV) affecting your well-being?", she replied:

> You can't be cold and clinical. You can't be impersonal and just pull somebody in a social worker; Okay, so how are you feeling today? Anybody that says that to me I tell them you know what? Kick your ass and go back out that door until you can come in and say hi! How are you? How's your day today? So ah what can I help you with? You know rather than somebody saying how are you feeling today? Are you suicidal? Do I need to phone the ambulance on you?

The failure on the part of care providers to deal with abuse issues could also contribute to women's lack of knowledge of available services regarding IPV and not knowing where to go when experiencing abuse. When asked why she did not want to address abuse, Janey said it was due to shame; the concept of shame raises other issues. Health care providers have repeatedly expressed a reluctance to address IPV with their patients. Identified barriers to screening for IPV include lack of effective interventions once patients are identified, fear of offending patients, lack of provider education, limited time to screen, patient nondisclosure and non-compliance and fear of repercussions (Erickson et al. 2001; Varcoe 2001; Gerbert et al. 2002; Zachary et al. 2002).

To understand why abuse is so difficult to address among both care providers and survivors of IPV, even more than other stigmatized issues such as HIV/AIDS, drug use and the sex trade, we must also understand the systemic impact of gender inequality. Heise et al. (1994: 1169) observe that "the results of several cross-cultural studies suggest that hierarchical gender relations – perpetuated through gender socialization and the socioeconomic inequalities of society – are integrally related to violence against women." In general, the health sector has been reluctant to implement gender analysis of health policies (Horne et al. 1999; Scott et al. 2001) as medicine is highly gendered and equality issues in training, retention and academic medicine have yet to be resolved (Miedzinski et al. 2003). Gender in organizations may be a critical issue in protocol implementation (Fulop and Linstead 1999). Gender plays a role, for instance, in defining work and working relationships.

4   Effects of HIV/AIDS and IPV Together

Having addressed surviving HIV/AIDS and surviving IPV separately through Janey's story, we return to addressing the interconnectedness of HIV/AIDS and IPV and how this impacts the lives of women. This brings together how surviving HIV/

AIDS and IPV affects physical, emotional and spiritual well-being, as well as general coping mechanisms. Experiences of abuse lead to a lack of self-worth and the inability to care for oneself. Maintaining relationships is difficult, especially with children, since one lacks the resources to care for oneself. Coupled with psychosocial, spiritual and physical impacts are medical complications that further interfere with day-to-day activities. These include chronic fatigue and depression.

A major connection between HIV and IPV is the loss of trust in others and the ability to form relationships. Lack of trust grew as a result of people using their HIV status against them, especially those they had trusted (i.e. partners and significant others):

> ...I haven't been exactly speaking my truth. I haven't been telling anybody anything. I don't talk to people anymore. I stopped talking to people for about three years now. I didn't trust anybody. I thought, certain people were after me and I was scared for my life.

The lack of trust is perpetuated by a system that treats them as a 'disease' rather than as a whole person:

> Well, there's nothing, there's nothing that anybody can really do about the way the agencies are and certainly nothing I can do and there's nothing I can suggest because everything is the way it is for a reason, I guess. And I just have to accept that for the way it is, right.

5 Conclusion

While HIV/AIDS and IPV as global epidemics are now receiving international recognition, myths, cultural beliefs and policies serve as barriers to considering the intersection of the two issues, undermining recognition of the impact on women's lives. The intersection of IPV and HIV infection impacts women's access to and use of health and social services. In addition to the anticipated progression of HIV to AIDS, women experiencing both situations are at risk of depression and high-level posttraumatic stress (Du Mont et al. 2005). There is evidence that HIV/AIDS and IPV are strongly related and women that are exposed to one have an increased risk of the other. Rooted in the complexity of this interaction is the socioeconomic and gender inequality between women and men as seen in women's higher unemployment, lower education and lower income (Krishnan et al. 2008). Some structural pathways have been identified in the literature for this interconnectedness and these include (a) childhood trauma resulting in patterns of sexual risk behaviors in the future, (b) traumatic forced sexual activities increasing women's risk for HIV, (c) violent experiences limiting women's ability to negotiate safer sex, (d) disclosure by HIV-positive women exposing them to abuse by their partners and (e) repeated violent experiences interfering with women's use of health care services, creating a cycle of abuse and difficulty in coping (Moreno 2007). Experiencing both conditions may impact all aspects of women's lives resulting in social, physical, psychological and spiritual disorders.

Janey's relationships with her children were disrupted more by her unresolved history of abuse than by her HIV status, although trying to disentangle the two at her age seemed pointless. It was difficult for us to focus on either HIV/AIDS or IPV and not to have the other issue immediately come into the picture. This reinforced the interconnectedness of these issues and underscored their complexity. Yet, care providers continue to make this separation in their work. To understand this intersection requires care that comes from a position of cultural safety. Cultural safety is a concept that incorporates an understanding of gender, the culture of the care providers and their institutions and the legitimacy of difference (Tupara 2001; Ramsden 2002), and it is essential in people-centred care (World Health Organization 2008). If cultural safety was the norm, we would expect that Janey's experiences may have been very different and her chances of reconciliation with her children much greater.

Many women may be experiencing challenges similar to those faced by Janey: feelings of incompetence as mothers, not having enough love to give or share with their children, their children being at risk of adopting the risky practises that they see their mothers doing and fear of losing their children to the state and strangers. Janey was never at peace with herself following separation from her children. She kept trying to stop her alcohol and drug use and to find a decent home where she could raise her children. She knew her children were not proud of who she was at the moment and hoped her efforts would change that. This hope gave her strength to go on. These experiences and hopes are a common discourse of motherhood.

References

Barroso J, Sandelowski M (2004) Substance abuse in HIV positive women. J Assoc Nurs AIDS Care 15(5):48–59

Beadnell B, Baker SA, Morrison DM, Knox K (2000) HIV/STD risk factors for women with violent male partners. Sex Roles 42(7–8):661–689

Bensing JM, Verhaak PFM, van Dulmen AM, Visser AP (2000) Communication: the royal pathway to patient-centered medicine. Patient Educ Couns 39(1):1–3

Bonomi AE, Thompson RS, Anderson M, Reid RJ, Carrell D, Dimer JA, Rivara FP (2006) Intimate partner violence and women's physical, mental, and social functioning. Am J Prev Med 30(6):458–466

Brach C, Fraser I (2000) Can cultural competency reduce racial and ethnic health disparities? A review and conceptual model. Med Care Res Rev 57(S1):181–217

Chandler MJ, Lalonde CE (2009) Cultural continuity as a moderator of suicide risk among Canada's First Nations. In: Kirmayer LJ, Valaskakis GG (eds) Healing traditions: the mental health of Aboriginal peoples in Canada. UBC Press, Vancouver, pp 221–248

Committee on HIV Prevention Strategies in the United States, Division of Health Promotion and Disease Prevention, Ruiz MS, Gable AR, Kaplan EH, Stoto MA, Fineberg HV, Trussell J (eds) (2001) No time to lose: getting more from HIV prevention. National Academy of Science, Washington, DC. http://www.nap.edu/catalog.php?record_id=9964. Accessed 3 July 2011

Du Mont J, Forte T, Cohen MM, Hyman I, Romans S (2005) Changing help-seeking rates for intimate partner violence in Canada. Women Health 41(1):1–19

Dunckle K, Jewkes R, Brown H, McIntyre J, Gray G, Harlow S (2003) Gender-based violence and HIV infection among pregnant women in Soweto. A technical report to the Australian Agency for International Development. Medical Research Council, Pretoria, Australia. http://www.mrc.ac.za/gender/women.pdf. Accessed 6 Sept 2011

Dunckle KL, Jewkes RK, Brown HC, Gray GE, McIntyre JA, Harlow SD (2004) Gender based violence, relationship power, and risk of HIV infection in women attending antenatal clinics in South Africa. Lancet 363(9419):1415–1421

Erickson MJ, Hill TD, Siegel RM (2001) Barriers to domestic violence screening in the pediatric setting. Pediatrics 108(1):98–102

Fulop L, Linstead S (1999) Management: a critical text. Macmillan Education, South Yarra

Gerbert B, Gansky SA, Tang JW, McPhee SJ, Carlton R, Herzig K, Danley D, Caspers N (2002) Domestic violence compared to other health risks. A survey of physicians' beliefs and behaviors. Am J Prev Med 23(2):82–90

Gielen AC, O'Campo P, Faden RR, Eke A (1997) Women's disclosure of HIV status: experiences of mistreatment and violence in an urban setting. Womens Health 25(3):19–31

Gielen AC, Fogarty L, O'Campo P, Anderson J, Keller J, Faden R (2000) Women living with HIV: disclosure, violence and social support. J Urban Health 77(3):480–491

Goldstein N, Manlowe JL (eds) (1997) The gender politics of HIV/AIDS in women: perspectives on the pandemic in the United States. New York University Press, New York

Green LW, Richard L, Potvin L (1996) Ecological foundations of health promotion. Am J Health Promot 10(4):270–281

Gupta GR (2000) Gender, sexuality, and HIV/AIDS: the what, the why, and the how. Can HIV/ AIDS Policy Law Rev 5(4):86–93. http://www.aidslaw.ca/publications/publicationsdocEN. php?ref=238. Accessed 29 Aug 2011

Heise LL, Raikes A, Watts CH, Zwi AB (1994) Violence against women: a neglected public health issue in less developed countries. Soc Sci Med 39(9):1165–1179

Horne T, Donner L, Thurston W (1999) Invisible women: gender and health planning in Manitoba and Saskatchewan and models for progress. Prairie Women's Health Centre of Excellence, Winnipeg, MB. http://www.pwhce.ca/invisibleWomen.htm. Accessed 29 Aug 2011

Jaffe PG, Wolfe DA, Wilson SK (1990) Children of battered women. Sage, Newbury Park

Johnson MP, Ferraro KJ (2000) Research on domestic violence in the 1990s: making distinctions. J Marriage Fam 62(4):948–963

Kathewera-Banda M, Gomile-Chidyaonga F, Hendriks S, Kachika T, Mitole Z, White S (2005) Sexual violence and women's vulnerability to HIV transmission in Malawi: a rights issue. Int Soc Sci J 57(186):649–660

Kirmayer LJ, Tait CL, Simpson C (2009) The mental health of Aboriginal peoples in Canada: transformations of identity and community. In: Kirmayer LJ, Valaskakis GG (eds) Healing traditions: the mental health of Aboriginal peoples in Canada. UBC Press, Vancouver, pp 3–35

Kleinman A, Eisenberg L, Good B (2006) Culture, illness and care: clinical lessons from anthropologic and cross-cultural research. Focus: J Lifelong Learn Psychiatry 4(1):140–149

Krishnan S, Dunbar MS, Minnis AM, Medlin CA, Gerdts CE, Padian NS (2008) Poverty, gender inequities, and women's risk of Human Immunodeficiency Virus/AIDS. Annu N Y Acad Sci 1136:101–110

Krishnatray P, Melkote SR, Krishnatray S (2006) Providing care to persons with stigmatised illnesses: implications for participatory communication. J Heal Manag 8(1):51–63

Levendosky AA, Graham-Bermann SA (2000) Behavioral observations of parenting in battered women. J Fam Psychol 14:18–94

Lewis S (2006) Race against time: searching for hope in AIDS-ravaged Africa. House of Anansi Press, Toronto

Medley A, Garcia-Moreno C, McGill S, Maman S (2004) Rates, barriers and outcomes of HIV serostatus disclosure among women in developing countries: implications for prevention of mother to child transmission programmes. Bull World Health Organ 82(4):299–307

Miedzinski LJ, Thurston WE, Lent B (2003) Gender equity: a solved problem or marginalized issue? CAME Newsletter 13(2):2–6. http://www.came-acem.ca/docs/newsletters/13_2/newsletter_13_2_en.pdf. Accessed 30 Aug 2011

Moreno CL (2007) The relationship between culture, gender, structural factors, abuse, trauma, and HIV/AIDS for Latinas. Qual Health Res 17(3):340–352

Navarro A, Voetsch K, Liburd L, Bezold C, Rhea M (2006) Recommendations for future efforts in community health promotion. Report of the National Expert Panel on Community Health Promotion. Centers for Disease Control and Prevention, Atlanta, GA. http://www.cdc.gov/chronicdisease/pdf/community_health_promotion_expert_panel_report.pdf. Accessed 30 Aug 2011

Piot P (1999) HIV/AIDS and violence against women. Speech from Panel on Women. http://www.thebody.com/content/art690.html. Accessed 30 Aug 2011

Public Health Agency of Canada (2006) The state of the HIV/AIDS epidemic in Canada. http://www.phac-aspc.gc.ca/media/nr-rp/2006/2006_05bk1-eng.php. Accessed 27 Aug 2011

Quinn TC, Overbaugh J (2005) HIV/AIDS in women: an expanding epidemic. Science 308(5728):1582–1583

Ramsden I (2002) Cultural safety and nursing education in Aotearoa and Te Waipounamu. Unpublished doctoral dissertation. Victoria University of Wellington, Wellington, New Zealand

Schleifer R (2004) Deadly delay: South Africa's efforts to prevent HIV in survivors of sexual violence. Human Rights Watch 16, 3(A). http://www.hrw.org/en/reports/2004/03/03/deadly-delay. Accessed 27 Aug 2011

Scott C, Horne T, Thurston W (2001) The differential impact of health care privatization on women in Alberta. In: Armstrong P, Amaratunga C, Bernier J, Grant K, Pederson A, Wilson K (eds) Exposing privatization: women and health care reform in Canada. Garamond Press, Aurora, pp 253–285

Smith DE (1999) Writing the social: critique, theory and investigations. University of Toronto Press, Toronto

Thurston WE, Vissandjée B (2005) An ecological model for understanding culture as a determinant of women's health. Crit Public Health 15(3):229–242

Trainor C (ed) (2002) Family violence in Canada: a statistical profile 2002 (Catalogue no. 85-224-XIE). Canadian Centre for Justice Statistics, Statistics Canada, Ottawa, ON. http://www.statcan.gc.ca/pub/85-224-x/85-224-x2000002-eng.pdf. Accessed 27 Aug 2011

Truth and Reconciliation Commission of Canada (2011) Reconciliation...towards a new relationship. http://www.trc.ca/websites/reconciliation/index.php?p=312. Accessed 24 Aug 2001

Tsosie E (2010) Native women and leadership: an ethics of culture and relationship. In: Suzack C, Huhndorf SM, Perreault J, Barman J (eds) Indigenous women and feminism: politics, activism, culture. UBC Press, Vancouver, pp 29–42

Tupara H (2001) Meeting the needs of Maori women: the challenge for midwifery education. N Z Coll Midwives J 25:6–9

UNAIDS (2004, November 23) Number of women living with HIV increases in each region of the world [Press Release]. http://www.thebody.com/content/art686.html. Accessed 29 Aug 2011

UNAIDS (2006) 2006 Report on the global AIDS epidemic: a UNAIDS 10th anniversary special edition. http://data.unaids.org/pub/GlobalReport/2006/. Accessed 29 Aug 2011

Varcoe C (2001) Abuse obscured: an ethnographic account of emergency nursing in relation to violence against women. Can J Nurs Res 32(4):95–115

Wagman J (2008) Twin pandemics in rural Uganda: intimate partner violence and HIV [Alumni Dispatches]. John Hopkins Public Health, Special Issue 2008 (online edition). http://magazine.jhsph.edu/2008/Spring/alumni_dispatch/jennifer_wagman/. Accessed 27 Aug 2011

Wilson S (2007) 'When you have children, you're obliged to live': motherhood, chronic illness and biographical disruption. Sociol Health Illn 29(4):610–626

Wingood GM, DiClemente RJ (1997) The effects of an abusive primary partner on the condom use and sexual negotiation practices of African-American women. Am J Public Health 87(6):1016–1018

World Health Organization (2008) The World Health Report 2008: primary health care – now more than ever. http://www.who.int/whr/2008/whr08_en.pdf. Accessed 27 Aug 2011

Zachary MJ, Schechter CB, Kaplan ML, Mulvihill MN (2002) Provider evaluation of a multifaceted system of care to improve recognition and management of pregnant women experiencing domestic violence. Womens Health Issues 12(1):5–15

Chapter 14
The Effects of Collective Action on the Confidence of Individual HIV-Positive Mothers in Vietnam

Pauline Oosterhoff and Tran Xuan Bach

1 Introduction

Studies from various parts of the world have reported how women's reproductive roles and identities as mothers and wives are key drivers of their biological vulnerability to contracting HIV (Amaro 1995; Clark et al. 2006; Hirsch et al. 2007). Recent research shows that in spite of socioeconomic disadvantages that increase women's vulnerability to contracting HIV (UNAIDS et al. 2004; Ojkutu and Stone 2005), women are actually often more privileged than men when it comes to accessing antiretroviral therapy (ART) (Braitstein et al. 2008; WHO 2008; Bila and Egrot 2009; Le Coeur et al. 2009). Among the reasons for this paradox are that general stigma about ill-health prevents men from seeking care (Bila and Egrot 2009), women have more interaction with health services due to their reproductive roles and duties, and in a context in which HIV/AIDS is driven by intravenous drug use (IDU), health staff favor women because they are seen as victims and more adherent to medical care (Le Coeur et al. 2009).

The recognition of a process that involves women's own agency and ability to act and to accomplish change is central to contemporary feminist discussions of empowerment. Naila Kabeer (1999: 437), for example, defines empowerment for women as "the expansion in people's ability to make strategic life choices in a context where this ability was previously denied to them." This dynamic approach to

P. Oosterhoff(✉)
Department of Development Health, Medical Committee Netherlands Vietnam, MCNV,
Weteringschans 32, 1017 SH Amsterdam, The Netherlands

Royal Tropical Institute, Mauritskade 63, 1092 AD Amsterdam, The Netherlands
e-mail: Pauline_Oosterhoff@yahoo.com; P.Oosterhoff@kit.nl

T.X. Bach
Institute for Preventive Medicine and Public Health, Hanoi Medical University,
No. 1 Ton That Tung St., Hanoi, Vietnam
e-mail: bach@hmu.edu.vn

P. Liamputtong (ed.), *Women, Motherhood and Living with HIV/AIDS:*
A Cross-Cultural Perspective, DOI 10.1007/978-94-007-5887-2_14,
© Springer Science+Business Media Dordrecht 2013

gender-based power relations, and the recognition of the need to build self-esteem to fight immobilizing "victimhood," has received considerable interest among academics and development practitioners (Evans 1980; Gillis and Perry 1991; Raphael 1993; Kling et al. 1999; Freire 2000; Malhotra et al. 2002).

Access to resources can be conceived as a result of or a condition for this empowerment (Malhotra et al. 2002). Support groups can enable women to articulate and reframe individual concerns into a shared public discourse. Historically, grassroots activism and support groups have been very important in improving access to ART in both resource-rich and resource-poor settings (Kalichman et al. 1996; Barbot 2006; Vanlandingham et al. 2006; Oosterhoff et al. 2007; Oosterhoff 2008, 2009; Liamputtong et al. 2009; Nguyen et al. 2009). Moreover, a number of studies have identified a strong connection between the ability of community groups to mobilize or gain access to resources and their ability to bring about social and political change (McCarthy and Zald 1977; Eisen 1994; Fawcett et al. 1995). Yet, although many social movements aim to improve access to goods and services, resources alone may not enable disenfranchized persons to change their situation at an individual level (Rifkin 1986; Malhotra et al. 2002; Laverack 2001; Kar and Pasteur 2005). Activists' success can eliminate their initial raison d'etre. Several countries such as France, the United States, and Australia saw a "normalization" of AIDS from the mid-1990s onwards, for example (Rosenbrock et al. 2000). This "normalization," which was due at least in part to the success of AIDS activists in improving access to effective medicine, also led to a decrease in AIDS grassroots mobilization in the countries involved (Barbot 2006). Hence, once the main goal of activists was achieved, they could return to "normal" life, and for many that also meant no longer engaging in the AIDS movement. However, this trend of "normalization" and associated disengagement were observed in countries like France and Australia and applying lessons on social mobilization from one context to another may be more complex than they immediately appear.

This chapter examines changes which occurred among members of support groups of HIV-positive mothers in Vietnam in a context where ART is becoming more widely available. We examine women's ability to accomplish their stated personal goals and priorities through group mobilization of resources and the effects of their efforts on reported self-esteem and confidence.

2   Vietnam

Vietnam provides an interesting case for research on HIV-positive motherhood, support groups, and empowerment. Vietnamese couples[1] invariably belong to an extended patriarchal family in which men have practical, social, and symbolic roles that are

---

[1] In this chapter, "Vietnamese" is a generalized term referring to members of the Kinh majority ethnic group.

grounded in a long historical Confucian cultural tradition. In these roles, Vietnamese men can be empowered or, alternatively, shamed, or dominated by other men (Harris 1998). The socialist government considers motherhood of national importance, and Vietnamese women's roles, identities, and choices are circumscribed by *thiên chức*, a "sacred motherhood mandate" (SRV 1984; Oosterhoff 2008). Many national policies support this cultural role (SRV 1984, 2002), providing wives and mothers with some social benefits that men do not enjoy, such as extended leave following the birth of a child and time off to take care of sick family members. However, *thiên chức* also brings familial and collective duties which are not borne by men, such as pressure to comply with population policies or being held responsible for the drug addiction or HIV-positive status of their children, as women are considered responsible for the good public moral image of the family. Further, the emphasis of *thiên chức* on the "motherhood mandate" implicitly excludes the rights of women to choose to stay single or childless.

HIV-positive mothers embody a social and ideological contradiction between the protection and obligations associated with *thiên chức* and the stigma and insecurity attached to an epidemic which is currently largely driven by IDU. Given the perceived relationship between HIV-positive status and drug use and sex work (both criminalized in Vietnam), HIV-positive women have to deal not only with their positive status but also with drug-related stigma, poverty, and in some cases drug-related domestic violence (see also Chaps. 9 and 13 in this volume).

Millions of Vietnamese women are already organized and represented in mass organizations, such as the Women's Union, and the Red Cross that are guided and controlled by the Communist Party of Vietnam, within the one-party state. Mass organizations are linked to the Communist Party and therefore support *thiên chức*. Only limited opportunities are available to independent local organizations and nongovernmental organizations (NGOs).

In 2004, some AIDS medicines for adults were available in Hanoi free of charge, but women were not accessing them. Doctors reported that women were fearful of visiting services because they feared stigma and other possible negative consequences for their children; hence, they were hiding and dying alone, leaving orphans behind while medicines were, in fact, available (Oosterhoff et al. 2007). To address this issue, an international nongovernmental organization, the Medical Committee Netherlands-Vietnam (MCNV), initiated a pilot program in April 2004 focusing on care and support for HIV-positive pregnant women and young mothers. A support group, the "Sunflowers," emerged, with the aim of providing prevention of mother-to-child transmission (PMTCT), helping HIV-positive mothers access available medicines for their children as well as other services needed by the family, based on their own assessment of their requirements. The group was founded following the four-pronged PMTCT model promulgated by the World Health Organization that included care and support for HIV-positive mothers and their children and families. It was the first organization for HIV-positive mothers in Vietnam. Although HIV-positive mothers belong to families that are often clearly different from the state's "cultural family" (*gia dinh van hoa*) ideal, this group (and their stated goals) was officially recognized by the state. Hundreds of similar and not so similar support groups for people living with HIV and AIDS have emerged since this time, with membership ranging from a dozen to hundreds of members. See also Chap. 15 in this volume.

A micro-credit intervention was developed in response to women's reported need to improve their income and of their being excluded from existing credit opportunities because of their HIV status. The program provided loans through the Women's Union, which had experience with supplying micro-credit through women's groups (though not HIV-positive mothers' groups) after a mostly successful trial period (Oosterhoff et al. 2008). To be eligible for loans, women were required to compose a business plan which was first reviewed on paper, followed by a visit to the proposed business site, often in the family's house, to assess familial support to the proposed plan, which is vital in multigenerational households.

In June 2004, the Bush administration named Vietnam the fifteenth "focus" country under the President's Emergency Plan for AIDS Relief (PEPFAR), which became an important source of funding for ART. With funding from PEPFAR and later the Global Fund, AIDS medicines became more available, with ART and other AIDS expenditure doubling from around USD 50 million in 2006 to USD 108.7 million in 2008, although 90% of funding was from international sources (National Committee for AIDS et al. 2010). As a result of these changes, in most provinces of Vietnam, HIV-positive people became increasingly able to access ART. However, failure to seek ART treatment still persists especially among young unmarried women and among those not in a support group (Nguyen et al. 2010). We were able to follow a group of HIV-positive mothers in support groups for several years, from just before the moment ART became more widely available in 2004 until June 2008. This provided us with an important opportunity to explore some of the actual and the perceived dynamics between these civil society groups, empowerment of members, and increased access to medicines.

3   The Study

The data on which this chapter is based were collected as part of a larger action research program on PMTCT, gender, and poverty in which the authors combined roles as researchers and program managers (Oosterhoff 2008, 2009). We conducted participant observation among Sunflower groups both during regular program activities and at almost all major meetings between group members and state authorities. The first group was founded in Hanoi in 2004, the second in Thai Nguyen City in the same year, and a third, fourth, and fifth group were established in 2005 in Dai Tu district in Thai Nguyen province, Cao Bang City in Cao Bang province, and Ha Long City in Quang Ninh province, respectively. In all locations, groups were established in a context where ART was available at some level.

For this study, we analyze data from personal development plans (PDP) made by HIV-positive mothers. When new members join a Sunflower group, they can independently complete a PDP as a means of helping them prioritize their medical, economic, and social needs. As part of this process, members identify a maximum of three "priority problems" for which they require assistance. Each Sunflower group has democratically elected "core members" who assist other members in thinking through their problems and identifying solutions and also link new member to services and individuals who can help them tackle their identified priority areas. The individual PDPs are kept by the women in their home or in a closed cupboard in the group office only accessible to elected core members. Each year, the PDP is evaluated by the member in question together with a core member, resulting in the establishment of a new plan. Based on the outcomes and evaluations of their plans, individual women can see if and how they have been able to make changes in their lives in the areas they identified as important, and draw their own lessons and conclusions regarding their accomplishments. The PDP evaluation contains both open (qualitative) and multiple-choice questions. These qualitative and quantitative data are entered into a computer using EPI Info. Codes are used to ensure members' anonymity. These data are analyzed and monitored in order to help group leaders and local authorities track any changes required in the services offered; at an aggregate level the data enable authorities to see if the service network of the group matches the needs of HIV-positive mothers, for example, and may prompt them to invite new partners to join the network.

In this chapter, we examine PDP data, including reported changes in the priorities, of 419 HIV-positive mothers/women in five Sunflower support groups across four provinces in North Vietnam between June 2004 and June 2008.[2] All except seven women made a new PDP after the evaluation of the results of their first.

4   Profile of the Women Who Joined the Group

The average (mean) age of the women studied was 30.2 years old. By the end of the study period, when the data were reviewed, they had been members of a Sunflower group for an average of 13.4 months. In Hanoi, the oldest and first group in the country, the average length of membership was almost double the average, at 21.4 months.

During the period studied, the total number of HIV-positive mothers who were members across the five groups increased from 4 to 557 members. Among the five groups, 80% of the total members had made a PDP by June 2008. Most of these 419 mothers included in the study sample decided to fill in the plan some months after they had joined a group (the average time members selected took to formulate a PDP was 8.4 months). The plan was filled in alone, with help from a fellow member or a representative of an authority supporting the group such as the Red Cross, according to each individual woman's preference. It was found that in groups where "core members" actively encourage and assist members, almost 90% of the HIV-positive

---

[2] Some other members joined as an exception. The total number of PDPs made by all members was 458 among whom mothers, 5 fathers of HIV+/affected children, 11 grandparents of HIV+/affected children, and 8 caregivers. This study focuses on the mothers.

Table 14.1 Number of HIV-
positive women by province

Province	Frequency	Percent
Thai Nguyen	180	42.96
Cao Bang	40	9.55
Hanoi	132	31.5
Quang Ninh	67	15.99
Total	419	100

mothers made a PDP, while in groups in which core members are not active and new members have to make the plan alone, just over half of members produce a PDP.

Over a third, 36.8% (154/419), of the mothers reported to be taking ART at the time of the first formalized evaluation of their PDP. Less than half, 43.9% (184/419), were living with HIV-positive male partners of whom just under half, 49.5% (91/184), were also on ART, while 28/419 (6.7%) lived with a partner who was either HIV negative or did not know his status. A total of 27 of the male partners were reportedly actively using drugs; of these, all but one were also HIV-positive.

There were many widows in all the groups, but the highest proportion of widows was found in the groups in Quang Ninh and Cao Bang provinces, possibly partly because in Quang Ninh ART arrived in 2006, a few years later than in Hanoi where small ART programs began in 2001 and PEPFAR scaled up in 2005. In Cao Bang, a mountainous province bordering China, internationally funded ART also arrived later in 2006.

In Hanoi and Cao Bang, most women lived in a more or less traditional multigenerational patrilocal arrangement with their husbands' families, either within a couple or as a widow. In the other two provinces, the majority of women – both those in a couple and widows – lived separately from the man's family in a nuclear family, in couples with the husband as the head of the household.

Although the groups are all located in urban areas, including the capital city, farming was found to be the most frequently reported profession of group members. Forty percent of the women (159; 36%) considered themselves farmers, while around 20% (87) reported being housewives and 83 (20%) were small shopkeepers (83) engaged in the sale of groceries, tailoring, food, hairdressing, and other services. Less than 10% (36) considered themselves laborers, around 5% (26) were directly involved in HIV-related work as counselors and peer educators, 14 were jobless, and 12 reported to be salaried and trained professionals such as working as a nurse, teacher, accountant, or government official. Two women did not provide information concerning their profession.

5   Increased Access to Medicines

The rapid scale-up and decentralization of ART services over the period studied is illustrated by the range of treatment service utilization at district level and provincial level of women reported by group members. In Hanoi and Thai Nguyen, women were able to access ART at central, provincial, and district levels, with district level the most common source. In Quang Ninh and Cao Bang, most women accessed medicine at provincial level (in Cao Bang treatment was rarely accessed outside of the provincial hospital). Few women (3/158) travelled to national-level facilities in Hanoi to obtain treatment, revealing that women managed to access ART at a local level (Table 14.2).

ART was not necessarily required for all members as it depends on their CD4 count. CD4 count refers to number of functioning CD4 cells that support the immune system. HIV damages the CD4 cells. Women who joined the group would receive a general health examination. If they did not know their CD4 count, they would also be supported to receive a CD4 count test through the health referral system to which the groups were networked. In addition, medical doctors were linked to each group and would visit regularly to discuss health issues such as when ART is required and where it is available. In Thai Nguyen, almost half the women (34/70) who were on treatment were already accessing ART when they entered the group and filled in their first PDP, while the rest received ART after they entered the group, reflecting close relationships between the health services and the support group.

In Hanoi, the group was instrumental in helping women to get access to ART and also provided women who had already access to medicines with adherence support and counseling from their Sunflower peers. In Hanoi, two-thirds of the women on ART accessed treatment after joining the group and stayed the longest in the group, almost 10 months, before getting ART. This suggests that the outreach work in Hanoi was particularly effective in helping women to join a group before they needed treatment and assisting them in accessing treatment at a decentralized level when required. The data suggest a diversity of roles that support groups can play in ART as for some women groups help them to overcome barriers to accessing available treatment and in others, such as in Thai Nguyen where women already were on ART support groups fulfill other needs such as adherence support.

Table 14.2 Decentralized access to ART: participants taking ART by level of health care providers and provinces

Levels of ART clinics	Thai Nguyen	Cao Bang	Hanoi	Quang Ninh	All
Central hospitals (N)	2	0	3	1	6
%	2.6	0	6.98	3.57	3.8
Provincial hospitals	10	8	16	24	58
%	12.99	80	37.21	85.71	36.71
Provincial health center	12	1	1	3	17
%	15.58	10	2.33	10.71	10.76
District health center	52	1	23	0	76
%	67.53	10	53.49	0	48.1
Hospice 09	1	0	0	0	1
%	1.3	0	0	0	0.63
All	77	10	43	28	158
	100	100	100	100	100

Table 14.3 Relationship between group membership and ART initiation

	Started ART after group involvement			Started ART prior to group involvement		
	N	Mean (months)	95% CI		N	Mean (months)	95% CI	
Thai Nguyen	36	4.6	3.1	6.1	34	0.9	−7.5	−3.8
Cao Bang	3	5.0	−8.1	18.1	6	1.8	−10.5	−1.5
Hanoi	37	9.6	6.2	12.9	11	1.2	−5.2	0.3
Quang Ninh	11	7.2	3.3	11.1	9	2.3	−12.2	−1.5
All	87	7.0	5.4	8.7	60	0.7	−6.7	−3.9

For some women, access to medicines was not a priority defined in their PDP because they were still feeling healthy, while others had already obtained ART in any case. Although health is an obvious concern for all HIV-positive mothers, these members also had other pressing social and economic needs, such as lack of access to micro-credit and/or fears about discrimination of their children in education which they tried to address by means of the linkages which existed between the groups and service providers (Table 14.3).

6   Changes in Social and Psychological Concerns of Women Who Received Support

With both access to health support including free ART and access to a network of social and economic services, one might assume women's confidence increased and reported stigma, including self-stigma, decreased.

Indeed, data analysis suggests that group membership helped HIV-positive mothers to reduce the stigma they feel from outsiders (Liamputtong et al. 2009; see also Chap. 15 in this volume). The sense of being discriminated by neighbors or family and reluctance to go out were found to decrease over time following group membership, but these were small reported concerns compared with women's perception of themselves. Women who joined the group had great concerns about being useful and suffered a lack of confidence in their own competencies and their contribution to social activities. These concerns diminished a little over time, but most women remained insecure about their ability to contribute or be useful to others. The vast majority (80%) reported having friends whom they felt they could share personal concerns with and these were not just friends who were also HIV-positive. For example, food plays a very central role in Vietnamese family life, and meals are usually shared among several close people (Marquis and Shatenstein 2005; Ochs and Merav 2006). Although 36% women did not share meals with other family members, this was attributed to a large proportion of those living in a nuclear family situation with a husband with an unstable social status and a distinct, complicated, stigmatizing background of IDU. About 90% of the women who were living with their own parents or their husband's family reported sharing their meals.

School access for children with HIV-positive parents was a concern that HIV-positive mothers raised in group meetings and is also a reported problem in many other countries. Therefore, this was an area of concern for the program. However, both an external evaluation and the PDP data showed that in fact most mothers were able to place their children in regular schools and could pay for the tuition fees for their children. We found no effect of micro-credit on the ability of women to send their children to school. Of the women who took out a loan, 80% said they could afford the tuition fees for children themselves. However, 87% of the children actually went to school. This reflects both the very high value that Vietnamese attach to education and the ability of mothers to mobilize support from other sources such as grandparents, aunts, or neighbors to enable their children to attend school.

7   Self-esteem, Social Concerns, Stigma, and Discrimination

There is a growing body and a wealth of literature and research available on HIV- and AIDS-related stigma and discrimination from all over the world (Herek and Capitanio 1998; Malcolm et al. 1998; Bond et al. 2003; Khuat Thu et al. 2004; Liamputtong 2012). Stigma and discrimination have important effects on almost all aspects of the epidemic notably on the demand and the provision of HIV testing and medical care and on the emotional well-being and quality of life of HIV-positive persons. Few long-term studies are available to show how HIV- and AIDS-related stigma and discrimination can change over time and if and how self-help groups contribute to positive changes (Oosterhoff 2008).

These findings all suggest that many HIV-positive mothers have at least some social support in important areas of daily life. However, their own lack of confidence, rather than external discrimination, seems to be a key challenge (Fig. 14.1).

8   Changing Priorities After Participation in a Support Group

When women first join the Sunflowers, they identify their problems, classifying them under social, economic, or health priorities, and discuss these with a core member and sometimes representatives of relevant authorities in order to identify what can be done to reduce or address these issues. Over time, it was found that social and health concerns reduced significantly and economic issues emerged as the main priority (Fig. 14.2).

The number of women who considered health a priority was substantially reduced after they joined the group. It was also observed that a large proportion of the women who had originally flagged social and health issues as a priority in their first PDP considered economics as their first priority when this first PDP was evaluated.[3]

---

[3] As already noted, seven women did not make a new PDP.

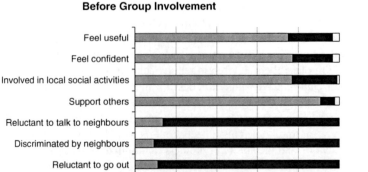

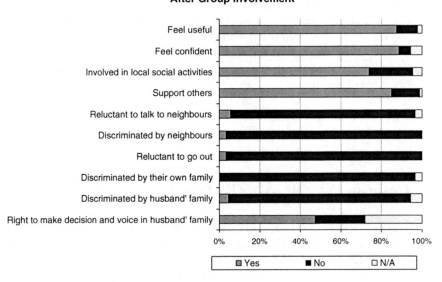

Fig. 14.1 Changes in self-reported social concerns, stigma, and discrimination before and after group involvement

The minority of women who still reported health as a main concern at their evaluation had access to ART and seemed to have been concerned for the health of others, such as their husband.

The shift between priorities, most notably from health to economics, suggests that certain concerns diminished in importance following, and at least partly, a result

Fig. 14.2 Changes in priorities among group members studied

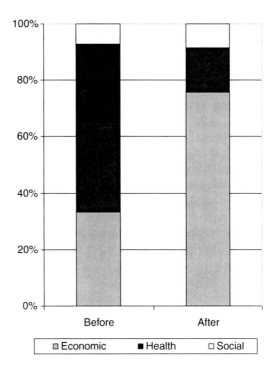

of group membership. No members mentioned low self-esteem issue as a priority area or as something that they wanted to work on in their personal development plan. Collectively, women do understand the gravity of the problem related to their lack of self-esteem, but as individuals, they seemed to feel unable to address this lack of self-esteem. At group meetings, women expressed often that a lack of confidence stopped them from taking actions and initiatives they wanted to take. Examples of activities that women wanted but reported not to feel confident about included applying for jobs, speaking out in public as an HIV-positive women about HIV/AIDS, and doing outreach in their community to reach other HIV-positive women. Women felt these activities were important to themselves and for others. The program, as a consequence of these concerns, had a number of group activities to address this lack of self-confidence. These included activities that helped women to participate in regular public activities just like other women: celebrating women's day, joining moon festival celebrations in the district, or, if this was too public, celebrating such occasions within the group. Other activities were specifically related to HIV/AIDS such as joining the celebration of world AIDS day, either in public or celebrating it more intimately depending on the group member's readiness to be public. Members who felt they wanted to come out in public received various types of communication training, including creative communication training, training on counseling, and hands-on training on making powerpoint presentations. The group was invited at many public events and made visits to parliament and UN agencies and received high-level visitors. Although core members were able to communicate with authorities at public events on behalf of the group, as a collective many of the members seemed to be psychologically immobilized to work on a problem they knew was holding them back.

Income-generating activities, facilitated by the micro-credit loans that were distributed to the support group members through the Women's Union, helped improve the income of those women who were eligible for such a loan based on their business plan. Of the women who received micro-credit, 67% reported an increase in income. This suggests that micro-credit can help HIV-positive mothers who have marketable skills and cannot access credit through regular channels to improve their economic situation. With the exception of Hanoi, where the transfer of responsibility for the repayment of loans moved between different levels of the Women's Union, causing confusion among borrowers, repayment of loans stood at more than 80% across all provinces, while more than 90% of members in Thai Nguyen repaid their loan.

9   Conclusion

As members of a support group for HIV-positive mothers, the women in our study were able to accomplish collective and individual changes such as the mobilization of health, social, and economic support. These occurred in a context where resources such as ART were also increasingly available. We found no clear evidence that the groups functioned as a catalyst for the mobilization of ART, nor that ART was a condition to group formation. Rather, we found a more dynamic and interactive process in which for people who already had access to ART, the group was a place to find additional health support. For others, the group provided an entry point for accessing ART. These processes also inevitably reflect more general contextual changes, including increased international funding to PMTCT, as members were referred to the groups from health facilities that had been provided with additional training, financial, and other resources. For both types of members, however, health was their key priority when they first joined the Sunflowers. And among both types, women reported a dramatic decrease in personal health-related concerns, but some women remained concerned about the health of their spouses. Women's health concerns were mostly replaced by economic concerns. In a few cases, women's pressing concerns disappeared altogether.

Our study confirms earlier findings that HIV-positive women who have marketable skills but cannot access formal credit channels because of discrimination are able to improve their income with targeted support. However, not all HIV-positive women in the groups had marketable and/or entrepreneurial skills but still expressed an interest in improving their income. This study suggests that, similarly to other grassroots and activist organizations, the Sunflowers will need to address the shifting focus towards economic concerns among members whose health and social situations improve, in order to remain meaningful to these members. Although the majority of these HIV-positive mothers live in urban areas where one might not expect farming to be a personal or a professional identity or as something important, agriculture still plays an important role in their lives. Most women reported to be farmers, which has implications for the types of economic activities that are likely to respond to their capacities and interests.

Arguably, improved access to ART, micro-credit, and other support expanded women's ability to make some strategic life choices that they previously lacked, but nonetheless this seemed to not have much effect on women's internal perception of themselves. They continued to have a low self-esteem even in familial and community environments that could not be reasonably categorized as nondiscriminating; women could largely live and eat with their families, they had friends outside their new circle of HIV-positive peers in support groups, and their children were attending school, for example. Mothers reported that the main concerns in their life that needed improvement were related to their individual feelings of being useless and own inability to join in normal social activities, rather than their family's or neighbors' behavior, but none of them made this a priority that they wanted to work on as individuals. These persistent concerns suggest that HIV-positive mothers who are active within a support group, have friends, and have access to a broad network of state-run services can still suffer from a self-inflicted and possibly psychologically immobilizing lack of self-esteem and a sense of circumstantial victimhood.

Of those women who initially reported feeling they had no right to make a decision and have their voice heard in their family, few reported an improvement in their situation. Hence, positive health and social changes in groups and the lives of members are not necessarily contributing to enhanced confidence in the capacity to act at an individual level. The study therefore confirms that an exclusive focus on material resources is unlikely to empower women in the sense of their perceived ability to make and act upon strategic decisions to enhance their lives, even if their context changes and they enjoy improved access to resources. The implications of these research findings for HIV-positive mothers in Vietnam are that they confirm that a combination of micro-credit and health support available through support groups can contribute to concrete, measurable, and experienced individual economic, sociocultural, health empowerment, as well as political empowerment of HIV-positive mothers as a group. Yet, psychological empowerment – confidence, self-esteem, and positive gender conceptions that legitimize their personal sense of dignity and self-respect – seems to continuously elude these HIV-positive mothers.

Acknowledgements   The authors are indebted to the HIV team of the MCNV and their counterparts and to the women at Sunflowers for their contributions as well as their moral support, to Joanna White for very helpful comments and editorial input, and to the main donors of the research and the PMTCT program, the Royal Netherlands Embassy and the Directorate General for International Cooperation (DGIS).

References

Amaro H (1995) Love, sex and power: considering women's realities in HIV prevention. Am Psychol 50:437–447

Barbot J (2006) How to build an "active" patient? The work of AIDS associations in France. Soc Sci Med 62(3):538–551

Bila B, Egrot M (2009) Gender asymmetry in health care-facility attendance of people living with HIV/AIDS in Burkina Faso. Soc Sci Med 69(6):854–861

Bond V, Chilikwela L, Clay S, Kafuma T, Nyblade L, Bettega N (2003) Kanayaka–"the light is on": understanding HIV and AIDS-related stigma in urban and rural Zambia. Zambart Project and KCTT, Lusaka

Braitstein P, Boulle A, Nash D, Brinkhof MW, Dabis F, Laurent C, Low N (2008) Gender and the use of antiretroviral treatment in resource constrained settings: findings from a multicenter collaboration. J Womens Health (Larchmt) 17(1):47–55

Clark S, Bruce J, Dude A (2006) Protecting young women from HIV/AIDS: the case against child and adolescent marriage. Int Fam Plan Perspect 32(2):71–78

Eisen A (1994) Survey of neighborhood-based comprehensive community empowerment initiatives. Health Educ Q 21(2):235–252

Evans S (1980) Personal politics: the roots of women's liberation in the civil rights movement and the new left. Alfred Knopf, New York

Fawcett SB, Paine-Andrews A, Francisco VT, Schultz JA, Richter KP, Lewis RK et al (1995) Using empowerment theory in collaborative partnerships for community health and development. Am J Community Psychol 23(5):677–697, Special Issue: Empowerment theory, research, and application

Freire P (2000) Pedagogy of the oppressed (trans: Ramos MB). The Seabury Press, New York

Gillis A, Perry A (1991) The relationship between physical activity and health promoting behaviors in mid-life women. J Adv Nurs Pract 16:299–310

Harris JD (1998) Incorporating men into Vietnamese gender studies. Vietnam Soc Sci 5(67):1–12

Herek GM, Capitanio GP (1998) Symbolic prejudice or fear of infection? A functional analysis of AIDS-related stigma among heterosexual adults. Basic Appl Soc Psychol Health Med 20(3):230–241

Hirsch JS, Meneses S, Thompson B, Negroni M, Pelcastre B, del Rio C (2007) The inevitability of infidelity: sexual reputation, social geographies, and marital HIV risk in rural Mexico. Am J Public Health 97(6):986–996

Kabeer N (1999) Resources, agency, achievements: reflections on the measurement of women's empowerment. Dev Chang 30:435–464

Kalichman SC, Sikkema KJ, Somlai A (1996) People living with HIV infection who attend and do not attend support groups: a pilot study of needs, characteristics and experiences. AIDS Care 8(5):589–599

Kar K, Pasteur K (2005) Subsidy or self-respect: community-based total sanitation. An update on recent developments. IDS working paper 257, IDS, Brighton. www.ids.ac.uk/ids/bookshop/wp/wp257. Accessed 20 June 2011.

Khuat Thu Hong, Nguyen Thi Van Anh, Ogden J (2004) Understanding HIV and AIDS-related stigma and discrimination. International Center for Research on Women (ICRW), Hanoi

Kling K, Shibley-Hyde J, Showers C, Buswell B (1999) Gender differences in self-esteem: a meta-analysis. Psychol Bull 125(4):470–500

Laverack G (2001) An identification and interpretation of the organizational aspects of community empowerment. Community Dev J 36(2):134–145

Le Coeur S, Collins IJ, Pannetier J, Lelievre E (2009) Gender and access to HIV testing and antiretroviral treatments in Thailand: why do women have more and earlier access? Soc Sci Med 69(6):846–853

Liamputtong P (ed) (2012) Stigma, discrimination and HIV/AIDS: a cross-cultural perspective. Springer, Dordrecht

Liamputtong P, Haritavorn N, Kiatying-Angsulee N (2009) HIV and AIDS, stigma and AIDS support groups: perspectives from women living with HIV and AIDS in central Thailand. Soc Sci Med 69(6):862–868

Malcolm A, Aggleton P, Bronfman M, Galvao J, Mane P, Verrall S (1998) HIV-related stigmatization and discrimination: its forms and contexts. Crit Public Health 8(4):347–370

Malhotra A, Schuler SR, Boender C (2002) Measuring women's empowerment as a variable in international development. Paper presented at the background paper for the World Bank workshop on poverty and gender: new perspectives, Washington DC

Marquis M, Shatenstein B (2005) Food choice motives and the importance of family meals among immigrant mothers. Can J Diet Pract Res 66(2):77–82

McCarthy JD, Zald MN (1977) Resource mobilization and social movements: a partial theory. Am J Sociol 82(6):1212–1241

National Committee for AIDS, Drugs, and Prostitution Prevention and Control (2010) The fourth country report on following up the implementation to the declaration of commitment on HIV and AIDS reporting period Jan 2008 – Dec 2009. Period report. National Committee for AIDS, Drugs, and Prostitution Prevention and Control, Hanoi

Nguyen TA, Oosterhoff P, Pham NY, Wright P, Hardon A (2009) Self-help groups can improve utilization of postnatal care by HIV-infected mothers. J Assoc Nurses AIDS Care 20(2):141–152

Nguyen T, Nam CB, Mogensen HO, Rasch V (2010) Factors associated with the failure to seek HIV care and treatment among HIV-positive women in a northern province of Vietnam. AIDS Patient Care STDS 24(5):325–332

Ochs E, Merav S (2006) The cultural structuring of mealtime socialization. New Dir Child Adolesc Dev 111(2):35–49, Special Issue: Family mealtime as a context of development and socialization

Ojkutu BO, Stone VE (2005) Women, inequality, and the burden of HIV. N Engl J Med 352:649–652

Oosterhoff P (2008) "Pressure to bear": gender, fertility and prevention of mother to child transmission of HIV in Vietnam. PhD thesis, Amsterdam Institute for Social Science Research, The Netherlands. http://www.mcnv.nl/uploads/media/Pressure_to_Bear.pdf. Accessed 30 Mar 2011.

Oosterhoff P (2009) Observations on action research with HIV-positive women and state service providers in northern Vietnam. Medische Antropologie 21(2):257–275

Oosterhoff P, Wright P, Nguyen TA, Pham NY, Hardon A (2007) Towards a continuum of care for mother and child: exploring prevention of mother to child transmission programs in Hanoi and Thai Nguyen. Medical Committee of Netherlands – Vietnam, Hanoi

Oosterhoff P, Nguyen TA, Pham NY, Wright P, Hardon A (2008) Can micro-credit empower HIV+ women? An exploratory case study in Northern Vietnam. Women's Health Urban Life 7(1). http://www.utsc.utoronto.ca/~socsci/sever/journal/contents7.1.html. Accessed 30 Mar 2011.

Raphael D (1993) Self-esteem & health: should it be a focus? The University of Toronto/Centre for Health Promotion, Toronto, Ontario, Canada

Rifkin SB (1986) Lessons from community participation in health programmes. Health Policy Plan 1(3):240–249

Rosenbrock R, Dubois-Arber F, Moers M, Pinell P, Schaeffer D, Setbon M (2000) The normalization of AIDS in Western European countries. Soc Sci Med 50(11):1607–1629

SRV (1984) Resolution no 176a-HĐBT on upholding the roles and abilities of women in the career of country's building and protection. http://vbqppl.moj.gov.vn/law/vi/1981_to_1990/1984/198 412/198412240003. Accessed 24 Sept 2011.

SRV (2002) Decision No 19/2002/QD-TTg ratifying the National Strategy for advancement of Vietnamese women till 2010. //vbqppl.moj.gov.vn/law/en/2001_to_2010/2002/200201/20020 1210002_en/lawdocument_view.Accessed 21 Jan 2011.

UNAIDS, UNFPA, UINIFEM (2004) Women and HIV/AIDS: confronting the crisis. http://www.unfpa.org/hiv/women/docs/women_aids.pdf. Accessed 30 Mar 2011.

Vanlandingham M, Im-Em W, Yokota F (2006) Access to treatment and care associated with HIV infection among members of AIDS support groups in Thailand. AIDS Care 18(7):637–646

World Health Organization (2008) Towards universal access: scaling up priority HIV/AIDS interventions in the health sector: progress 640 report 2008. http://www.who.int/hiv/pub/ towards_universal_access_report_2008.pdf. Accessed 30 Mar 2011.

Chapter 15
Women, Motherhood, and Living Positively: The Lived Experience of Thai Women Living with HIV/AIDS

Pranee Liamputtong, Niphattra Haritavorn, and Niyada Kiatying-Angsulee

1 Introduction

The HIV/AIDS epidemic has entered its fourth decade and continues to be a major public health problem worldwide (Norman et al. 2009). It has now tremendously affected women around the globe (Zhou 2008). Of the 33.4 million people worldwide who are living with HIV/AIDS in 2008, 15.7 million were women (The Joint United Nations Programme on HIV/AIDS (UNAIDS) AIDS epidemic update, 2009). In Asia, the AIDS epidemic continues to grow, and compared with 1.7 million in 2003, at the end of 2005, the number of women living with HIV was estimated at two million (UNAIDS 2005). Thailand is one of the Asian countries that have been hit hard by the epidemic of HIV/AIDS.

Ever since the diagnosis of the first case of AIDS in 1984, the epidemic has risen rapidly and now it has affected people from injecting drug users, sex workers, heterosexual men, their wives, and sexual partners to the infants of infected mothers (Singhanetra-Renard et al. 2001). Currently, about one million Thai people are living with HIV/AIDS (UNAIDS/World Health Organization (WHO) 2008). Although Thailand has successfully reduced the spread of HIV among female and

P. Liamputtong (✉)
School of Public Health, La Trobe University,
Kingsbury Drive, Bundoora, VIC 3086, Australia
e-mail: pranee@latrobe.edu.au

N. Haritavorn
Faculty of Public Health, Thammasat University,
Rangsit Road, Rangsit, Patoomthani 12121, Thailand
e-mail: niphattraha@yahoo.com

N. Kiatying-Angsulee
Social Research Institute (CUSRI), Chulalongkorn University,
Bangkok 10330, Thailand
e-mail: niyada.k@chula.ac.th

P. Liamputtong (ed.), *Women, Motherhood and Living with HIV/AIDS:*
A Cross-Cultural Perspective, DOI 10.1007/978-94-007-5887-2_15,
© Springer Science+Business Media Dordrecht 2013

male sex workers and their clients (McCamish et al. 2000), the number of HIV seroprevalence among pregnant women has steadily increased (Ruxrungtham and Phanuphak 2001). In 1998, there were approximately 23,000 HIV-positive women who gave birth in Thailand (Siriwasin et al. 1998), and around 26 % of HIV-infected women in Bangkok had HIV-negative partners. In 2007, there were 250,000 HIV-positive women, aged 15 and over, living in Thailand (UNAIDS/WHO 2008). Similarly to women in other parts of Asia (Ainsworth et al. 2003), Thai women contracted HIV from having sex within monogamous relationships with partners who engaged in high-risk behavior (Siriwasin et al. 1998; Liamputtong et al. 2009).

Living with HIV/AIDS signifies the need to deal with numerous emotional challenges resulting from compound losses, anxieties, fears, self-blame, and social stigmatization (Plattner and Meiring 2006). Culturally, HIV in Thai society is still perceived as a "death sentence." Because physical and moral appearances are important in Thai society, shame is therefore experienced by Thai people infected with HIV/AIDS (Bennetts et al. 1999; Liamputtong et al. 2009). The continuing high rates of HIV/AIDS and the shame and stigmatization attached to the epidemic are due mainly to inadequate knowledge and understanding of the infection and its transmission among Thai people.

Although living with an incurable illness and feeling uncertainty about one's own health condition is a very stressful experience, many HIV-positive individuals are able to maintain their emotional well-being (Pakenham and Rinaldis 2001). This begs the question of what strategies these individuals employ to allow them to do so (Plattner and Meiring 2006). In this chapter, we examine the strategies that Thai women who are mothers and living with HIV/AIDS use to deal with their health condition. In doing so, it is essential that we must situate our discussion within a theoretical framework, and the theory which is relevant to our research question examined in this chapter is the living positively discourse that we discuss below.

2   Living Positively Discourse: Theoretical Framework

Living positively discourse has been adopted to explain positive living among those with disabilities and illnesses, but it is particularly advocated for people living with HIV/AIDS. The discourse makes use of a specific "narrative account of life with HIV" to alter the damage, which is brought to one's life by an HIV diagnosis, into a rational story (Levy and Storeng 2007: 56). The narrative is not just "a creative story making" but a means for an individual living with HIV/AIDS to reconcile the new reality within the existing prospect of his/her life. It emphasizes the ability of an individual living with HIV/AIDS to boost "self-fulfillment" in spite of the hardship associated with being diagnosed and living with a life-threatening health condition. This can be accommodated through changed actions and understandings characterized as "positive living advice" (Levy and Storeng 2007: 56).

For many individuals, in particular those who lack or have limited access to sufficient health care, adopting positive living advice offers a possible means to change the course of HIV/AIDS. It is suggested that healthy diet, exercise, sufficient sleep, stress decrease, preventive actions (such as using condoms to prevent the reinfection of HIV), and proper health-care seeking will enhance immune functioning of the body and hence postpone the inception of opportunistic infections and AIDS. Within the positive living discourse, it is theorized that the potential for individuals to participate in these behaviors is made possible by their "open and accepting attitude toward HIV" (Levy and Storeng 2007: 56). This can be achieved by revealing one's HIV status to others such as family members and friends and participating in AIDS support groups where the discourses of positive living are often discussed and emotional and social support can be obtained. The living positively discourse contests not only "the image of the culpable AIDS sufferer" but also "the assumption that an HIV diagnosis leads to an inevitably rapid demise" (Levy and Storeng 2007: 56).

Living positively is essential for people living with HIV/AIDS because it contests the disapproving social interpretations of the disease. It is now known that HIV/AIDS has "a polysemic concept" (Levy and Storeng 2007: 59). The disease produces the disruption of the "embodied experience" of those living with it. It implies not just a continuing decline of the bodily immune reaction but has dealt with diverse meanings connected with sexuality, class, gender, and ethnicity. This has led Treichler (1988) to refer to AIDS as "an epidemic of signification." Moral judgments such as good and bad, right and wrong, and responsibility and danger have been implanted within the social interpretations of HIV/AIDS (Levy and Storeng 2007). All too often, being infected with HIV is connected with promiscuity, unruly behavior, and other types of discriminated "risky" conducts (Levy and Storeng 2007: 59). As such, AIDS is seen as being produced by "a moral failure" of the individual (Brandt and Rozin 1997). Once labeled as such, these individuals are disconnected from other identity groups (Schoepf 2001). By definition then, they are despoiled and stigmatized (Levy and Storeng 2007). Living positively allows individuals living with HIV/AIDS to fight against the negative images of the disease and hence be able to deal with their conditions and environments in a more positive way.

Nevertheless, we contend that to be able to live positively, individuals are required to make meaning of their life circumstances. Here, the discourse of "meaning making" (Plattner and Meiring 2006) becomes relevant. The concept of meaning making was theorized by Park and Folkman (1997) within the broader framework of stress and coping theory. According to Park and Folkman, meaning making is "a psychological process" which elucidates how individuals construe acutely traumatic and potentially destructive incidents that occur to them. Often, on encountering a shocking and stressful experience, people would pose the question why it happened to them. In the process of looking for underlying explanations, people "construct meaning from the event." Park and Folkman (1997) theorize that meaning making can be perceived as both "part of coping" and "an outcome of the coping process" which individuals experience when dealing with stressful incidents. Meaning making can be different and change over time. This depends on the person's broad outlook toward life and the personal significance that an event has for him/her. However, it is only through meaning making that people are equipped to cope with stressful life-changing events. Those who cannot make meaning out of specific experiences would have difficulties dealing with them (Park and Folkman 1997). According to Plattner and Meiring (2006), meaning-making discourse assists us to understand how individuals handle the situations of living with HIV/AIDS.

3   The Study

This chapter is based on our larger project on the experiences of women living with HIV and AIDS who have participated or are participating in drug trials in Thailand (see also Liamputtong et al. 2009). Because of the epidemic of HIV infection and AIDS in the country, numerous clinical trial centers have been established in Thailand. These trials are supported by international organizations and agencies in developed nations, mainly the United States. The HIV/AIDS Collaborative Centre was established in 1990 within the Ministry of Public Health in Nonthaburi, located on the periphery of Bangkok. It is a joint venture of the United States Centers for Disease Control and Prevention and the Ministry of Public Health of Thailand. Most clinical trials in Thailand are carried out in general and specialist hospitals and medical schools at the provincial, regional, and national levels (Chokevivat 1998).

A qualitative approach is adopted in this study. This approach is appropriate because qualitative researchers accept that, to understand people's behavior, we must attempt to understand the meanings and interpretations that people give to their behavior. This approach is particularly appropriate when the researcher has little knowledge of the researched participants and their world views (Padgett 2008; Liamputtong 2013).

Because we aimed to examine the lived experiences of women living with HIV and AIDS, descriptive phenomenology was adopted as our methodological framework. Descriptive phenomenology allows researchers to understand the issues under study from the experiences of those who have lived through it (Carpenter 2010; Norlyk and Harder 2010). Hence, this permitted us to examine the experiences of HIV-positive women and how they dealt with HIV and AIDS in our study. Within the phenomenological framework, in-depth interviews are usually adopted by qualitative researchers. In this study, in-depth interviews and some participant observations were conducted with 26 Thai women.

Purposive sampling technique (Morse 2006; Liamputtong 2013) was adopted; that is, only Thai women who had experienced HIV and AIDS and who were participating, or had participated, in HIV clinical trials were approached to participate in the study. The participants were recruited through advertising on bulletin boards at hospitals where drug trials have been undertaken and personal contacts made by the Thai coresearchers, who have carried out a number of HIV and AIDS research projects with Thai women. In conducting research related to HIV and AIDS, the recruitment process needs to be highly sensitive to the needs of the participants (Liamputtong 2007; Stevens et al. 2010). The sensitivity of this research guided our discussion of how we would approach the women and invite them to take part in this research. We only directly contact potential participants ourselves after being introduced by our network or gatekeepers. Because of the sensitive nature of this study, we also relied on snowball sampling techniques, that is, our previous participants suggested others who were interested in participating (Liamputtong 2013). We enlisted the assistance of leaders of two HIV and AIDS support groups to access the women in this study. We also took part in the activities of the groups as part of the methodology of our study.

The number of participants was determined by theoretical sampling technique, which is to stop recruiting when little new data emerges, and this signifies data saturation (Patton 2002; Liamputtong 2013). The sociodemographic characteristics of the women are as follows. The majority of the women were aged between 31 and 40 years. Four were under 30 years of age and five were over 40. Most (25) are Buddhist and one is Muslim. Nineteen women were living with their new partners at the time of the interview, one was married, two were divorced, two were widowed, and another two were single mothers. Twelve women had only primary school education, 11 finished secondary school education, and three had vocational college training. At the time of the interview, seven women worked as outreach health workers, six were self-employed, four were office workers, five had casual employment, one was unemployed, and three women performed home duties. All the women, except one, were mothers: 13 women had 2 children and 11 had only 1 child. One woman was pregnant when she was interviewed. Twenty-three women had children who were HIV negative and three women did not know about the HIV status of their children. Twelve women had family income of less than 5,000 baht (about US$160) per month and 12 received income of between 5,000 and 10,000 baht (US$160 and $322). Only two women had a family income of more than 10,000 baht. Eighteen women were covered by the "30 baht scheme" health insurance (under the coverage of the government), seven were under the "Social Security scheme," and one has no health insurance coverage.

Interviews were conducted in the Thai language to maintain as much as possible the subtlety and any hidden meaning of the participant's statements (Liamputtong 2010). Prior to the commencement of the study, ethical approval was obtained from the Faculty of Health Sciences Human Ethics Committee, La Trobe University, Australia, and Ethics Committee at Chulalongkorn University, Thailand. Before making an appointment for interviews, the participant's consent to participate in the study was sought. After a full explanation of the study, the length of interviewing time, and the scope of questions, the participants were asked to sign a consent form. Each interview took between 1 and 2 h. Each participant was paid 200 Thai baht as a compensation for their time in taking part in this study. This incentive is necessary for a sensitive research because it is a way to show that research participants are respected for their time and knowledge.

When we participated in women's activities, they were informed that it was part of our research and there was no separate informed consent obtained for this method. We used participant observation as a means of field observations.

With permission from the participants, interviews were tape-recorded. The tapes were then transcribed verbatim in Thai for data analysis. The in-depth data was analyzed using a thematic analysis (Braun and Clarke 2006; Liamputtong 2013). This method of data analysis aims to identify, analyze, and report patterns or themes within the data. Initially, we performed open coding where codes were first developed and named. Then, axial coding was applied which was used to develop the final themes within the data. This was done by reorganizing the codes which we have developed from the data during open coding in new ways by making connections between categories and subcategories. This resulted in themes, and they were used to explain the lived experiences of the participants. The emerging themes are presented in the findings section. In presenting women's verbatim responses, we used their fictitious names to preserve confidentiality of the women's identity.

Several themes emerged from the interview data. These themes are discussed according to the sequence of events which reflect the lived experiences of the participants. They are presented below.

4   Learning About HIV-Positive Status

As Singhanetra-Renard and colleagues (2001) and Maman and associates (2009) have shown in their studies, most women in our study too learned about their HIV status through their contacts with health services (see also Chaps. 3, 4, 16, and 17 in this volume). Most often, it was during their pregnancies when they went for an antenatal care checkup, referred to as *fak thong* in Thailand, that they were told by health professionals that they *pen AIDS* (have AIDS):

> I knew about it when I was two months pregnant. Because I came to *fak thong* at hospital that I learned that I *pen AIDS*. When I was told about it, I first felt so sad because it should not have happened to me like this. (Ajchara)

Nataree was suspicious of her illness about 13 years ago when her husband was still alive, but she never went for a blood test. Even after his death, she was still unsure if she had contracted the disease from her husband. After living with a new partner, she became pregnant, and it was through antenatal care that she learned about her HIV status:

> I became pregnant with my new partner's child so I went for a checkup. After the checkup, they told me to come back for a counseling session, and that was the time they told me that I had a virus and they asked me if I wanted to take antiretroviral drugs which will prevent me passing the disease to my baby.

Other women learned about the HIV status through contact with health professionals for other health issues. One woman had to have an operation to remove a lump in her uterus. After a blood test, she was told that she has AIDS. Other women only came to know about their HIV status when their husbands/partners became very ill.

5 Women's Feelings Once Learned

The inevitability of being confronted by death, sooner or later, and the stigma attached to HIV/AIDS make the disease "one of the most feared of all diseases" (Plattner and Meiring 2006: 241). Hence, being informed that one is HIV-positive is often met with feelings of shock and emotional devastation, and for many, they also have ideas of suicide (Jirapaet 2001; Maman et al. 2009; Ross et al. 2007a; see also Chaps. 3 and 12 in this volume). In the study conducted by Maman and colleagues (2009: 967), many participants were "emotionally unprepared" when informed about the diagnosis of HIV-positive status. Sanders (2008) also found in her research in the USA that most women were extremely shocked, frightened, and sorrowful on learning about their HIV status. This was mainly because of the fact that they believed they would die soon. In our study, Puangchompoo said she was so shocked about the bad news and she cried for three nights because she believed she would die very soon. Meena too said that:

> When I knew the result that I was HIV-positive, I was so shocked. I walked out without any real feelings but only the thought that I had no more hope in this life. I could not speak and *nam ta tok nai* (my tears were coming down inside me). I went home and told my husband that the doctor found AIDS in me. He was also shocked and said nothing, just kept quiet.

For these women, being told that they had HIV was a disruption of "the taken-for-granted conceptions of self" (Levy and Storeng 2007: 58). The positive diagnosis of HIV status produces what Pierret (2000: 59) has referred to as a "watershed" that unravel the "before" and "after" life of most HIV-positive people. Kesaree remarked:

> I could not say a word after hearing what the doctor told me. I only cried and cried because I could not accept it. It was my first pregnancy. And I was only selling my groceries at home, never went out to mix with people. I could not accept that I have the disease. From that day on, I could not eat even though I was pregnant. And I was so stressed out. I was losing weight because I could not eat and because of the stress.

All the women also felt puzzled about their HIV status. They were housewives who stayed home to look after family and had never been promiscuous; they could not have contracted a serious disease like HIV. When Naree, who was told about her HIV status when she went for the antenatal check up of her first child at a hospital, was asked how she felt when she was told, she remarked that:

> It was impossible and I did not want to believe it. I never had sex with other men and never went to bars or clubs to drink, only work and look after home. How could I believe that I got it?

Many women have thought of or attempted suicide after being diagnosed with HIV. Plattner and Meiring (2006) found in the study that the participants considered committing suicide after learning about their HIV serostatus. In Thailand,

Bennetts and colleagues (1999), Jirapaet (2001), and Ross and Srisaeng (2005) suggested that shame, despair, and suicidal thoughts were common among pregnant women and mothers of young children who were HIV-positive. Some women in our study became so distressed that they wanted to end their lives:

> When the doctor told me about it, I cried because I was so sad that why it happened to me. I was so sad because I did not expect that I would get the disease. I was afraid that people would know about my illness and then *rang kiat* (discriminate) me. I did not know what I should do, so I *kit san* (think of shortening her life). (Ajchara)

For Sinjai, she went further than Ajchara in trying to kill herself. She jumped from the second floor of her house. But, she and the baby survived:

> I walked out from the hospital and I did not cry. When I got home, I did not think about anything else. On the way home, in a train, my husband asked me what was the matter with me, but I said nothing. I was thinking about what the nurse said to me, that I must be the one who got the disease and passed it on to my husband. I was thinking a lot. When my husband went outside the house, I jumped from the second floor. I was seven months pregnant then, but nothing happened.

6 Living Positively: Dealing with the Illness

Once it is confirmed that they had HIV, women attempted to deal with HIV/AIDS in diverse ways. Plattner and Meiring (2006: 243), in their study, contended that although the women still felt disturbed and troubled and their financial and social burden might continue, all of them had eventually accepted that "they were HIV-positive." The women in our study too had attempted to live positively once they have accepted their illness status.

6.1 Taking Care of Self

Once they were sure that they had HIV, most women would try to take care of themselves to prolong their lives. Eating healthily, exercising, and not thinking too much about the health condition and life were means to live positively. Wasana said that she would do a few things to look after her own self:

> If I have got time, I will rest. I will take rice and milk on schedule. I will eat fruits and vegetables, in fact anything that will make me healthy. I used to have CD4 166 but now it has increased a lot. Now, it is 400. It has come up a lot because the doctor advises me to eat lots of vegetables, fish, meat and milk. I have and my CD4 has increased a lot. My doctor says that I was great.

Some women would attempt to do anything to make themselves better and, for some women, to cure the illness:

> My cousin took my husband to take *ya tom samoon prai* (brewed herbal medicines). If people told us that there were good medicines somewhere, even it is far away from my

home, my cousin would take him there and I would also go because I wanted to be cured from this disease. It was like all eight corners of my world were so dark that I did not know what to do to recover from this disease, so when people say there were good medicine, we would go to find them. (Pensri)

6.2 Accepting Faith

Thai Buddhists see HIV/AIDS as "a disease of Karma (*rok khong khon mee kam*)" (Jirapaet 2001: 26). Research in Thailand revealed that people living with HIV/ AIDS (PLWHV) believed that their suffering from AIDS was the consequence of their own karma (Kobotani and Engstrom 2005; Ross et al. 2007a, b; Balthip et al. 2012; see also Chap. 12 in this volume). Most women in our study perceived that their HIV status was brought on by their own *wen kam* (karma). In Thai culture, *wen kam* refers to a bad or evil deed that the person has committed and therefore causes disastrous consequences. The law of karma is that every action, be it good or bad, has its consequences. The outcomes are inescapable but might happen immediately after one has performed or long afterward, or even in subsequent lives (Ross et al. 2007a). From the strong belief in the law of karma among Buddhists, it follows that the state of an individual's present existence is the consequence of his/her karma accumulated in previous lives (Klunklin and Greenwood 2005). The more good deeds are accumulated from a past life, the better and happier the state of being will be experienced in the present one. The opposite holds true for bad deeds, and usually these result in *wen kam* of an individual.

Meena talked about this when she told us about how she contracted HIV. She was a single woman and working in Bangkok until the death of her father. Because there was no one to take over the rubber plantation in the south of Thailand, she returned to her father's home. As a single woman, it became difficult for her to look after the plantation. Her nephew introduced her to her husband who was at that time a single man, and after a few meetings, she decided to marry him and expected to have children soon afterward. However, her dream was shattered when she contracted HIV from her husband. She spoke about her *wen kam* that:

It is really my *wen kam* that I come across terrible experience like this. I was living in Bangkok for a long time and nothing bad happened to me, but when I returned to the south and married, I have to deal with this huge problem until I gave birth to my son.

However, Kobotani and Engstrom (2005) suggest that their participants' belief in karma also assisted them to accept that their AIDS was the part of life which is seen as suffering in Buddhism. Connecting their AIDS to karma signifies that they were not the only ones who are suffering; other human beings who live in this life are also suffering. Buddhist teachings are employed as a means to help individuals living with HIV/AIDS to "understand and make sense of what AIDS is and how to cope" (Kobotani and Engstrom 2005: 18). In their study, Ross and colleagues (2007b) also suggested that all Thai women believed that their belief in karma permitted them to embrace the reality of their health status, feel more at peace with their condition, take care of themselves, and continue their lives (see also Balthip et al. 2013; Chap. 12 in this volume).

Wen kam assisted many women in our study to deal with their life-threatening illness better. In the case of Sinjai, who attempted suicide by jumping from the second floor of her house, the doctor consoled her and told her not to think too much about the disease. In a way, the doctor promoted the "positive living" discourse (Levy and Storeng 2007: 59); he offered her some ways that she could deal with the diagnosis and HIV:

> The doctor told me that we, as a human being, always get something in our life. If we do not contract one disease now, one day we will get another one. He told me not to think too much about my HIV and he gave me a lot of counseling and support. He gave me good information about the disease and how to take care of myself. Because of this doctor, I then decided not to kill myself and also accept my situation. So, I can now live with the disease.

The doctor also suggested that it was her own *wen kam* that she contracted HIV. The doctor and nurses were all supportive of her and this helped her not to give up her life and to deal with her illness better. She also realized that she has already got the virus and she would not be able to recover from it, so she had to deal with it as best as possible, and this has stopped her from thinking of committing suicide.

The women also suggested that to reduce their own *wen kam* in this life and the next, they must perform more good deeds in their present life. This is part of the beliefs in Thai Buddhism. Ross and colleagues (2007b) have also suggested that the women in their study believed that doing good things in the present life would allow them to be better off later on in this present or next life. Hence, the women in their study performed many good deeds such as giving alms to Buddhist monks, freeing animals, and giving out money to unfortunate people. These simple actions are commonly carried out by Thai people including the women in our study.

6.3 Disclosure to Family Members

Literature suggests that people living with HIV/AIDS tend to conceal their health status for fear of being discriminated against and rejected (Anderson and Doyal 2004; Varga and Brookes 2008; Medley et al. 2009; Greeff 2013; Ho and Mak 2013; see Chaps. 8 and 16 in this volume). Somsri said:

> I can't tell anyone about my HIV. I don't want to tell anyone anyway because people will *rang kiat* (discriminate against) me and they would not want to have anything to do with me. People still have a lot of fears about HIV and AIDS in my community. If they know I have AIDS, I and my family will have a lot of problem living around here.

However, some would disclose it to their significant others, particularly family members (Baumgartner 2007; Dageid and Duckett 2008). Some women in our study dealt with the illness by telling their extended family members, and most often, the women would confide in their mothers. For Nataree, for example, her mother was the first person who knew about her illness:

I told my mother as the first person. We talked about the illness and other things. My mother did not *rang kiat* (discriminate against) me, but gave me *kam lang jai* (emotional support). I told her when I was very sick. I did not take any medication and I had viral infection in my mouth, so I went home and told my mother about it.

Ross and associates (2007a), in their study, suggested that the disclosure of their HIV status to family members or partners led to gaining support from them. We asked the women who said they had informed their family members about their feelings on this. Most women expressed that revealing the status of their illness to family members helped them to deal with their health and other issues better than trying to keep it secret. It also made them feel more relieved and less frustrated. Sinjai elaborated:

I feel *sabai jai* (relieved) from living with the feelings of frustration about not being able to talk about it. It also makes me stronger about my life. If I say anything, they understand my points. They used to question me about what I do and why I do it my ways, like when I was sick often, they thought that I was *sam oi* (being too weak and too lazy to do anything). But, now if I am sick or have headaches and can't get up to do anything, or if I am tired often, they understand my situations.

Yardtip too said that telling family members about the illness had helped her to deal with the illness better because she received more support from them:

When I was *kread* (too much emotional stress to deal with), my symptoms became worse. I could not eat and I lost a lot of weight; I was down to 38 kgs. Virus started to creep in and every evening I would have bad headache. It was so terrible and I was so thin. So, I decided to tell my sister. After I told her, it was much better. From trying to ignore each other before, we are now much closer. Because she knew about my HIV, she has looked after me. She would ring me often. When I was having side effects from ARV, she came to stay and look after me. I think telling your family is good. Before, I would keep everything inside my chest. Now, I can just ring her and talk about my health problems.

6.4   Joining AIDS Support Groups

Joining AIDS support groups has been employed by many people living with HIV/AIDS (PLWHA) as a means to counteract stigma about their conditions and lives (Levy and Storeng 2007; Liamputtong et al. 2009; Lyttlteon et al. 2007; see also Chap. 14 in this volume). This strategy was also used by some women in our study. Belonging to an AIDS support group helped the women to be able to reverse the shame and stigma that come with HIV and AIDS. Collectively, a support group was a means that the women employed to fight against stigma and discrimination that they felt or experienced (see Chap. 14).

Because of the issue of disclosure and social acceptance, most PLWHA tend to seek emotional support from people who share similar conditions such as other PLWHA, rather than close friends and family (Liamputtong et al. 2009). Belonging to a support group allows PLWHA to access more emotional support from their peers (Levy and Storeng 2007). In our study, PLWHA support groups provided emotional support to many women. Kanokwan felt relieved after joining an HIV/

AIDS group because it allowed her to talk to *puag diew kan* (people who have similar experiences). Learning more about others in the group also made women emotionally stronger about their own HIV status. Wasana too remarked that:

> Joining the group activity is good because I can meet many of my friends there. Everyone in the group looks good [no negative physical appearances], and this makes me have more emotional strength that it is not only me who has got this disease in the world.

Support groups offered women more knowledge about the illness and how to deal with it better. As Foucault (1980) theorizes, with more knowledge, individuals believe that they have more power to deal with their situations. Support groups also provided women with a sense of belonging. Women got to know more about others who were in the same situation as themselves. By joining the group, it made them realize that they were not alone in the world living with HIV and AIDS. With more knowledge and a greater sense of belonging, support groups offered the women emotional strength to deal with stigma and their health conditions. Joining support groups created collective power for all women, and this collective power allowed the women to defend their conditions and view themselves in a more positive light (see also Chap. 14).

7 Living Positively: Constraints

Although the living positively discourse is seen as a positive attempt to assist women to deal with their HIV/AIDS, it is not without constraints. As discussed above, disclosure had resulted in more support from family members and others. But, we also found that some women who disclosed their HIV status to family were discriminated and rejected by those around them. Orachorn told us that:

> When I told my mother about my HIV, she stopped talking to me. She would avoid me as much as she could. She would separate kitchen utensils and she would not wash her clothes in the same tub as me. She would eat in a separate room. I felt so sad when my own mother *rang kiat* me like this.

In their study, Plattner and Meiring (2006) revealed that some of the participants who disclosed their HIV status to family members and friends received harsh rejection from those whom they told. Ugandan women in Withell's study (2000) were also rejected by their family after the disclosure of their HIV status. See also Greeff (2013) for a review of this issue.

Most often, the rejection of family members in our study stemmed from the lack of understanding about HIV/AIDS. Isara's brother and sister-in-law, for example, did not wish to be close to her and her children for fear of being contaminated by HIV. Her children were HIV-negative. She remarked:

> Talking about my family, I cannot touch my niece. My sister invited my brother and the family for dinner at a restaurant and my children went with my sister. My brother would not eat anything that day and after that he rang my sister and scolded her for taking my children to the dinner. My brother has good education and work as a manager but he is very afraid of this

disease. He is afraid that my children would pass it onto his child. My sister told him that my children won't pass anything onto his child, but he does not believe her. When I was in hospital, my children wanted to see me and asked my sister to take them. My brother told my sister not to take the children to visit me because they might contract the disease from me.

Living positively requires one to take care of oneself by eating healthily and adhering to medication (Levy and Storeng 2007). However, the maintenance of this lifestyle can be challenged by the living reality of the person, particularly for those with little resources available to them. Having good nutrition is claimed to be one of the efficacious means to maintain sufficient immune functioning (Levy and Storeng 2007). However, many people living with HIV/AIDS are, as Singhanetra-Renard and colleagues (2001: 174) refer to them, people who *ha chao kin kham* (earn in the morning and eat in the evening) or subsist on day-to-day wage employment in Thailand. For the same reason, some of the women in our study found their attempts to obtain nutritious food for good health met with difficulty. Their living condition could also impact on the adherence of medication and they had less time to take care of themselves.

Additionally, only some women had the luxury to join AIDS support groups. Many others in our study could not do so because of their family commitment and work. Hence, the living positively discourse can be a constraint for some women living with HIV/AIDS.

8   Discussions and Conclusion

Living with HIV/AIDS signifies the need to deal with numerous emotional challenges resulting from not only feelings of losses, fears, and self-blame but also social stigmatization (Plattner and Meiring 2006). However, many HIV-positive individuals, including the women in our study, are able to maintain their emotional well-being (Pakenham and Rinaldis 2001). We have discussed some of the strategies that the women in our study adopted as a means to deal with their health conditions. These include taking care of own self, accepting one's own faith, disclosure of their HIV status to family members, and joining AIDS support groups. These strategies can be situated within the "living positively" discourse theorized by Levy and Storeng (2007). Living positively creates "a sense of optimism about combating the HIV epidemic" (Levy and Storeng 2007: 56) among the women in our study.

The women in our study not only took an active role in ensuring their own health by taking care of themselves but also employed more positive attitudes about their life as a way to deal with their HIV status (Levy and Storeng 2007). Many women used their religious beliefs to cope with their health condition more positively. According to Plattner and Meiring (2006: 244), for those living with HIV/AIDS, ascribing their HIV-positive status to religion and faith made their health status more meaningful. This ascription not only brings "a purpose to their infection but also hope." The women in our study also attributed their HIV status to their own karma. Religion can be a means for individuals to cope with difficulties in their lives when there is no other hope left for them (Plattner and Meiring 2006). Religion performs a crucial role in the process of meaning making (Park and Folkman 1997). Ascribing health conditions to something beyond one's control, such as karma, is a mechanism that makes the reality of one's life more meaningful and comprehensible (Plattner and Meiring 2006). The belief that their HIV status was the result of their own *wen kam* was a good rationality for allowing the women in our study to also develop their hope by doing good deeds. Hope allowed them to be able to focus on their future. This was crucial because it made them not give up on life (Plattner and Meiring 2006).

The living positively discourse dictates that individuals must accept their HIV status and be open about their condition (Levy and Storeng 2007). This can be achieved by revealing one's HIV status to significant others such as family members and friends because this disclosure could also lead to support from them (Ross et al. 2007a). This was the experiences of many of the women in our study. Participating in AIDS support groups where positive living is often discussed and emotional and social support can be obtained is another salient aspect of the living positively discourse. Many women in our study joined AIDS support groups for this reason. The AIDS support groups in Thailand can be seen to provide "strength" to the positive living dictum. AIDS support groups in Thailand not only act as "a panacea for stigma and alienation" (Lyttlteon et al. 2007: S49) but are also "the site of communication and empowerment" (Levy and Storeng 2007: 62). Support groups offer those living with HIV/AIDS a space to socialize with others who are in the same situation and form groups which Alonzo and Reynolds (1995) refer to as "a community of 'own'." Within this new community, people realize that despite their health condition, they are able to assist other HIV-positive individuals with emotional support and knowledge that they have generated from their lived experiences. This creates the opportunity for them to see themselves as "individuals with strengths and resources" rather than as "victims" of HIV/AIDS (de Jager and Kirk 1998; Levy and Storeng 2007: 62).

Nevertheless, not all women in our study were able to follow the living positively discourse. Implicitly, the dictum anticipates that individuals would take responsibility to live healthily without considering the social and structural constrictions that might impact on the behaviors of these individuals (Levy and Storeng 2007). A simple task such as consuming nutritious food can be a formidable task for those who are poor. As we have pointed out, although the women in our study attempted to adhere to "openness rhetoric of disclosure" (Levy and Storeng 2007: 61), in reality, for some women, disclosure led to rejection instead of support from their significant others. Joining AIDS support groups might seem like a simple thing to do, but not all women could do so because of their family commitment and other constraints in their everyday life.

Notably, after the initial shock of learning about their HIV status, most of the women in our study had accepted this reality. The acceptance of their HIV status played an essential role in the meaning-making process because it assisted individuals living with the infection to be able to sustain the equilibrium of their emotional well-being (Plattner and Meiring 2006). According to Park and Folkman (1997), acceptance is "a means of resolution" because it propitiates a traumatic life event with the purposes, beliefs, and cultural norms of the individuals. Acceptance allows them to be able to manage their conditions because it is they who decide to "make 'peace' with their life circumstances" (Plattner and Meiring 2006: 243).

In conclusion, we have shown in this chapter that the living positively discourse is a persuasive narrative strategy adopted by a group of Thai women who are mothers and living with HIV/AIDS. Its power and efficacy is due partly to the social context in which these women are located. Thailand, as with many other poor nations, has been a site for drug and treatment testing, and this has produced space and hope for positive living (Levy and Storeng 2007). Because most women had participated in drug trials for combating AIDS and some were on antiretroviral therapy when this study was undertaken, most were relatively healthy with few HIV symptoms. Many of them were also mothers who were given an opportunity to take part in the Prevention of Mothers-to-Child Transmission program and therefore gave birth to healthy babies. Hence, the women in our study are situated in a fertile ground that allows them to embody the positive living discourse.

Our findings add an extra layer of interest to examine how the living positively discourse functions in the Thai society. It reveals that these women are not passive victims but that they act in their own agencies to counteract any negativity they might encounter. As such, it provides a theoretical understanding about the ways that women in non-Western culture deal with their HIV/AIDS which can be adopted as a means to provide culturally sensitive HIV/AIDS care for women living with HIV/AIDS in Thailand and elsewhere.

Acknowledgments We thank the Faculty of Health Sciences, La Trobe University, who provided a research grant to enable this study. An earlier version of this chapter was published in *Qualitative Health Research* (2011). We thank Sage for giving a permission to include this chapter in this book.

References

Ainsworth M, Beyrer C, Soucat C (2003) AIDS and public policy: the lesson and challenges of 'success' in Thailand. Health Policy 64:13–37

Alonzo AA, Reynolds NR (1995) Stigma, HIV and AIDS: An exploration and elaboration of a stigma trajectory. *Social Science & Medicine,* 41(3):303–315

Anderson J, Doyal L (2004) Women from Africa living with HIV in London: a descriptive study. AIDS Care 16(1):95–105

Balthip Q, Boddy J, Siriwatanamethanon J (2013) Achieving harmony of mind: moving from experiencing social disgust to living with harmony in people with HIV/AIDS in the Thai context (Chapter 21). In: Liamputtong P (ed) Stigma, discrimination and HIV/AIDS: a cross-cultural perspective. Springer, Dordrecht

Baumgartner LM (2007) The incorporation of the HIV/AIDS identity into the self over time. Qual Health Res 17(7):919–931

Bennetts A, Shaffer N, Manopaiboon C, Chaiyakul P, Siriwasin W, Mock P, Klumthanom K, Sorapipatana S et al (1999) Determinants of depression and HIV–related worry among HIV–positive women who have recently given birth, Bangkok, Thailand. Soc Sci Med 49(6): 737–749

Brandt A, Rozin R (1997) Introduction. In: Brandt A, Rozin P (eds) Morality and health. Routledge, New York, pp 1–11

Braun V, Clarke V (2006) Using thematic analysis in psychology. Qual Res Psychol 3:77–101

Carpenter C (2010) Phenomenology and rehabilitation research. In: Liamputtong P (ed) Research methods in health: foundations for evidence-based practice. Oxford University Press, Melbourne, pp 123–140

Chokevivat V (1998) The current status of clinical trials in Thailand. Paper presented at the DIA workshop, "Recent development in clinical trials in the Asia Pacific Region", Taipei, Taiwan, Republic of China, 2–3 Oct 1998

Dageid W, Duckett F (2008) Balancing between normality and social death: black, rural, South African women coping with HIV/AIDS. Qual Health Res 18(2):182–195

De Jager W, Kirk J (1998) Using groups to help people. In: Baumann S (ed) Psychiatry and primary health care: a practical guide for health care workers in southern Africa. Juta, Cape Town, pp 423–432

Foucault M (1980) The politics of health in the eighteenth century. In: Gordon C (ed) Power/knowledge. Selected interviews and other writings, 1972–1977. The Harvest Press, Brighton, pp 166–182

Greeff M (2013) Disclosure and stigma: a cultural perspective (Chapter 5). In: Liamputtong P (ed) Stigma, discrimination and HIV/AIDS: a cross-cultural perspective. Springer, Dordrecht

Ho CYY, Mak WWS (2013) HIV-related stigma across cultures: adding family into the equation (Chapter 4). In: Liamputtong P (ed) Stigma, discrimination and HIV/AIDS: a cross-cultural perspective. Springer, Dordrecht

Jirapaet V (2001) Factors affecting maternal role attainment among low-income, Thai, HIV-positive mothers. J Transcult Nurs 12(1):25–33

Klunklin A, Greenwood J (2005) Buddhism, the status of women and the spread of HIV/AIDS in Thailand. Health Care Women Int 26(1):46–61

Kobotani T, Engstrom D (2005) The roles of Buddhist temples in the treatment of HIV/AIDS in Thailand. J Sociol Soc Welf 6, XXXII(4):5–21

Levy JM, Storeng KT (2007) Living positively: narrative strategies of women living with HIV in Cape Town, South Africa. Anthropol Med 14(1):55–68

Liamputtong P (2007) Researching the vulnerable: a guide to sensitive research methods. Sage Publications, London

Liamputtong P (2010) Performing qualitative cross-cultural research. Cambridge University Press, Cambridge

Liamputtong P (2013) Qualitative research methods, 4th edn. Oxford University Press, Melbourne

Liamputtong P, Haritavorn N, Kiatying-Angsulee N (2009) HIV and AIDS, stigma and AIDS support groups: perspectives from women living with HIV and AIDS in central Thailand. Soc Sci Med 69(6):862–868

Lyttlteon C, Beesey A, Sitthikriengkrai M (2007) Expanding community through ARV provision in Thailand. AIDS Care 19(Supplement 1):S44–S53

Maman S, Cathcart R, Burkhardt G, Ombac S, Behets F (2009) The role of religion in HIV-positive women's disclosure experiences and coping strategies in Kinshasa, Democratic Republic of Congo. Soc Sci Med 68(5):965–970

McCamish M, Storer G, Carl G (2000) Refocusing HIV/AIDS interventions in Thailand: the case of male sex workers and other homosexually active men. Cult Health Sex 2(2):167–182

Medley A, Kennedy CE, Lunyolo S, Sweat MD (2009) Disclosure outcomes, coping strategies, and life changes among women living with HIV in Uganda. Qual Health Res 19(12):1744–1754

Morse J (2006) Strategies of intraproject sampling. In: Munhall PL (ed) Nursing research: a qualitative perspective, 4th edn. Jones and Bartlett Publishers, Sudbury, pp 529–539

Norlyk A, Harder I (2010) What makes a phenomenological study phenomenological? An analysis of peer-reviewed empirical nursing studies. Qual Health Res 20(3):420–431

Norman LR, Abreuc S, Candelariad E, Sala A (2009) The effect of sympathy on discriminatory attitudes toward persons living with HIV/AIDS in Puerto Rico: a hierarchical analysis of women living in public housing. AIDS Care 21(2):140–149

Padgett DK (2008) Qualitative methods in social work research, 2nd edn. Sage Publications, Los Angeles

Pakenham KI, Rinaldis M (2001) The role of illness, resources, appraisal, and coping strategies in adjustment to HIV/AIDS: the direct and buffering effects. J Behav Med 24(3):259–279

Park CL, Folkman S (1997) Meaning in the context of stress and coping. Rev Gen Psychol 1:115–144

Patton M (2002) *Qualitative research and evaluation methods* (3rd ed.). Thousand Oaks, CA: Sage.

Pierret J (2000) Everyday life with AIDS/HIV: surveys in the social sciences. Soc Sci Med 50(11):1589–1598

Plattner IE, Meiring N (2006) Living with HIV: the psychological relevance of meaning making. AIDS Care 18(3):241–245

Ross R, Srisaeng P (2005) Depression and its correlates among HIV-positive pregnant women in Thailand. A paper presented at the Sigma Theta Tau international: 38th biennial convention, Indianapolis, Indiana

Ross R, Sawatphanit W, Draucker CB, Suwansujarid T (2007a) The lived experiences of HIV-positive, pregnant women in Thailand. Health Care Women Int 28(8):731–744

Ross R, Sawatphanit W, Suwansujarid T (2007b) Finding peace (*kwam sa-ngob jai*): a Buddhist way to live with HIV. J Holist Nurs 25(4):228–235

Ruxrungtham K, Phanuphak P (2001) Update on HIV/AIDS in Thailand. J Med Assoc Thai 84(supplement 1):S1–S17

Sanders LB (2008) Women's voices: the lived experience of pregnancy and motherhood after diagnosis with HIV. J Assoc Nurses AIDS Care 19(1):47–57

Schoepf B (2001) International AIDS research in anthropology: taking a critical perspective on the crisis. Annu Rev Anthropol 30:335–361

Singhanetra-Renard A, Chongsatitmun C, Aggleton P (2001) Care and support for people living with HIV/AIDS in northern Thailand: findings from an in-depth qualitative study. Cult Health Sex 3(2):167–182

Siriwasin W, Shaffer N, Roongpisuthipong A, Bhiraleus P, Chinayon P, Mangclaviraj Y, Wasi C, Singhaneti S, Chotpitayasunondh T, Chearskul S, Pokapanichwong W, Mock W, Weniger BG, Mastro TD (1998) HIV prevalence, risk factors and partner serodiscordance among pregnant women, Bangkok, Thailand. J Am Med Assoc 280(1):49–54

Stevens MM, Lord BA, Proctor M-T, Nagy S, O'Riordan E (2010) Research with vulnerable families caring for children with life-limiting conditions. Qual Health Res 20(4):496–505

The Joint United Nations Programme on HIV/AIDS (2009) AIDS epidemic update, December 2009. The Joint United Nations Programme on HIV/AIDS, Geneva. http://data.unaids.org/pub/Report/2009/JC1700_Epi_Update_2009_en.pdf. Accessed 25 Mar 2010

The Joint United Nations Programme on HIV/AIDS (UNAIDS) (2005) AIDS epidemic update-December 2003. The Joint United Nations Programme on HIV/AIDS, Geneva

The Joint United Nations Programme on HIV/AIDS & World Health Organization (2008) Epidemiological fact sheet on HIV and AIDS, 2008 update: Thailand. http://apps.who.int/globalatlas/predefinedReports/EFS2008/full/EFS2008_TH.pdf. Accessed 25 Mar 2010

Treichler P (1988) AIDS, gender, & biomedical discourse: current contests for meaning. In: Fee E, Fox D (eds) AIDS: the burdens of history. University of California Press, Berkeley, pp 190–266

Varga C, Brookes H (2008) Factors influencing teen mothers' enrollment and participation in prevention of mother-to-child HIV transmission services in Limpopo Province, South Africa. Qual Health Res 18:786–802

Withell B (2000) A study of the experiences of women living with HIV/AIDS in Uganda. Int J Palliat Nurs 6:234–244

Zhou YR (2008) Endangered womanhood: women's experiences with HIV/AIDS in China. Qual Health Res 18(8):1115–1126

Chapter 16
Scaling Up HIV/AIDS Care Among Women in Sub-Saharan Africa: Cross-Cultural Barriers

Damalie Nakanjako, Florence Maureen Mirembe, Jolly Beyeza-Kashesya, and Alex Coutinho

1 Introduction

HIV/AIDS is one of the major cross-cultural ailments affecting women's health, with up to 20 million women living with HIV/AIDS (WLHIV) and more than two million pregnancies occur among HIV-positive women annually (McIntyre 2005). The HIV/AIDS epidemic wears a predominantly female face as evidenced by the exceptionally high women's vulnerability to HIV infection particularly in the sub-Saharan Africa (SSA) region. Women and girls continue to be affected disproportionately by HIV infection relative to men and boys, and they account for approximately 60% of the estimated HIV infections worldwide (UNAIDS 2008). In Kenya, young women between 15 and 19 years are three times more likely to be infected than their male counterparts, while in Uganda this age group is estimated to have six times more HIV infection among women compared to the same age group of young men HIV (UNAIDS 2009). Similarly, in southern Africa, the HIV prevalence among young women aged 15–24 years is three times higher than among men of the same age (Gouws et al. 2008). The risk of becoming infected is

D. Nakanjako (✉)
Department of Medicine, Makerere College of Health Sciences, Makerere University, Mulago Hospital Complex, P.O. Box 7072, Kampala, Uganda
e-mail: drdamalie@yahoo.com

F.M. Mirembe • J. Beyeza-Kashesya
Department of Obstetrics and Gynaecology, Makerere College of Health Sciences, Makerere University, Mulago Hospital Complex, P.O. Box 7072, Kampala, Uganda
e-mail: flomir2002@yahoo.com; jbeyeza@yahoo.com

A. Coutinho
Infectious Diseases Institute, Makerere College of Health Sciences, Makerere University, Mulago Hospital Complex, P.O. Box 22418, Kampala, Uganda
e-mail: acoutinho@idi.co.ug

P. Liamputtong (ed.), *Women, Motherhood and Living with HIV/AIDS: A Cross-Cultural Perspective*, DOI 10.1007/978-94-007-5887-2_16,
© Springer Science+Business Media Dordrecht 2013

disproportionately high for girls and young women not only because of the known women's greater physiological and biological susceptibility to heterosexual transmission but also because of the compromised environment that increases their vulnerability relative to their male counterparts. Women in the developing world confront serious socio-cultural, economic, and gender disadvantages that influence the dynamics of the HIV/AIDS epidemic among females. It is critical, therefore, to have strategies to provide culturally appropriate HIV prevention, care, and treatment for women. This may, however, require a challenge of the accepted cultural norms (like wife inheritance or polygamy) that put women at risk.

The scale-up of HIV treatment and care among women in resource-limited settings faces several challenges, many of which are unique to the cultural context of women. The substantial diversity of national epidemics underscores not only the need to tailor prevention strategies to local needs but also the importance of decentralizing responses to the HIV/AIDS pandemic (UNAIDS 2009). Over the last three decades of the HIV epidemic, there is so far no generic HIV/AIDS prevention and treatment package that has met all the needs of people living with HIV (PLHIV) across all geographical/cultural boundaries. There is a need to put the HIV/AIDS prevention and treatment interventions into the variable socio-cultural contexts in order to model innovative society-tailored interventions that will effectively control the epidemic worldwide.

In this chapter, we review the cross-cultural perspectives, norms, and practises around motherhood that present unique challenges to the scale-up of HIV prevention, care, and treatment interventions in SSA. We consider socio-cultural issues surrounding pregnancy and child birth, family planning and infertility, disclosure of HIV serostatus and HIV sero-discordance, conflict and war situations, and how these have affected the uptake and scale-up of HIV/AIDS prevention, treatment, and care programs. We tackle specific vulnerable groups of girls/women such as adolescents and orphans and how these groups have increased vulnerability to HIV infection in the African socio-cultural context. We also highlight some strategies to make the current prevention, care, and treatment interventions adaptable to the specific socio-cultural settings of the HIV/AIDS epidemic.

2 Theoretical Framework

Figure 16.1 presents a summary of the socio-cultural differences that influence women's HIV/AIDS care and treatment choices. The arrows to these factors are two way because whereas the listed factors influence women's HIV/AIDS care and treatment choices in general, in return the variable unique socio-cultural norms affect women's responses to these challenges. This chapter explains in detail how each of these factors affects women's responses to the HIV/AIDS epidemic and the reverse, within the African socio-cultural context. The proposed solutions include innovations to improve HIV/AIDS care delivery to women. These require a combination of improved health-care delivery systems in general, improvement of maternal child care facilities,

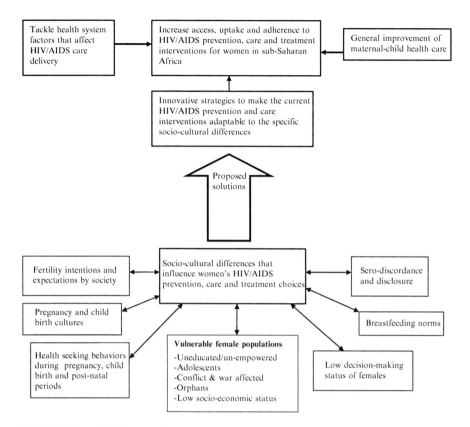

Fig. 16.1 Theoretical framework

and targeted interventions that put into consideration the gender-specific sociocultural differences discussed herein. It is important to note that this chapter is limited to the socio-cultural barriers to the access, uptake, and adherence to HIV/AIDS prevention, care, and treatment programs in sub-Saharan Africa.

3 Pregnancy and HIV/AIDS

Across cultures worldwide, pregnancy and motherhood are valued normal milestones of life and society expects every woman to successfully go through them (Echezona-Johnson 2009; Radcliffe 2009). Therefore, safe motherhood is of cross-cultural importance. In the developed world, people celebrate pregnancies as early as conception. However, in the developing world, because many cultures are unsure of the pregnancy outcomes and the associated high risks for the mother and baby, the norm is to celebrate pregnancy after a safe delivery. As a result, many pregnancies are not announced until it becomes obvious that the woman is undeniably pregnant or after delivery, lest the pregnancy becomes unsuccessful. Numerous biological factors affect pregnancy directly and these include anemia, undernutrition, infectious diseases such as tuberculosis, malaria, and HIV/AIDS, the majority of which are preventable.

In Africa, mothers have an honored social position (Mama 2002; Arnfred 2003). Women are valued for being able to get pregnant and deliver children to propagate the next generation but more importantly to produce heirs for the continuation of the linage of their spouses and for the women's own security later in life (Beyeza-Kashesya et al. 2009, 2010). Theoretically, women want to attain the prestige associated with motherhood (Oyewumi 2003). In some cultures, especially the patriarchal societies, the women attain status and power in the home only when they have sons (Kandiyoti 1988). Similarly, in some cultures, a man's virility is measured by his ability to have a child (Helman 1994) and infertile men are "nonexistent" (Hollos and Larsen 2008). The societal expectations for childbearing lead to high fertility rates in Africa (5–7 births/woman) (United Nations 2010) and make childlessness/infertility highly stigmatized (Hollos and Larsen 2008; see also Chap. 1 in this volume). Unfortunately, these childbearing expectations remain the same in HIV-infected women/couples. These socio-cultural expectations, together with the inherent desire of women to have children, have put women in a vulnerable position. Sometimes, WLHIV are not willing to use birth control methods lest they be named infertile (see case study 1). This social pressure contributes to nondisclosure of HIV serostatus and noncompliance to safe sex practises like condom use. Women may practise high-risk sexual behavior in the attempt to fulfill the socio-cultural expectations, have a sense of belonging, and avoid the stigma associated with childlessness (Nakayiwa et al. 2006; Hollos and Larsen 2008; Beyeza-Kashesya et al. 2009, 2011) consequently increasing the risk of maternal-to-child transmission of HIV (MTCT) and transmission to partners. Similarly, children that acquire HIV through MTCT are not exempt from these socio-cultural norms/expectations when they grow into adulthood.

Case Study 1

Mary Anne (not real name) is a 36-year-old lady who got married 5 years ago. She was diagnosed with HIV 3 years ago when she was nursing her husband in hospital. Mary Anne started HAART 2 years ago and so did her husband. She said: "I was advised not to have children since I have advanced HIV disease. However, my in-laws have advised my husband to marry another woman who can bear children. We have not disclosed to them our HIV status so they think I am infertile." Mary Anne is here to ask her doctor if she and her husband have a chance to have a baby and dispel the in-laws' misconception about her failure to have children.

Case study 1 presents a snap shot of the socio-cultural dilemmas facing HIV-infected couples. Whereas the couple above has overcome the battle of disclosure to each other, they are still faced with the challenge of disclosing to other family members. The husband is under pressure from his family to have concurrent sexual partners and bear children. This contributes to the high-risk heterosexual networks in Africa. Although advances in prevention of mother-to-child transmission of HIV (PMTCT) have given hope to HIV-infected couples to have uninfected children, there is still need to support couples and care providers to deal with the societal stigma associated with HIV infection and fertility.

4 Adolescence and HIV/AIDS

Across the globe, there is a renewed emphasis on developing HIV prevention interventions that take into consideration the local realities among adolescents and young people (UNICEF 2009). Adolescent sexuality and teenage pregnancies are highly stigmatized in many cultures (Arnfred 2003; Nakayiwa et al. 2006; Bakeera-Kitaka et al. 2008) and this interferes with the young people's rights and freedom to access support on safe sex practises and family planning services. In addition, there has been a gap in the availability of culturally appropriate interventions in the area of HIV prevention and sexual risk reduction in this target group (Bakeera-Kitaka et al. 2008). Furthermore, there is limited emphasis on education of the girl children in many African cultures. Many drop out of school and are exposed to early marriages and the related high-risk sexual behaviors. Similarly, sexual relations between young women and men who are 5 or more years older are the major factors in the spread of HIV to the younger generation in African countries (UNICEF 2009). Therefore, there is an urgent need to develop a culture of openness with adolescents about their sexuality and the challenges they may have in order to understand and address the greater HIV risks to girls such as multiple concurrent partnerships, intergenerational sex, transactional sex, and violence against women and girls. Both in and out of school adolescents should be empowered to make appropriate and safe sex decisions to avoid HIV infection. Sexually active young people need support in order to avoid multiple partnerships and in using condoms consistently. In addition, the young people who are not sexually active need support to delay sexual initiation.

On the other hand, adolescents living with HIV/AIDS face unique challenges of social discrimination. As highly active antiretroviral therapy (HAART) becomes increasingly available, young people living with HIV are growing into adulthood. However, many are orphans and have suffered recurrent illnesses and subsequently limited education. It is challenging to support them through adolescence and adulthood in the context of the prevalent stigma in schools, homes, and communities. There is a need to prepare society to receive them and be mindful of their unique needs. In an effort to support the transition from pediatric to adult HIV/AIDS clinics, the Infectious Diseases Institute (IDI) in Kampala, Uganda, has pioneered a transition clinic that caters for HIV-infected children at a time when they seem too old to attend the pediatric HIV clinics yet too young to be comfortable in the adult HIV clinic. The transition clinic is designed to meet the unique needs of adolescents living with HIV/AIDS (ALHIV), and peer counselors have been shown to influence the attitudes and practises of adolescents and encourage them to cope with the challenges of sexuality, dating, disclosure, lifelong HAART, and adherence to ongoing HIV/AIDS care among ALHIV (Bakeera-Kitaka et al. 2008). Similarly, there is a need to integrate family planning services into routine support for adolescents in order to prevent unwanted and unsafe pregnancies and the associated complications. Therefore, HIV prevention practises; should address the unique needs of WLHIV in the context of their socio-cultural expectations of motherhood and provide for safe options for women to have children with the reduced risk of MTCT. The entry point to this strategy is through scaling up HIV testing to all women in the reproductive age group (15–45 year) who constitute the majority of PLHIV in SSA (Were et al. 2006; UNAIDS 2009) that are potentially fueling the new HIV infections.

5   The HIV/AIDS Epidemic Among Women in Conflict-Affected Areas

Many countries in sub-Saharan Africa have been affected by war in the last three decades of the HIV epidemic, and the overlap of conflict and HIV gives the epidemic unique dynamics. Sexual violence and rape are believed to fuel the epidemic in countries affected by conflict. It is hypothesized that the high incidence of rape and forced displacement that accompany conflicts/wars increase the risk of HIV transmission within the affected population. The increasing incidence of rape in South Africa (Ostergard and Tubin 2008) is reported to be associated with increased HIV transmission, and the reverse is also true since the high prevalence of HIV infection is also reported to be in part responsible for the increasing incidence of rape. In particular, young people who suspect that they are HIV positive have developed an inclination to spread the disease (Ostergard and Tubin 2008). Therefore, HIV/AIDS care programs and health services in general should consider availing postexposure prophylaxis services for rape victims (Population Council 2011) in addition to increasing antirape campaigns in conflict-affected areas. Furthermore, HIV prevention strategies should be an essential component of the amnesty programs because refugees are likely to transmit or acquire HIV infection within the host communities as well as among themselves (Spiegel et al. 2007). On the other hand, conflicts and war are also responsible for an increased number of orphans who face various socio-cultural disadvantages including poverty, poor or no education, lack of love and social support, early marriages, and rape, all of which make them more vulnerable to HIV infection. Similarly, there is a scarcity of health-care services in many war-stricken areas thereby posing a challenge to the scale-up of HIV/AIDS care and treatment services. Therefore, the war-affected areas need specific HIV prevention interventions to address this unique situation that is prevalent in many parts of Africa. Innovative ways are critically needed to deliver essential health services including HIV care and treatment to this vulnerable population.

6 Orphans and Motherhood in Africa

Besides the wars, HIV/AIDS has exponentially increased the number of orphans and vulnerable children in SSA which is the home for 77% (11.6 M) of the 15 million children under 18 years that have been orphaned by AIDS worldwide. Even with the scale-up of HIV treatment, it is estimated that by 2015–2020, the number of orphaned children will still be overwhelmingly high (Foster and Williamson 2000; UNAIDS 2009). In Africa, the roles of motherhood are not limited to biological mothers since members of the extended family such as grandmothers, cousins, and aunties traditionally take on the roles of mothering parentless children thus offering an "extended family safety net"(Foster and Williamson 2000; UNAIDS 2009). However, with the upsurge of orphans due to the HIV/AIDS epidemic, the extended families are overstretched and under stress to handle the large number of orphans. Hence, some children slip through the safety net and are exposed to vulnerable situations that expose them to HIV infection such as child-headed households, child labor, prostitution, rape, violence, and poverty. However, there are also reports of child abuse by the very relatives who act as guardians of these children. Therefore, global and national responses to the HIV/AIDS epidemic need to support and preserve the "extended family safety net" that is more culturally acceptable in communities that maintain the tradition of child fostering. In urbanized communities where the "extended family safety net" is weakened, there is a need to develop other alternatives for orphans such as institutions, children's villages, and adoption placements. However, institutional responses are often unsustainable and may be viewed as inappropriate by community members who recognize their potential to undermine existing coping mechanisms (Drew et al. 1998; Foster and Williamson 2000). Therefore, HIV/AIDS prevention and care interventions for orphans and vulnerable children (OVC) should be tailored to the existing norms and practises and designed to strengthen family and community capacities to care for OVC.

7 Scaling Up of HIV Testing for Mothers and Linkage to Comprehensive HIV/AIDS Care

The entry point to HIV care and treatment for mothers is universal knowledge of HIV serostatus (Musoke 2004; Nassali et al. 2009; UNAIDS 2009). HIV testing, counseling, and prevention services in antenatal settings offer an excellent opportunity not only to prevent newborns from becoming infected but also to protect and enhance the health of HIV-infected women while enhancing the prevention of infection among those found to be HIV negative (Nguyen et al. 2008; Nassali et al. 2009). Recent evidence suggests that inadequate testing rates impede national AIDS responses and contribute to delayed entry HIV/AIDS care programs as well as inadvertent HIV transmission (UNAIDS 2009). By 2008, up to 60% of HIV-infected pregnant mothers were unaware of their HIV serostatus (UNAIDS 2009) and therefore missed opportunities to access HIV treatment and PMTCT interventions. The documented factors that hinder mother's access to HIV testing include lack of money to transport them to the testing centers, failure to leave their homes because they are taking care of children while the men are at work, and fear of the stigma associated with HIV infection and motherhood in addition to the fear of having to disclose their results to spouses (Nguyen et al. 2008; Visser et al. 2008; Nassali et al. 2009), all compounded by the failure of health system to offer routine HIV tests. Many of these reasons stem from the socio-cultural norms and beliefs pertaining to the position of the woman in society. For example, women in Africa stay at home and look up to the men as the sole breadwinners and decision makers including taking decisions for mothers to seek health care. In addition, African women are not empowered enough to make choices on safe sexual practices like condom use (Visser et al. 2008; Lifshay et al. 2009) mainly for fear of violence, abandonment, and loss of security since most women own no property.

8   HIV Sero-Discordance

A unique evolution of the mature HIV epidemic in SSA is that the majority of the HIV infections are attributable to heterosexual transmission and discordance of HIV serostatus. This is emerging as a major risk factor for new infections particularly among marriage relationships (Dunkle et al. 2008), more so because the majority of the discordant couples are not aware of their HIV discordant status. In a community-based study that provided home-based HIV testing in rural Uganda, 43% of the spouses of patients on HAART were HIV negative (Were et al. 2006). Unfortunately, the confluence of high rates of discordance within marriage, low ability of women to make choices of safe sex practises, and the low rates of condom use contribute to the increasing new HIV infections within the marriage setting (Dunkle et al. 2008). Data shows that women in discordant relationships have often had unprotected sex for the sake of having children (Nakayiwa et al. 2006; Beyeza-Kashesya et al. 2009, 2011). Furthermore, women face more discrimination if they are the positive partner because society seems to condone or justify high-risk sexual behaviors among men. Moreover, the gender of the HIV-positive partner influences childbearing differently. Couples where the woman is the positive partner were more than two times more likely to want to have more children than couples where the man is the positive partner (Beyeza-Kashesya et al. 2010).

> **Case Study 2**
> Jane (not real name) is a 30-year-old woman who was diagnosed with HIV infection 2 years ago. She is afraid of telling her husband because she imagines he will kick her out of the house. For the same reason, she has not enrolled into any HIV/AIDS care programs since she tested HIV positive. As a result, she usually accepts to have unprotected sex. Moreover, she is unaware of her husband's HIV serostatus. She is pregnant and she is at Makerere College of Health Sciences to know whether her child is at risk of HIV infection.

Case study 2 is an example of a typical woman living with HIV/AIDS (WLHIV) that walks into the adult infectious diseases clinic at Makerere College of Health Sciences that offers free HIV/AIDS care to over 20,000 PLHIV in Uganda. Amidst the long patient queues at many HIV clinics in Africa, the care providers have to attend to several of these situations. The concept of HIV sero-discordance is both scientifically and socially complex for both the health worker and the patients. It is even more complicated in the polygamous African society. We recommend evidence-based interventions that target heterosexual couples in order to promote counseling and testing for couples and create a culture that encourages disclosure of HIV serostatus to sexual partners. There is a need for HIV care providers to further study the determinants of HIV sero-discordance and consider innovative interventions, for example, preexposure prophylaxis, that can be tailored to the prevalent socio-cultural norms and practises in Africa.

9 Disclosure of HIV Status and Its Consequences

The social stigma associated with being HIV disease hinders PLHIV from disclosing their HIV serostatus to spouses and other family members. Many WLHIV do not disclose their serostatus to their partners, family members, and friends, thereby creating potential barriers to prevention of sexual transmission of HIV to partners and MTCT (Visser et al. 2008). A study in South Africa reported that 78% of recently diagnosed patients with HIV infection did not disclose their serostatus to their partners and 46% did not know their partner's serostatus (Olley et al. 2004). In a hospital-based HIV clinic in South Africa, nondisclosure to partners was up to 21% and disclosure was not associated with availability of HAART (Skogmar et al. 2006). Disclosure of positive test results is still challenging for mothers who usually receive HIV testing during pregnancy (Visser et al. 2008; Nassali et al. 2009; see also Chaps. 3, 4, 15, and 17 in this volume). Many mothers in developing countries do not disclose because of the fear of blame, accusation of infidelity, fear of abandonment by partners, rejection, stigmatization, emotional and physical abuse, and most of all loss of economic support from the partner (Karamagi et al. 2006; Visser et al. 2008). Unfortunately, lack of disclosure creates barriers to preventing sexual transmission to partners and limits access to prevention of maternal-to-child transmission (PMTCT) programs as well as subsequent linkage to comprehensive HIV/AIDS care including HAART for the mother and baby (Nguyen et al. 2008; Visser et al. 2008; Nassali et al. 2009). However, prevention of HIV infection to the unborn baby is a strong motivator for mothers to take up HIV testing and PMTCT services during pregnancy (Varga et al. 2006; Nassali et al. 2009). Unfortunately, only one-third of the mothers are estimated to return for follow-up HIV/AIDS care post delivery (Nassali et al. 2009). This means, therefore, that most mothers miss the current PMTCT strategies where mothers are supposed to receive prolonged HAART (up to 6 months post delivery) to reduce HIV transmission to the baby through breastfeeding (Visser et al. 2008; WHO 2009) as well as specific treatment for the mothers.

Evidence shows that the majority of the mothers who disclose their positive HIV serostatus to spouses receive acceptance and social support (Visser et al. 2008; Nassali et al. 2009). For pregnant women in South Africa, voluntary disclosure ultimately resulted in a supportive response for 70% of the women (Varga et al. 2006). Focusing on the positive outcomes of disclosure is critical in the development of effective post-test counseling practises to increase uptake of comprehensive HIV/AIDS care. Mothers should be empowered to disclose their HIV results to spouses and close family members/friends as nondisclosure has serious implications for HIV transmission to the child at the time of birth and through breastfeeding (Visser et al. 2008). We, therefore, need campaigns to support mothers to weigh the anticipated consequences and benefits of disclosure in order to make the appropriate decision to disclose to sexual partners and family members.

The low male involvement in HIV testing has been sighted as an important hindrance for mothers to disclose and access testing and care as well as the required follow-up and support services (Nguyen et al. 2008; Nassali et al. 2009). It is, therefore, critical to advocate for couple counseling and testing so that disclosure issues are made easier for the women. In addition, there is a need to tailor HIV testing services to reach the men who are usually at their workplaces in order to improve male access (Nassali et al. 2009). It is also important to modify the HIV testing facilities for women to accommodate the accompanying spouses.

Case Study 3
Mary (not real name) is a 21-year-old woman in the transition clinic at the Infectious Diseases Institute in Uganda. She was diagnosed with HIV infection at the age of 6 years when she lost 2 of her siblings to HIV/AIDS and subsequently lost both parents. She was raised by her maternal grandmother. On two occasions, she has disclosed her HIV status to her boyfriend and they rejected her and terminated the relationship. She knows she has a right to her sexuality and she would like to have children in order to fulfill her long-time dream to be a mother. She also admits that she prefers a partner who is HIV negative in order to reduce the chances of infecting her baby.

Case study 3 represents some hindrances to disclosure of positive HIV serostatus. It is important to empower health workers with knowledge and skills to show a nonjudgmental attitude and build the patients' trust in order to encourage disclosure to the health worker which contributes to continuity of care since patients are encouraged to return (Nassali et al. 2009). Peer counselors have been found to play an important role in modifying the perspectives of HIV to newly diagnosed mothers and articulate the needs and practises of PLHIV and their communities. Mothers are the best vehicles to support other mothers. However, it is important to dispel misconceptions so that they are not passed on, for example, in this case where the mother thinks that a negative partner reduces the risk of MTCT. The mother-to-mother (m2m) program in South Africa has been helpful to meet the much-needed psychological support for women who have learned they are HIV positive so that they can both accept their HIV status and adhere to the medical recommendations for PMTCT (Mother2mother 2007). Peer women/mother support groups are very instrumental in developing a socio-cultural acceptance of HIV infection among women with consideration of the unique needs of PLHIV and their role in prevention of HIV transmission.

10   Prevention with Positives

HIV prevention by PLHIV is emerging as a fundamental component of HIV prevention in developing countries although appropriate prevention with positives (PWP) guidelines are not yet implemented widely (Lifshay et al. 2009). Following a positive HIV test and enrollment into HIV/AIDS care, PLHIV are reported to increase condom use and reduce the number of sexual partners (Bunnell et al. 2008; Lifshay et al. 2009). A household survey in Uganda indicated that HIV-infected individuals who knew their HIV serostatus were more than three times likely to use a condom during their last sexual encounter compared with those who did not know their status (Bunnell et al. 2008). In rural Zimbabwe, women who tested HIV-positive reported increased consistent condom use with primary partners although individuals testing negative reported an overall increase in risky sexual behavior (Sherr et al. 2007), thus underscoring the need to intensify HIV prevention services among PLHIV to accompany initiatives to promote knowledge of HIV serostatus. The PWP strategy has potential to change the tide of the epidemic since it inherently caters for the specific beliefs, challenges, and needs of PLHIV (King et al. 2009). Similarly, HIV prevention programs should raise awareness about the gender-power inequalities that continue to increase the risk of HIV infection among the uninfected partners such as male dominance of practical sex options like condom use, domestic violence, lack of socio-economic support for WLHIV (Nguyen et al. 2008; Nassali et al. 2009), and the social blame towards the women who test positive first within a relationship (Lifshay et al. 2009). There is, therefore, a need to work out innovative, culturally acceptable interventions tailored to improve women's negotiations for lower-risk sexual practises.

11 Child Delivery and PMTCT

Globally, coverage of PMTCT services rose from 10% in 2004 to 45% in 2008 (UNAIDS 2009). SSA has made remarkable strides in expanding access to PMTCT services. Evidence shows that mother-to-child transmission of HIV (MTCT) is contributing a declining proportion of new infections in countries with a high HIV prevalence. As PMTCT services are brought to scale, the annual number of new HIV infections among children has declined fivefold in Botswana, from 4,600 in 1999 to 890 in 2007 (Stover et al. 2008), and administration of HAART during pregnancy and breastfeeding has reduced MTCT rate to less than 2% (Marazzi et al. 2011). In 2008, 45% of HIV-infected pregnant women received antiretroviral drugs for the prevention of HIV transmission to their newborns, compared with 9% in 2004 (UNAIDS 2009). However, reaching all mothers with HIV testing, PMTCT and HIV treatment and care for both mothers and children remains a big challenge in developing countries where access to health facilities is limited due to various socio-cultural factors that affect women's health-seeking behavior.

In many cultures in the subregion, home is the primary place for childbirth, and worldwide, over 90% of the people alive today were born at home (Denomme 2009). This is probably one of the main reasons why we still have up to 60% of mothers in SSA who deliver babies without assistance from skilled birth attendants. This situation greatly increases the risks of complications, contributing to greater maternal and child death and disability (Kimani 2008). It is, therefore, worthwhile to expand HIV testing and PMTCT services outside health facilities and make them more accessible to mothers within the community setting.

In addition to interventions to reduce MTCT through vaginal delivery, elective caesarian section as a mode of delivery has been proven to reduce the intrapartum risk of MTCT during labor that otherwise contributes 60–75% of MTCT HIV infections (Perez-Then et al. 2003; Musoke 2004; Nassali et al. 2009). However, this intervention continues to face challenges in communities where normal labor is considered a measure of bravery, strength, and real womanhood (Echezona-Johnson 2009; Radcliffe 2009). In addition to the substantial risks associated with cesarean deliveries in resource-limited settings, the procedure is not readily available or accessible to the majority of the women at primary health-care facilities. Therefore, HIV-infected mothers may opt for normal labor because of limited availability, cost, as well as the fear of the social stigma associated with failure to attempt normal labor thereby putting the unborn baby at risk of MTCT. Thus, there is a need to educate mothers, families, as well as communities in order to create understanding, acceptance, and value for mothers who opt for cesarean section to prevent MTCT to their unborn babies.

12 Breastfeeding and Prevention of Mother-to-Child Transmission of HIV

In 2008, an estimated 430,000 new HIV infections occurred among children below 15 years, most of which stem from transmission in utero, during delivery, or post-partum as a result of breastfeeding (UNAIDS 2009). Breastfeeding accounts for up to 20% of MTCT in predominantly breastfeeding populations (Musoke 2004) without any interventions. Persistence of the breastfeeding cultures affects the uptake of postnatal PMTCT interventions. For example, artificial (bottle) feeding is difficult to implement as a strategy for PMTCT because most of the mothers cannot afford to supplement appropriately and this could result in accelerated infant mortality and morbidity that is often due to diarrheal diseases. Secondly, inability to breastfeed is associated with stigma in most African communities where breastfeeding is valued as a sign of motherhood and is implemented in almost 100% of all mothers. In many African cultures, breastfeeding in public is socially acceptable and bottle-feeding is considered to be for orphans (007 Breasts, 2009). Elsie from Ghana said that "once your baby cries and you do not breast feed your baby, people draw a conclusion that the baby is not yours" (007 Breasts, 2009). This inadvertently translates to discrimination of biological mothers who choose not to breastfeed their children. Adelaide from Zimbabwe also remarked that "breastfeeding in public is the norm, in fact if your baby is crying and you do not give him/her the breast you are frowned upon and told off by people" (007 Breasts, 2009). Therefore, mothers who opt for artificial feeding may be tempted to practise mixed infant feeding in order to avoid the societal stigma and discrimination associated with bottle-feeding (Oyewumi 2003; Carr and Gramling 2004; Nguyen et al. 2008), more so if the mother has not disclosed her HIV serostatus. In this case, mothers may be better off opting for exclusive breastfeeding for 6 months to reduce MTCT. All this emphasizes the need for interventions like highly active antiretroviral therapy (HAART) for the mother during pregnancy and breastfeeding to reduce MTCT in communities where mothers cannot do without breastfeeding. It is in response to this challenge that trials are ongoing in Africa to study the risk of MTCT through breastfeeding when the mother receives prolonged HAART (up to 6 months post delivery). This strategy is in line with the 2010 WHO PMTCT guidelines that include HAART for mothers from 14 weeks of pregnancy until 1 week after cessation of breastfeeding or lifelong HAART for those with CD4 counts <350 cells/μL. See also Chaps. 1, 10, 11, 19, and 20 in this volume.

13 Impact of HAART on Motherhood

Provision of antiretroviral drugs to HIV-positive pregnant women has averted about 200,000 cumulative new HIV infections in the past 12 years. The biggest impact has been in SSA with 134,000 averted infections compared with 33,000 in Asia and 23,000 in Western Europe and North America where HIV prevalence rates are lower (UNAIDS 2009). There is data to show that administration of HAART decreases MTCT rates to less than 2% when given to mothers during pregnancy and breastfeeding irrespective of CD4 counts or stage of HIV disease (WHO 2009; Marazzi et al. 2010, 2011). However, most countries have not yet reached all pregnant women with these PMTCT services and the maternal treatment regimens used for PMTCT vary markedly across resource-limited settings (UNAIDS 2009). It is important to note that HAART improves pregnancy outcomes, reduces HIV-related maternal mortality, prolongs the lives of the mothers (Marazzi et al. 2010, 2011), and ultimately prolongs the lives of children since having a mother plays a big role in the child's welfare and survival (Oyewumi 2003; Skinner et al. 2006). On the other hand, HAART reduces the HIV RNA viral load and reduces the risk of transmission of HIV infection to partners and unborn babies. Therefore, HAART has provided women the security to have more babies with the reduced risk of MTCT and has thus restored the mothers' role in society as a mother and caretaker of her children and entire household (Oyewumi 2003). However, the success of HAART for mothers in SSA depends largely on disclosure to improve adherence and continued HIV treatment post delivery, throughout breastfeeding (Nassali et al. 2009), and thereafter as lifelong therapy (Ware et al. 2006). Therefore, amidst the challenges facing the scale-up of HIV treatment in resource-limited settings, mothers with HIV/AIDS should be prioritized for timely initiation of HAART. Similarly, culturally and socially acceptable strategies should be utilized to improve continuity/adherence of mothers to comprehensive HIV prevention, care, and treatment services.

14   Conclusion

Various socio-cultural factors influence motherhood and increase women's vulnerability to HIV infection in addition to increasing the risks of HIV transmission to their partners and the unborn babies. Women's access, uptake, and adherence to comprehensive HIV/AIDS prevention care and treatment programs including PMTCT and HAART are hampered by numerous socio-cultural constraints including the socio-economic status, power-gender inequalities, male dominance of women's decision-making processes, and continuous pressure on women to conform to the society expectations and prestige surrounding motherhood. Therefore, women/mothers remain central in the responses to the HIV/AIDS epidemic. In order to reach all the women in need of HIV/AIDS care and change the tide of the HIV/AIDS epidemic, the prevention and treatment interventions should be tailored to the socio-cultural perspectives, norms, and practises of the communities affected by the epidemic. We recommend a large base of operational research in the different socio-cultural settings in order to develop evidence-based local solutions for site-specific problems and challenges.

Acknowledgements The authors acknowledge the Sewankambo scholarship program at the Infectious Diseases Institute, Makerere College of Health Sciences, that has made it possible for Damalie Nakanjako to undertake this review.

References

Arnfred S (2003) Images of 'motherhood' – African and Nordic perspectives. J Cult Afr Women Stud 4:80. Online journal: http://www.africaknowledgeproject.org/index.php/jenda/article/view/80

Bakeera-Kitaka S, Nabukeera-Barungi N, Nostlinger C, Addy K, Colebunders R (2008) Sexual risk reduction needs of adolescents living with HIV in a clinical care setting. AIDS Care 20(4):426–433

Beyeza-Kashesya J, Kaharuza F, Mirembe F, Neema S, Ekstrom AM, Kulane A (2009) The dilemma of safe sex and having children: challenges facing HIV sero-discordant couples in Uganda. Afr Health Sci 9(1):2–12

Beyeza-Kashesya J, Ekstrom AM, Kaharuza F, Mirembe F, Neema S, Kulane A (2010) My partner wants a child: a cross-sectional study of the determinants of the desire for children among mutually disclosed sero-discordant couples receiving care in Uganda. BMC Public Health 10:247

Beyeza-Kashesya J, Kaharuza F, Ekstrom AM, Neema S, Kulane A, Mirembe F (2011) To use or not to use a condom: a prospective cohort study comparing contraceptive practices among HIV-infected and HIV-negative youth in Uganda. BMC Infect Dis 11:144

Breastfeeding in public around the world (2009) http://www.007b.com/public-breastfeeding-world.php. Accessed 22 Aug 2011

Bunnell R, Opio A, Musinguzi J, Kirungi W, Ekwaru P, Mishra V et al (2008) HIV transmission risk behavior among HIV-infected adults in Uganda: results of a nationally representative survey. AIDS 22(5):617–624

Carr RL, Gramling LF (2004) Stigma: a health barrier for women with HIV/AIDS. J Assoc Nurses AIDS Care 15(5):30–39

Denomme S (2009) Let's talk about the cultures of childbearing. http://pregnancy.families.com/blog/lets-talk-about-the-cultures-of-childbearing. Accessed 15 Dec 2009

Drew RS, Makufa C, Foster G (1998) Strategies for providing care and support to children orphaned by AIDS. AIDS Care 10(Suppl 1):S9–S15

Dunkle KL, Stephenson R, Karita E, Chomba E, Kayitenkore K, Vwalika C et al (2008) New heterosexually transmitted HIV infections in married or cohabiting couples in urban Zambia and Rwanda: an analysis of survey and clinical data. Lancet 371(9631):2183–2191

Echezona-Johnson C (2009) Rituals for honoring pregnancy in different cultures. http://www.helium.com/items/852948/-rituals-for-honoring-pregnancy-in-different-cultures. Accessed 15 Dec 2009

Foster G, Williamson J (2000) A review of current literature on the impact of HIV/AIDS on children in sub-Saharan Africa. AIDS 14(Suppl 3):S275–S284

Gouws E, Stanecki KA, Lyerla R, Ghys PD (2008) The epidemiology of HIV infection among young people aged 15–24 years in southern Africa. AIDS 22(Suppl 4):S5–S16

Helman CG (1994) Culture, health and illness: an introduction to health professionals. http://www.amazon.com/Culture-Health-Illness-Cecil-Helman/dp/0723608415. Accessed 22 Aug 2011

Hollos M, Larsen U (2008) Motherhood in sub-Saharan Africa: the social consequences of infertility in an urban population in northern Tanzania. Cult Health Sex 10(2):159–173

Kandiyoti D (1988) Bargaining with patriarchy. Gend Soc 2(3):274–290

Karamagi CA, Tumwine JK, Tylleskar T, Heggenhougen K (2006) Intimate partner violence against women in eastern Uganda: implications for HIV prevention. BMC Public Health 6:284

Kimani M (2008) Investing in the health of Africa's mothers. Afr Renew 4:8

King R, Lifshay J, Nakayiwa S, Katuntu D, Lindkvist P, Bunnell R (2009) The virus stops with me: HIV-infected Ugandans' motivations in preventing HIV transmission. Soc Sci Med 68(4):749–757

Lifshay J, Nakayiwa S, King R, Reznick OG, Katuntu D, Batamwita R et al (2009) Partners at risk: motivations, strategies, and challenges to HIV transmission risk reduction among HIV-infected men and women in Uganda. AIDS Care 21(6):715–724

Mama A (2002) Gains and challenges: linking theory and practice. www.gwsafrica.org/knowledge/mama. Accessed 21 Aug 2011

Marazzi MC, Liotta G, Nielsen-Saines K, Haswell J, Magid NA, Buonomo E et al (2010) Extended antenatal antiretroviral use correlates with improved infant outcomes throughout the first year of life. AIDS 24(18):2819–2826

Marazzi MC, Palombi L, Nielsen-Saines K, Haswell J, Zimba I, Magid NA et al (2011) Extended antenatal use of triple antiretroviral therapy for prevention of mother-to-child transmission of HIV-1 correlates with favorable pregnancy outcomes. AIDS 25(13):1611–1618

McIntyre J (2005) Maternal health and HIV. Reprod Health Matters 13(25):129–135

Mother2mother (2007) AIDS counselling from mother to mother. http://www.sagoodnews.co.za/health_and_hiv_aids/aids_counselling_from_mother_to_mother.html. Accessed 22 Aug 2011

Musoke P (2004) Recent advances in prevention of mother to child (PMTCT) of HIV. Afr Health Sci 4(3):144–145

Nakayiwa S, Abang B, Packel L, Lifshay J, Purcell DW, King R et al (2006) Desire for children and pregnancy risk behavior among HIV-infected men and women in Uganda. AIDS Behav 10(4 Suppl):S95–S104

Nassali M, Nakanjako D, Kyabayinze D, Beyeza J, Okoth A, Mutyaba T (2009) Access to HIV/AIDS care for mothers and children in sub-Saharan Africa: adherence to the postnatal PMTCT program. AIDS Care 21(9):1124–1131

Nguyen TA, Oosterhoff P, Ngoc YP, Wright P, Hardon A (2008) Barriers to access prevention of mother-to-child transmission for HIV positive women in a well-resourced setting in Vietnam. AIDS Res Ther 5(7). http://www.aidsrestherapy.com/content/pdf/1742-6405-5-7.pdf. Accessed 12 Oct 2011

Olley BO, Seedat S, Stein DJ (2004) Self-disclosure of HIV serostatus in recently diagnosed patients with HIV in South Africa. Afr J Reprod Health 8(2):71–76

Ostergard R, Tubin M (2008) Rape and the HIV/AIDS epidemic: evidence from South Africa. Paper presented at the ISA's 49th annual convention, bridging multiple divides, San Francisco, CA, USA

Oyewumi O (2003) Abiyamo: theorizing African motherhood. J Cult Afr Women Stud 4:79. Online journal: http://www.africaknowledgeproject.org/index.php/jenda/article/view/79

Perez-Then E, Pena R, Tavarez-Rojas M, Pena C, Quinonez S, Buttler M et al (2003) Preventing mother-to-child HIV transmission in a developing country: the Dominican Republic experience. J Acquir Immune Defic Syndr 34(5):506–511

Population Council (2011) The prevention and management of HIV and sexual and gender-based violence: responding to the needs of survivors and those-at-risk. http://www.popcouncil.org/pdfs/2011_HIVSGBVBrief.pdf. Accessed 22 Aug 2011

Radcliffe R (2009) Rituals for honoring pregnancy in different cultures. http://www.helium.com/items/852948/-rituals-for-honoring-pregnancy-in-different-cultures. Accessed 15 Dec 2009

Sherr L, Lopman B, Kakowa M, Dube S, Chawira G, Nyamukapa C et al (2007) Voluntary counselling and testing: uptake, impact on sexual behaviour, and HIV incidence in a rural Zimbabwean cohort. AIDS 21(7):851–860

Skinner D, Tsheko N, Mtero-Munyati S, Segwabe M, Chibatamoto P, Mfecane S et al (2006) Towards a definition of orphaned and vulnerable children. AIDS Behav 10(6):619–626

Skogmar S, Shakely D, Lans M, Danell J, Andersson R, Tshandu N et al (2006) Effect of antiretroviral treatment and counselling on disclosure of HIV-serostatus in Johannesburg, South Africa. AIDS Care 18(7):725–730

Spiegel PB, Bennedsen AR, Claass J, Bruns L, Patterson N, Yiweza D et al (2007) Prevalence of HIV infection in conflict-affected and displaced people in seven sub-Saharan African countries: a systematic review. Lancet 369(9580):2187–2195

Stover J, Fidzani B, Molomo BC, Moeti T, Musuka G (2008) Estimated HIV trends and program effects in Botswana. PLoS One 3(11):e3729

UNAIDS (2008) Report on the global AIDS epidemic. http://www.unaids.org/en/dataanalysis/epi
demiology/2008reportontheglobalaidsepidemic/. Accessed 14 Mar 2011

UNAIDS (2009) AIDS Epidemic update. http://www.unaids.org/en/dataanalysis/epidemiology/20
09aidsepidemicupdate/. Accessed 14 Mar 2011

UNICEF (2009) Children and AIDS: third stocktaking report advocates early HIV testing. http://
www.unicef.org/eapro/media_9720.html. Accessed 14 Mar 2011

United Nations (2010) The UN total fertility ranking 2005–2010. List of countries and territories
by fertility rate. http://en.wikipedia.org/wiki/Total_fertility_rate. Accessed 22 Aug 2011

Varga CA, Sherman GG, Jones SA (2006) HIV-disclosure in the context of vertical transmission:
HIV-positive mothers in Johannesburg, South Africa. AIDS Care 18(8):952–960

Visser MJ, Neufeld S, de Villiers A, Makin JD, Forsyth BW (2008) To tell or not to tell: South
African women's disclosure of HIV status during pregnancy. AIDS Care 20(9):1138–1145

Ware NC, Wyatt MA, Tugenberg T (2006) Social relationships, stigma and adherence to antiretroviral therapy for HIV/AIDS. AIDS Care 18(8):904–910

Were WA, Mermin JH, Wamai N, Awor AC, Bechange S, Moss S et al (2006) Undiagnosed HIV
infection and couple HIV discordance among household members of HIV-infected people
receiving antiretroviral therapy in Uganda. J Acquir Immune Defic Syndr 43(1):91–95

World Health Organization (2009) Rapid advise: use of antiretroviral therapy drugs for treating
pregnant women and preventing HIV infection in infants. www.who.int/hiv/pub/mtct/rapid_
advice_mtct.pdf. Accessed 14 Mar 2011

Chapter 17
Mothers with HIV: A Case for a Human Rights Approach to HIV/AIDS Care in Northeastern Brazil

Jessica Jerome

1 Introduction

Brazil is the national center of the HIV/AIDS epidemic in South America and accounts for 57% of all AIDS cases in Latin America and the Caribbean (Berquo 2005). It is also virtually unique among both developing and developed countries in its highly centralized, rights-based, publicly funded, and internationally lauded HIV/AIDS program. Some of its more innovative approaches include framing the need for antiretrovirals (ARVs) as a human right and providing free and universal access to AIDS drugs through the establishment of a series of HIV/AIDS clinics throughout the country (Biehl 2007). In an attempt to reduce high rates of perinatal HIV transmission, in 1996, the Brazilian Ministry of Health mandated universal HIV testing for all pregnant women, free antiviral drugs for HIV-positive women and newborns, as well as formula feeding for newborns during the first 6 months of life (Knauth et al. 2003). These and other policies have been hailed globally and seen as responsible for a 70% reduction in both AIDS mortality and the use of AIDS-related hospital services (Biehl 2007). The perinatal transmission rate of HIV has fallen to less than 5%, making it comparable with the US rate (Mofenson 2003; Kreitchmann et al. 2004).

Given the strong emphasis Brazil has placed on human rights in respect to the HIV/AIDS crisis and the international excitement generated over particular programs, such as those for mothers with HIV, I sought to examine the experiences of a group of HIV-positive mothers with their HIV care and treatment more than a decade after the establishment of such programs. What were the lived experiences of HIV-positive mothers, on the ground, getting treatment, I wondered?

J. Jerome (✉)
St. John's College, 1160 Camino Cruz Blanca, Santa Fe 87501, NM, USA
e-mail: jsjerome@sjcsf.edu

P. Liamputtong (ed.), *Women, Motherhood and Living with HIV/AIDS:*
A Cross-Cultural Perspective, DOI 10.1007/978-94-007-5887-2_17,
© Springer Science+Business Media Dordrecht 2013

What kinds of medical, institutional, or familial support did these women feel they had, and how did their experiences compare to what was being praised in the press as a "the best national AIDS program in the developing world"? (Biehl 2007).

The study was based in Fortaleza, a large urban center in Northeastern Brazil, which had adopted the national standards of HIV care by the early 2000s and maintained a large infectious disease hospital that devoted an entire wing to HIV treatment and care, including the care of mothers with HIV. Despite these advances, in 2008, Fortaleza was the second capital in the nation for number of pregnant women with HIV (Maia 2008). Understanding how to reduce the risk of these women passing HIV onto their children became a priority of the city's health services.

For this study, I conducted semi-structured in-depth interviews with a small group of Fortaleza mothers about their feelings and experiences regarding pre-natal care, HIV testing, disclosure of HIV status, and about the kinds of support they received in coping with an HIV diagnosis. Based on the results, I argue that aspects of Brazil's Universal HIV treatment program, as well as more traditional forms of support such as family networks, provided mothers in Fortaleza with a strong foundation to accept and continue HIV treatment and care. This chapter further suggests that particular forms of health care, such as the human rights-based approach Brazil has taken to HIV/AIDS, may improve patient-provider relationships.

2   Theoretical and Methodological Frameworks

This study relies on recent scholarship and theoretical innovation in the area of human rights and public health (Gostin 1997; Farmer 2003; Parker and Aggleton 2003; Galvao 2005; Taket 2012) in order to critically examine Brazilian women's experiences with HIV/AIDS care and treatment. Human rights can be defined as a set of fundamental claims to life, liberty, and equality of opportunity that cannot be taken away by government, persons, or institutions (Gostin 1997; Taket 2012). Although human rights and public health may present complementary approaches to advancing peoples' well-being, only recently has human rights discourse begun to encompass health-related entitlements (Gostin 1997). Recognizing health as a human right, rather than simply a moral claim, suggests that state should be obligated to respect, defend, and promote that right (Taket 2012). Brazil was one of the first countries to acknowledge the explicit link between human rights and health care and enshrined the right to health in their 1988 constitution. While other studies on HIV/AIDS in Brazil have focused on the legal ramifications of a human rights approach to health care (Galvao 2005), my interest was in the perceptions and feelings of HIV-positive Brazilian women and how, for example, patient-doctor relationships were experienced within a health care system that had taken a human rights-based approach.

Table 17.1 Sample population

	Fortaleza
Median age	33 (23–43)
Living below the poverty line in their respective countries	18/18
Finished high school	3/18
Every formally employed	7/18
Children (mean and range)	3 (1–7)
Routine prenatal care	12/18
Number of mothers with HIV-positive children	1/18

The study used qualitative interviews and data analysis techniques with a group of 18 HIV-positive mothers from Fortaleza, Brazil, in order to elucidate responses to four main topic domains: prenatal care, HIV testing, revealing HIV status, and forms of support used in coping with HIV diagnosis. Initial interviews were conducted with public health workers, advocacy groups, nongovernmental organizations, and mothers with HIV. These interviews, in addition to a review of the literature on perinatal HIV transmission in Brazil, served as a framework for constructing the interview instrument and the theoretical frameworks. Interviews with the mothers were conducted in the summer and fall of 2007.

In order to identify HIV-positive mothers most similar to those known to have given birth to HIV-positive children in Fortaleza, the HIV-positive mothers in my study were all identified through the sole public hospital for infectious diseases in the state. The hospital is the primary referral and treatment center for all infectious disease cases in the state, including HIV/AIDS. The selection criteria included all women between the ages of 18 and 45 years, who had given birth to at least one child with knowledge of their HIV status. Eighteen women were identified, all of whom agreed to participate. For a more detailed description of the characteristics of these women, please see Table 17.1.

These women gave a 2-h interview and were provided with transportation and/or transportation reimbursement. The hospital ethics board in Fortaleza prohibited direct financial payment to respondents. A proxy interviewer was used in order to protect the respondents' confidentiality. Respondents were provided with the option of using a pseudonym, and neither the interviewer personnel nor the researchers knew the respondents' identity. Consent was obtained for both written and audio recording of the interview. Two institutional review boards granted human subjects protection approval for this study, including the University of New Mexico IRB and the IRB of the Hospital Sao Jose in Fortaleza.

Following the interviews, the transcripts were analyzed using the grounded theoretical approach for the emergence of common themes (Liamputtong 2013). These were then coded and inputted into Atlas TI, a data management program. Open coding and investigator and theory triangulation were also used as validation techniques to achieve theme saturation. Direct quotes from the women are identified by a pseudonym.

3   Results

3.1   Social and Demographic Characteristics

Like the majority of women living with HIV in Fortaleza, the 18 women in my study shared the common life circumstances of coming from one of the peripheral neighborhoods (*favelas*) of Fortaleza and living in conditions of social and economic marginalization. Specifically, the women in this study were relatively young (the median age was 33), had typically left school before graduating from high school, had not experienced consistent employment, and generally reported a household income of less than 2 minimum wages per month (the minimum monthly salary in 2007 was approximately 400 real – or about 240 dollars).

Nearly all of the women I interviewed lived in rented homes or apartments that were shared with family members or friends. The mean number of children was three, and only one of the mothers with whom I spoke had a child living with HIV. This profile (undereducated, underemployed, and weak household resources) is typical of low-income residents throughout Brazil who make up the majority of the population. Despite economic challenges at home and in other areas of their daily lives, our interviews showed that women were able to mobilize substantial institutional and familial resources to interact positively with the medical system and to adhere to a relatively stable routine of HIV treatment and care.

3.2   Experiences with HIV Treatment and Care: Prenatal Care, Testing, and Disclosure of HIV Status

I began by asking the mothers I interviewed to comment on the amount of prenatal care they received during their pregnancies. As I have noted in the introduction, prenatal care was made freely available to pregnant HIV-positive women in Brazil in 1996. Despite reporting occasional difficulties in arranging childcare or transportation, nearly two thirds of the women received routine prenatal care, and the remaining five reported at least intermittent medical visits and care (cf. Chap. 4 in this volume).

I found that the women were also likely to receive an HIV diagnosis in the context of a prenatal care appointment (see also Chaps. 3, 4, 15, and 16 in this volume). A total of 13 out of 18 women received a diagnosis of HIV during the prenatal exam. The remaining women either arrived at a health clinic with illness complaints, or had watched boyfriends or partners struggle with the disease, and were subsequently tested for HIV. The number of times doctors reached out to the women in this study to inquire about taking an HIV test was particularly striking. For example, two of the women reported that doctors had sought them out and asked them if they would be willing to be tested for HIV after their boyfriends or partners had tested positive for the disease. In another case, a respondent reported that she had presented at a local health clinic with a severe case of boils. The attending doctor asked about her background and, in the course of their conversation, suggested that she take an HIV test, in addition to being seen by a dermatologist.

Although I did not ask women to comment specifically on the quality of their visits with doctors regarding the HIV test, nearly all of the women in my study voluntarily described details about these interactions that showed their doctors in a positive light. For example, Isabel reported that

> I had a fever, and I got the chicken pox. I went to the doctor, and when I showed him my arm, he said, "Oh my child, we're going to examine you for HIV. You might have this virus, should we make a test?" And I said okay because it is better to know.

Another woman, Solange, reported that her doctor "looked at her with concern" when she said her boyfriend had HIV and asked her "well what do you think? Should we make a test too?" The majority of the women used words such as *bonita* (lovely) or *simpatico* (nice) to describe the doctor or medical caregiver who performed the HIV test.

Stories of positive interactions with doctors surfaced again when I asked women to describe their feelings and experiences revealing their HIV status. Most of the women in this sample revealed a willingness to tell doctors and other medical professionals about their HIV status and reported doing so with a measure of tranquility. In total, 13 out of 18 women reported that fear of revealing their HIV status did not act as a barrier to care, while 5 women stated that fear of stigma sometimes prevented them from revealing their HIV status.

> Joelma's comment was typical of the many responses I received:
>
> I reveal my HIV status in health clinics when necessary. I don't have fear of revealing my positive status on necessary occasions since after my diagnosis, many things went right for me, and with the knowledge of Jesus and God, I've been given more of a chance of victory.

Other women simply stated that they "always reveal their status when necessary." When asked to describe why they did not have a problem disclosing their HIV status, most often, the women referred to the positive attitudes of the health care workers they interacted with. For example, Linda stated:

> I don't fear revealing my status in health clinics because I think they [the staff] are given an orientation about how to behave. When they found out about my status, they gave me support and didn't treat me any differently.

Another woman, Manuela, acknowledged that the behavior of her doctors actually motivated her to disclose her status. She said:

> There's just no way to hide. The doctor needs to know, and what motivates me to speak is that I need treatment... I've never feared telling people I'm HIV-positive. When I go get the medicine and they see the prescriptions, they don't ask any kind of questions. Maybe they're curious to know, but they don't ask.

A notable minority of Fortaleza women did report a fear of disclosure (6 out of 16). However, for these women, this fear surfaced most often in the context of a local health center where they were worried that they would be recognized by friends or family members. One woman, Angela, said, for example,

> I would reveal my status if necessary in a big hospital, but never in the health center in my neighborhood, because I have a fear of prejudice from my neighbors.

Another woman stated that

> For me, the big issue is telling someone I have feelings for that I'm HIV-positive. But telling the doctor is no big deal.

Only one of the women in the Fortaleza group, Francinete, reported to be fearful in all contexts, stating, "If I reveal my status, I'll be prejudiced against. I'm afraid of speaking about it even in hospitals."

Several of the women I interviewed linked the quality of care they received and the lack of stigmatization they experienced with the fact that they were being treated in a hospital where doctors and caregivers were used to dealing with people with HIV. For example, Vanessa said:

> They know exactly how to treat you here; they know what you're going through and don't make you feel like you're alone.

However, other women consistently used the phrase *meu amigo* (my friend) to describe their doctor and to explain why they did not experience stigma in revealing their HIV status. Andressa, for example, suggested that

> Even now the doctor is the person that I trust, I get along very well with him; he's my doctor, my friend.

Another woman, Analouisa, commented that

> The doctors are very attentive, and they have the desire to talk to you like you are a professional. I feel very comfortable during the appointment. I talk to my doctors about everything.

The most negative experiences women reported did not concern stigma but were rather about having to wait for medical appointments. Maria Jose, for example, stated that her doctor was often late for her appointments, whereas if she herself were to show up late, they would tell her to come back another day. However, she ended the story by commenting that in general, the doctors were excellent and that now she "really likes the doctor."

3.3   Coping with an HIV Diagnosis: Depression Following HIV Diagnosis and Motivation to Accept Treatment

Once I had elicited responses regarding women's experiences with early HIV medical care and treatment, I wanted to know more about how they coped with an HIV diagnosis once they had received it and what role doctors, medical institutions, and family networks played in their ability to accept and continue with treatment routines. I found that women consistently mentioned more traditional forms of support from their family, friends, religious faith, and in conjunction with medical care professionals and institutions as crucial to their attempts to overcome depression following HIV diagnosis and in their motivation to accept HIV treatment (see also Chaps. 12, 14, and 15 in this volume).

More than one half of the women I interviewed were living with a partner (9 out of 16 women reported living with a spouse or partner), and 8 out of 16 were married. Although these women reported living in "small" or "cramped" houses, often with large numbers of family members (as many as 9), they reported no incidents of physical, sexual, or mental abuse, nor did they tend to comment negatively on their living situations in general. When asked, "who helps in taking you to meetings with doctors or other hospital visits?," in almost every case, the women provided detailed lists of specific family members who would accompany them to the hospital, who could stay home with their children, and who could come to stay with them on overnight visits. There was not a strict uniformity in terms of which family members played which roles; rather, mothers, grandmothers, sisters, partners, in-laws, and children were all listed as possible, and often interchangeable, helpers.

In addition, despite the fact that most of these women had left school early (more than half of the women in the study had a 6th grade education or below) and fewer than half of them were employed at the time of the interview, they did report being embedded in multiple social settings that facilitated positive social bonds. For example, almost all of the respondents went to church at least once a week, and a third of them went three or more times per week.

A significant number of the women also described a particular medical institution (most often the infectious disease hospital) as helping to facilitate their HIV treatment. For example, Vanessa described always bringing her children with her to her medical consults. She stated: "The doctors never said this was a problem; they're always welcoming." "I even bring my 3-year-old," she continued, "he stays at the *casa de apoio* [nongovernmental 'houses of support' which provide food and lodging to those in need], when I don't have someone to stay with him." Another woman, Manuela, pointed out that in the absence of strong family relations, she counted on her medical clinic to provide the necessary support. She remarked that

> One time, I stayed in the hospital, and they talked to me and paid for my children to stay. It is a marvelous institution. I can't count on anyone from my family to do this, so I depend on these institutions.

Thus, in the context of our interviews, relationships with family members, friends (who in certain cases were incorporated into family structures), church groups, and medical institutions were all reported to provide a strong basis of social support and solidarity.

The existence of strong social and institutional embeddedness appeared to play a significant role in women's responses to being diagnosed with HIV and in their motivations to accept HIV treatment. For example, although the majority of Fortaleza mothers reported having significant episodes of depression after learning that they were HIV-positive, these women also reported mobilizing social and institutional connections to help cope with their reactions. Irene offered a typical response to her feelings after being told she was HIV-positive:

I wanted to cry all the time; I didn't have the motivation to do anything; I didn't feel like eating. Finally, someone from my family came to see me and made sure I was able to get out of bed and start living again.

Another woman, Glicia, remarked:

When I was diagnosed, I was depressed; I stayed 15 days alone in the house, and I didn't want to see anyone … I passed 15 days crying all the time. After this time, a friend of mine took me to the hospital, and a doctor talked to me and told me about the medication I could take and that everything was going to be okay.

In total, 17 out of 18 women from the study reported significant episodes of depression, followed by sustained attempts to overcome this depression through the help of religion, family, friends, or medical caregivers.

When asked to describe in detail how they coped with their depression, most often, the women invoked their religious faith. For example, Francinete commented:

Soon after the HIV diagnosis, I became depressed. During this time, I asked for the help of God, and you know, if it hadn't been for God, I would have gone crazy. I recovered from this crisis with divine intervention.

Another woman, Bruna, replied:

I came here [to the local health clinic] to be assisted for HIV, I asked God for help, and He helped me. He told me – every three months to have an appointment with the doctor. The birth [of my child] was a victory; God provided me with strength and courage; I was fearless.

The narration of religious experiences often took up several pages of interview notes and became a focal point in women's descriptions of their reactions to an HIV diagnosis. For example, Nezia began a long story about her religious involvement when she was asked to describe her HIV diagnoses. She said:

After the diagnosis, I knew that I had to accept Jesus and have faith in God.…I stayed in my house for 15 days, and I was only listening to the voice of Senhor, talking with him all the time, why have you done this – I asked him. In Isaiah, it says this, and I went to church, and then I put it [religion] in my soul – I am cured, today I am cured.

In cases where religious faith was not mentioned, several women reported turning to their doctors immediately following their diagnosis. Rosalena remarked that

The day I got my diagnosis [that I was HIV-positive], I was all day with a psychologist; I only thought to kill myself, when I discovered that I was pregnant. I was very sad, but then after 3 months, I began treatment.

When asked to clarify why she began the treatment, she answered:

The doctors knew I didn't want my baby to get this. At first, I said no to the treatment, but then the doctors said that it was better for me to make the treatment, so that there was a chance my baby wouldn't have the disease. Also, one of my aunts came to talk to me and told me that I should go home that being with my family would be important.

Another woman, Jucylena, confirmed the role of her doctor in helping her to accept her diagnosis. She told me that

> When I was diagnosed, it was at the local health post. I felt that they were very professional when they gave me my result. Before this, the doctor told me he was my friend; I had known him from before – he had been my doctor for another pregnancy, and he came with me to the diagnosis; he was a very good friend. And then, afterwards, I got counseling from the doctors.

In total, nearly half of the women in the study reported relying on their doctor in some way, and in only one instance did a woman report having no one to turn to for emotional support following her HIV diagnoses.

With regard to the question of their motivations to accept HIV treatment, the women I interviewed indicated ambivalence about taking antiretroviral drugs and sometimes expressed contradictory feelings about their effects. For example, Fernanda stated that she was not going to take any drugs because "they just make you die quicker – they make you worse." Similarly, Angela said that "I just don't like swallowing pills, and I have fear of the effects of the medication – it doesn't sit with my body." However, all of these women also acknowledged their desire to go on living for their family members.

A striking aspect of my results was the number of times women mentioned multiple family members in their responses. Vanesa's response, which was typical of this trend, illustrated this:

> My former partner, my bosses, and my former sister-in-law encouraged me to get medical assistance, and they encouraged me in the routine of going to the hospital.

Another woman, Andresa, included her child in her response, stating that

> When I arrived here [at the hospital], I didn't want to stay at all, but my aunt and mother talked to me a lot, they talked with me when I wanted to get treatment about the rest of my life, and I wanted to have more time for life, I wanted to see my son grow up. So, I tried to stay getting treatment. I think this is what motivated me to get treatment. The care of my child and my partner, my mother – I didn't want to abandon them.

Almost all of the women in the study expressed a profound sense of faith in the future. For example, Irene said that

> Before I had the test, I felt full of fear of death. But afterwards, I began to use the ARVs. With the treatment, I decided to get help because I wanted to live longer. If you begin treatment, it is in order to have force to live. If you give up the problem, you don't have love of life; you commit suicide. I have received support from my family and friends who know that I am sick. It helps that my family knows that I'm positive. My motivations to go are for my family.

4 Discussion

As part of Brazil's highly innovative response to the HIV/AIDS crisis and in accordance with the legal requirement to provide all citizens who are HIV-positive with access to anti-HIV treatment, a number of measures have been made available to women in order to reduce mother-to-child transmission of the disease. These include the offer of HIV testing to all pregnant women, the administration of antiretroviral drugs to pregnant HIV-positive women and their babies, testing for viral loads, and a free milk supply to replace breastfeeding (Knauth et al. 2003). Scholars have been careful to warn of the complexities involved in coordinating such a large-scale delivery system of ARVs and to insist that access does not necessarily guarantee delivery of or adherence to medication (Biehl 2007). Nonetheless, a number of studies have demonstrated that the efforts made on behalf of pregnant women with HIV have brought about significant reductions in the number of perinatal HIV cases (Bergenstrom and Sherr 2000; Matida and Silva 2005; de Brito 2006; Turchi et al. 2007).

In the case of my study, despite coming from poor neighborhoods and experiencing logistical difficulties and complications in arranging to attend prenatal care appointments, the majority of mothers I interviewed both routinely received prenatal care and were likely to receive an HIV test during their prenatal appointments. In trying to understand why these particular women were successfully in getting care, what stood out for me was the number of respondents who went out of their way to praise their doctors and medical caregivers, particularly around the issue of HIV testing. The number of times women characterized their doctors as "warm" or "good," and connected this description to their doctor's decision to reach out to them and ask them about taking an HIV test, was striking. I cannot offer a conclusive interpretation of this finding, but it appears that in the case of my study, Fortaleza doctors clearly felt comfortable actively reaching out to their patients, asking them if they wanted to be tested, and soliciting conversations about the disease. Brazil's universal HIV testing policy, which requires doctors to offer women the opportunity to be tested during their prenatal care appointments and excludes requirements such as consent forms and pretest counseling, may act as an incentive to doctors to establish the kind of warm and active relationships with their patients that the mothers in our study valued.

Another important finding of this study was that women directly linked a willingness to reveal their HIV status to their doctors' warmth, friendliness, and the lack of stigma they felt exposed to. Specifically, women stated that the attitudes of medical professionals made them feel comfortable about their own HIV-positive status and thus more willing to disclose it. These responses stand in direct contrast to studies conducted in other countries, which have shown that women exhibit an unwillingness to reveal their HIV status because of the disrespectful, stigmatizing attitudes they encountered when interacting with medical caregivers (Painter et al. 2004; Lindau et al. 2006).

Why would stigma about being HIV-positive be less likely to have been felt by the women in Fortaleza? One possible response to this question may be to point to research that has suggested that Brazil's human rights approach to the HIV/AIDS crisis has lead to a decrease in the stigmatization of AIDS. Studies have noted, for example, that both doctors and patients report that access to free treatment has positively transformed the general public attitude toward HIV in Brazil (Cseste 2001; Galvao 2005; Okie 2006; Biehl 2007). One doctor working with HIV patients explained that "Previously people with HIV infection hid it from their families and at work. Now they tell everybody that they have the virus. They claim their rights, they know they can have the medicines, so they reveal themselves, to live better" (Okie 2006: 1980).

These claims are consistent with the kinds of comments I heard when speaking to a number of HIV-related nongovernmental organizations in Fortaleza. Nearly all of them described the connection Brazil has drawn between human rights and health as explicitly improving the public attitude toward AIDS and the people who have it. For example, in an interview with the head of APROCE (Associação das Prostitutes do Ceará), we discussed the connection between respecting the rights of marginalized populations and increasing the support for AIDS treatment; she told me that

> The HIV epidemic is aided by social exclusion – marginalized populations are the most vulnerable to HIV infection....Breaking this cycle of social exclusion is thus crucial both to preventing transmission, and to maximizing the care and support available to people living with HIV/AIDS. This is perhaps the key to the tremendous impact of Brazil's 1996 decision to guarantee constitutionally access to ARV therapy. Not only has this decision led to an enormous increase in the number of Brazilians with access to the drugs, it also sent the signal that people with HIV/AIDS were valued citizens who were entitled to medical care, and should not be stigmatized. (Interview, 6/8/2007)

Linking the reduction of stigma to the implementation of a human rights-based social policy recalls Parker and Aggleton's (2003) plea that research about the stigma surrounding HIV should go beyond describing stigmatizing attitudes and stereotypes and focus instead on the structural conditions that produce exclusion from social and economic life (see also Liamputtong 2013). My study cannot confirm a causal link between Brazil's rights-based HIV programming and the relatively stigma-free environment that many of the women in my study reported, but it is significant that women consistently reported a willingness to disclose their HIV status because of their doctors' open, nonjudgmental attitudes. I suggest that future research pursues this link between the adoption of particular health policies and the reduction of stigma regarding HIV/AIDS.

In addition to describing the importance of doctors' positive attitudes during prenatal care and HIV testing, the women I interviewed also brought up more traditional support systems when discussing their behavior following an HIV diagnosis. Nearly all of the women I spoke with described elaborate kinship networks often made up of extended family members or friends, whom they depended on for economic, social, and medical support when confronting their HIV diagnosis and making decisions about HIV treatment and care. This support appears to have been offered both in times of crises and in day-to-day activities and interactions. Although educational and employment institutions were often lacking in these women's lives, they reported extremely strong ties to religious institutions, frequently citing their relationship to God as a primary motivation to accept their HIV diagnosis and treatment.

These findings are consistent with studies that have demonstrated the strength of kinship networks in Northeastern Brazil (Borges 1992; Rebhun 1999). In particular, scholars have pointed to extended family members' willingness to stand in for one another, forming makeshift "families" which shift and change depending on circumstance (Scheper-Hughes 1992).

Other scholars of Northeastern Brazil have noted the tremendous power of Catholic and evangelical religious faith to orient action and to help mobilize, even in extremely poor settings, social resources for health care needs (Borges 1992; Scheper-Hughes 1992). Key to this power has been the proliferation of local churches and faiths, which appeal to lower class needs and concerns. During the past three decades, small religious establishments of both Catholic and Protestant faiths have appeared throughout working class neighborhoods in Northeastern Brazil and attracted a loyal audience by embracing a wide range of issues, including HIV/AIDS (Biehl 2007). It is likely that the explicit inclusion of lower and working concerns in religious sermons has encouraged the women I interviewed to maintain a strong connection to religious institutions and to understand faith as a potent response to HIV diagnosis and treatment. In a book-length treatment on the topic of HIV/AIDS in Brazil, medical anthropologist, Joao Biehl, identifies religion as part of the "economy of survival" of the poor, Northeastern Brazilian AIDS patients he interviewed. "Religion," he writes, "provided them with an alternative value system that made them more than a social and statistical void – that is, they now had a proxy community, hope, and a real chance at life" (Biehl 2007: 320).

While these cultural features of northeastern life were clearly extremely important in helping mothers cope with episodes of depression and in their attempts to develop healthy routines, to take medications, or simply to find reasons to continue living, I want to emphasize that these struggles occurred in a context of a particular set of health policies and practises, which appeared to provide additional levels of support for these women. Even with regard to more personal topics following an HIV diagnosis, a number of women mentioned either their doctors or medical caregivers as an important source of support. Several women even mentioned the hospital in which they received care as an institution that would, for example, allow their children to spend the night if they were receiving medical treatment. I contend that further research should be undertaken to elucidate how family members and religious organizations can work in tandem with medical caregivers and institutions to provide a broad umbrella of support for mothers with HIV.

5   Conclusion

Despite a steep decline in the overall prevalence of perinatal HIV transmission in Brazil, data from the city of Fortaleza indicates that economically marginalized HIV-positive women remain at risk for the transmission of HIV to their infants and that health care providers must be vigilant in making sure that women with HIV continue to have both access to treatment and the support necessary to take advantage of this treatment (Maia 2008). Using a human rights-based theoretical approach, I have argued here that one of the key factors in ensuring that women actually take advantage of the medical treatment and care they are offered is doctors' attitudes and the overall environment of care in which they disclose their HIV status and receive treatment. The women I interviewed consistently linked their perceptions of doctors' attitudes and the overall environment in which they received care with their willingness to attend prenatal care appointments, take an HIV test, disclose their HIV status to caregivers, and even to continue to adhere to treatment regimes – all crucial steps in reducing perinatal HIV transmission.

This study reveals the need for more research that explicitly investigates the link between ideologies of health care, such as a human rights approach to health, and the quality of doctor-patient relationships. A continuing decrease in the levels of mother-to-child HIV transmission, particularly among the world's most vulnerable populations of mothers, cannot occur without attention to both the social and institutional forces that encourage women to disclose their HIV status and accept care.

References

Bergenstrom A, Sherr L (2000) A review of HIV testing policies and procedures for pregnant women in public maternity units of Porto Alegre, Rio Grande do Sul, Brazil. AIDS Care 12(2):177–186

Berquo E (2005) Comportamento sexual e percepcoes da populacao Brasileira sobre o HIV/AIDS. Programa Nacional de DST e AIDS, Brasilia

Biehl J (2007) Will to live: AIDS therapies and the politics of survival. Princeton University Press, Princeton

Borges D (1992) The family in Bahia, Brazil, 1870–1945. Stanford University Press, Stanford

Cseste J (2001) Several for the price of one: right to AIDS treatment as link to other human rights. Conn J Int Law 17:263–272

de Brito AM (2006) Trends in maternal-infant transmission of AIDS after antiretroviral therapy in Brazil. Rev Saude Publica 40(Suppl):9–17

Farmer P (2003) Pathologies of power: health, human rights and the new war on the poor. University of California Press, Berkeley

Galvao J (2005) Brazil and access to HIV/AIDS drugs: a question of human rights and public health. Chic J Public Health 95(7):1110–1116

Gostin L (1997) Human rights and public health in the AIDS pandemic. Oxford University Press, Oxford

Knauth D, Barbosa R, Hopkins K (2003) Between personal wishes and medical prescription: mode of delivery and post-partum sterilisation among women with HIV in Brazil. Reprod Health Matters 11(22):113–121

Kreitchmann R, Fuchs S, Suffert T, Preussler G (2004) Perinatal HIV-1 transmission among low income women participants in the HIV/AIDS control program in southern Brazil: a cohort study. BJOG 11:579–584

Liamputtong P (2013) Qualitative research methods, 4th edn. Oxford University Press, Melbourne

Liamputtong P (ed) (2013) Stigma, discrimination and HIV/AIDS: a cross-cultural perspective. Springer, Dordrecht

Lindau ST, Jerome J, Miller K, Monk E, Garcia P, Cohen M (2006) Mothers in the margins: implications for eradicating perinatal HIV. Soc Sci Med 62:59–69

Maia J (2008) Fortaleza e a 2nd capital do Pais em gravidas com HIV. Diario Do Nordeste. Sabado, 13 de Setembro

Matida L, Silva M (2005) Prevention of mother-to-child transmission of HIV in Sao Paulo State, Brazil: an update. AIDS 19(Suppl 4):37–41

Mofenson LM (2003) Tale of two-epidemics – the continuing challenge of preventing mother-to-child transmission of human immunodeficiency virus [comment]. J Infect Dis 187(5):721–724

Okie S (2006) Fighting HIV- lessons from Brazil. N Engl J Med 354:1977–1981

Painter T, Diaby K, Matia DM, Lin LSL, Sibailly TS, Kouassi MK et al (2004) Women's reasons for not participating in follow up visits before starting ARVs for prevention of mother to child transmission of HIV: qualitative interview study. Br Med J 339(7465):543

Parker R, Aggleton P (2003) HIV and AIDS-related stigma and discrimination: a conceptual framework and implications for action. Soc Sci Med 57:13–24

Rebhun LA (1999) The heart is unknown country: love in the changing economy of north eastern Brazil. Stanford University Press, Stanford

Scheper-Hughes N (1992) Death without weeping. University of California Press, Berkeley

Taket A (2012) Health and social justice (Chapter17). In: Liamputtong P, Fanany R, Verrinder G (eds) Health, illness and well-being: perspectives and social determinants. Oxford University Press, Melbourne

Turchi M, Durate L, Martelli M (2007) Transmissao vertical do HIV: fatores associados e perdas de oportunidades de intervencao em gestantes atendidas dem Goiania, Goias, Brasil. Cad Saude Publica 23(3):1–12

Chapter 18
The MOMS (Making Our Mothers Stronger) Project: A Culturally Tailored Parenting Intervention for Mothers Living with HIV in the Southern USA

Susan L. Davies, Herpreet Kaur Thind, and Jamie L. Stiller

1 Introduction

African Americans represent a small proportion (13.6%) of the US population; however, they accounted for 50.3% of the HIV diagnosis in adolescents and adults during 2005–2008 in 37 US states (CDC 2010a). Further, the rates of HIV infection have increased among African American women; in 2006, it was approximately 15 times as high as that of Caucasian women (CDC 2010a). The estimated lifetime risk of being diagnosed with HIV is 1 in 30 for African American women compared to 1 in 588 for White females (Hall et al. 2008), making it the third leading cause of death among 35–44-year-old African American women (CDC 2010b).

1.1 HIV in the Southern USA

The Deep South region of the United States has had the highest increase of new HIV/AIDS cases among all regions in the country (Reif et al. 2006). In the six states that collectively make up the Deep South (Alabama, Georgia, Louisiana, Mississippi,

S.L. Davies (✉)
Department of Health Behavior, School of Public Health,
University of Alabama at Birmingham, Birmingham, AL 35294-0022, USA

UAB Center for AIDS Research, University of Alabama at Birmingham,
Birmingham, AL 35294-0022, USA

Center for the Study of Community Health, University of Alabama at Birmingham,
Birmingham, AL 35294-0022, USA
e-mail: sdavies@uab.edu

H.K. Thind • J.L. Stiller
School of Public Health, University of Alabama at Birmingham,
Birmingham, AL 35294-0022, USA
e-mail: herpreet@uab.edu; jstiller@uab.edu

P. Liamputtong (ed.), *Women, Motherhood and Living with HIV/AIDS:*
A Cross-Cultural Perspective, DOI 10.1007/978-94-007-5887-2_18,
© Springer Science+Business Media Dordrecht 2013

North Carolina, and South Carolina), HIV incidence rates increased 36% from 2000 to 2005, while comparable rates decreased 6% in the other regions of the USA over the same period (Pence et al. 2007). In addition, the Deep South's HIV epidemic is exponentially higher among African Americans, women, and residents of rural communities than other regions of the country (McKinney 2002). Among females in the South, African American women accounted for 70% of all HIV diagnoses during 2005–2008 (CDC 2011). Moreover, in Alabama, African American women accounted for 22% of all HIV/AIDS diagnoses and 73% of female diagnoses in 2009. Many women living with or at risk for HIV infection do not engage in high-risk sexual behaviors; their increased vulnerability stems from the risk behavior of their male partners (Kojic and Cu-Uvin 2007; amfAR 2008).

The HIV epidemic in southern states is so unique to the rest of the country. In fact, it has been said to have more in common with those of developing countries. Reasons for this are many and complex but include the fact that these states are significantly poorer compared to other states, stigma and ostracism are more common, and conservative values predominate (Konkle-Parker et al. 2008). Peterman and colleagues (2005) examined US counties with reported increases in AIDS incidence rates. Of 20 counties with this disturbing trend, 18 of them were in the southeast. These counties had a higher proportion of households headed by a single mother, a higher proportion of persons with less than a 9th grade education, a larger proportion of the population that was African American, and lower overall literacy levels. Further, these counties with the largest increases in AIDS incidence also had higher incidence rates of syphilis, age-adjusted mortality and infant mortality, and more low-birth-weight infants.

These trends will be difficult to reverse given the region's concomitant rates of poverty and uninsured individuals, which further hinder HIV prevention and treatment efforts. Adimora and colleagues (2002) examined the role of various contextual factors (including racism, discrimination, limited employment opportunity, and resultant economic and social inequality) that may promote HIV transmission in this population. They posit that the social and economic environment of many African American communities in the Deep South discourages long-term monogamy and promotes concurrent sexual partnerships, which may, in turn, fuel the HIV epidemic in this population.

1.2 Heightened HIV-Related Stigma in the African American Community

In addition to the concerns about physical health and death, the main issue faced by the people living with HIV (PLWH) is stigma (see Liamputtong 2013; Chap. 1 in this volume). Research has shown that stigma associated with HIV/AIDS is greater than many other stigmatizing conditions such as mental illness and physical health problems (Crawford 1996; Corrigan et al. 2000). Moreover, HIV-related stigma is found to be significantly higher among African Americans compared to Whites

(Emlet 2007). In a study in New York City, black men living with HIV/AIDS reported that stigma marks them as "just one more body" within medical and social institutions. The dynamics of stigma is so severe that it leaves those experiencing it feeling that they are "stuck in the quagmire of an HIV ghetto" (Haile et al. 2011).

Stigmatizing attitudes are associated with misconceptions and lack of knowledge of the mechanism of HIV transmission (Sengupta et al. 2010; see also Liamputtong 2013) and overestimating the risk of casual contacts (Price and Hsu 1992; Herek and Capitanio 1994). People feel uncomfortable having direct contact with PLWH. This feeling of discomfort leads to avoidance or discrimination (Herek et al. 2002). For example, in a national telephone survey, one-third respondents said they would avoid shopping at a grocery store if the owner had AIDS (Herek et al. 2002). Studies have indicated that religious beliefs can also instigate discrimination against PLWH (Fullilove and Fullilove 1999). Especially for African American women, high religiosity beliefs are associated with higher stigma since HIV/AIDS is associated with immoral behaviors and considered a curse or punishment from God (Muturi and An 2010).

Fear of HIV-related stigma is a barrier to testing among African Americans (Hutchinson et al. 2004; Payne et al. 2006; Wallace et al. 2011). It also impedes them from seeking health care and adhering to antiretroviral medication (Konkle-Parker et al. 2008). Especially in smaller communities and rural areas, the fear of being seen at a HIV clinic by someone from their neighborhood prevents them from attending HIV clinics for treatment (Kempf et al. 2010). PLWH do not disclose their status to protect themselves from stigma. However, not disclosing prevents them from receiving education, medical care, and the needed social support (Serovich 2001; Hudson et al. 2001). Lack of access or delayed access to care further results in disease progression, which increases HIV/AIDS morbidity and mortality in this population (Sengupta et al. 2010).

HIV-related stigma has several consequences that affect the physical, psychological, and social health of PLWH. It leads to feelings of loneliness, isolation, and social exclusion (Sayles et al. 2007; Vyavaharkar et al. 2010). Studies have indicated that depression is much higher among PLWH compared to the general population (Ciesla and Roberts 2001). Further among PLWH, depression is much higher among women, especially African American women (Moneyham et al. 2000; Phillips et al. 2011). Women living with HIV face extreme stress in excess to their coping abilities, which results in adverse psychological outcomes (Vyavaharkar et al. 2010).

1.3   HIV in Women and Mothers

Women, minorities, and low-income persons are more likely to contract HIV. As a result, these groups, which are already compromised by discrimination, stigma, and inadequate health insurance, experience higher mortality rates than those in other sociodemographic groups. African American low-income women are a highly vulnerable group that have the greatest unmet needs and who are also less likely to seek treatment for their HIV.

Women are already more likely than men to delay HIV medical care for themselves; having children in the household strengthens this association (Stein et al. 2000). Mothers living with HIV (MLWH) in the Deep South face a number of barriers that preclude their ability to receive optimal medical and mental health care. Lack of childcare and transportation are common obstacles to care among low-income women in the South. These structural and financial barriers are compounded by psychosocial barriers of inadequate support systems, concerns about confidentiality and heightened stigma for MLWH in the South. Stigma fuels the HIV epidemic by increasing denial and decreasing testing and treatment seeking in those living with or at high risk for HIV. High levels of perceived stigma have been associated with lower physical, psychological, and social functioning in MLWH (Clark et al. 2003; Murphy et al. 2006), as well as lower levels of disclosure (Clark et al. 2003). Stigma has a particularly strong impact on MLWH, and while this population could benefit immensely from social support, too often, they experience rejection and exclusion from their social networks (Ciambrone 2002; see Chap. 1). Limited perceived social support significantly predicts distress in MLWHs (Hudson et al. 2001). The South's conservative, religious culture exacerbates these problems and inhibits communities from actively addressing this growing crisis.

1.4 Issues Faced by MLWHs and Their Children

While MLWHs often perceive motherhood to be their most important role, they also report that it is a significant source of their stress (Andrews et al. 1993; Van Loon 2000). Being both a primary caregiver and a patient with a condition that others do not know about puts MLWH at several disadvantages. First, they do not receive the social support that they need from family members and friends, either because others do not know of their status, and MLWHs keep them from getting too close because of their "secret," or because others are aware of their HIV status, and choose not to provide support because of their own misguided concerns and beliefs about HIV transmission. Second, as HIV affects an individual physically, mentally, emotionally, and spiritually, MLWHs are likely to have many HIV-specific needs that they cannot meet on their own. Finally, having to keep something so significant hidden from those who could provide the needed support and resources is a very difficult task. While the disease itself rarely threatens maternal mortality for those with access to the antiretroviral therapy (HAART), the psychological toll of holding a secret so powerful that it can bring immediate ostracism, discrimination, unemployment, and even eviction and a host of other catastrophes if it were revealed, not only to oneself but to one's children and family, is often too painful to acknowledge. Denial brings its own adverse outcomes, both physiologic and emotional.

The persistent stressors faced by the MLWHs can complicate their HIV management through the direct effects that stress can have on the immune system (Glover et al. 2010). Studies have shown that stress can influence immune system functioning and also affect the HIV symptom severity and progression of disease (Kopnisky et al. 2004; Glover et al. 2010). Other negative outcomes been reported by MLWHs with increased stress include depression and substance abuse, which further compromise their health condition (Glover et al. 2010).

A mother's depression rarely leaves her children unscathed. Rather, maternal depression often spills over to adversely impact the family. Depression in MLWHs has also been associated with increased disruptive behaviors in their children (Pilowsky et al. 2003). Maternal depression brought on by social isolation, economic worries, and concern over children's future well-being can significantly affect the children. An inverse relationship has been shown between levels of depression and amount of caregiver involvement, whether the parents are living with HIV or not (Webster-Stratton and Hammond 1990; Stormshak et al. 2002).

In addition to the direct toll that stress can have on MLWHs, it can have indirect adverse effects by compromising their parenting skills and general coping abilities. Poorer parenting skills in turn lead to increased child behavior problems (Tompkins and Wyatt 2008). However, research has shown that positive parenting and family management practises by MLWHs are associated with better child outcomes (Murphy et al. 2010). Further, studies have shown that a coping style of seeking social support is associated with increased survival among parents living with HIV (Lee and Rotheram-Borus 2001). These studies point to the need to strengthen parenting skills and build social support systems among MLWHs to decrease their stress and improve their functioning.

One of the most daunting barriers to participation in psycho-educational and/or support group sessions for MLWH is the fear of disclosure. Less HIV disclosure to children has also been associated with missing medical appointments (Mellins et al. 2002). MLWHs would rather miss appointments if childcare was not available than bringing their children to their clinic appointment (Kempf et al. 2010). Further, low levels of HIV disclosure to children have been associated with higher externalizing behaviors, internalizing symptoms, and increased distressing life events (Nöstlinger et al. 2006). Nonetheless, research suggests that disclosure may be protective against maternal depression (Wiener et al. 1998; Murphy et al. 2011). Disclosure may result in better mental and physical health (Pennebaker et al. 1990), in that keeping a secret may stress one's body as well as their mind (Pennebaker et al. 1987; Imber-Black 1998). Increasing awareness and reducing concerns about stigma can help prepare MLWHs to disclose their status to their children and other support systems.

1.5 Parenting Interventions

Although the structure of families has changed dramatically over time, societal expectations of parents have not. Society still expects the parent(s) to be competent in performing its essential functions despite formidable stressors and challenges (McCubbin et al. 1997). Unfortunately, many of today's families are inadequately prepared or unable to equip their children with essential skills to thrive within and/or outside the family. Many parents today lack effective parenting skills for optimal parent, child, and family functioning. Until these skills are learned, unconstructive patterns of behavior and interaction are repeated and reinforced. Their impact takes a significant toll on the child (i.e., anger, shame, diminished self-concept, self-regulation, social, and emotional skills), the parent (guilt, exhaustion, social isolation), and family unit (chaos, disruption, disintegration, reduced communication).

Families in every culture have the same basic goals and functions that are critical to both health and quality of life. Just like all mothers, MLWHs want the best for their children, including the opportunity to realize their fullest potential and live a healthy, safe, and satisfying life. And, just like all mothers, MLWHs struggle to protect their children from the daily assaults from poverty and violence to loneliness and fear that threaten their health and well-being (Boyce 2009). While MLWHs often report experiencing significant parenting-related stress, they also report that their children are a source of comfort for them (Wood et al. 2004). Therefore, improving parent–child connectedness could not only protect children from risk behaviors but can also benefit MLWHs by reducing their stress and improving their quality of life.

Parent-training interventions have been shown to be effective in numerous settings and populations. Reid and colleagues (2001) used home observations of parent–child interactions and parent reports of parenting practices and child behavior problems to demonstrate that a parent-training intervention showed positive changes in both mothers (more positive, less critical, more consistent, and more competent in their parenting) and children (exhibited fewer behavior problems) in a large multiethnic population of families enrolled at a Head Start Center. This is important because changing these interactions early will continue to shape more positive future interactions throughout the lifespan.

In summary, being a mother while living with HIV can be both rewarding and a significant source of stress. HIV-related stressors and life adversities faced by the MLWHs can compromise immune function, complicate HIV management, increase risk for depression, decrease parenting skills, and reduce coping abilities. Poorer parenting skills in turn lead to increased child behavior problems, which exacerbates maternal stress. Thus, it is crucial for MLWHs to limit stressors and learn more adaptive ways to cope with adversities that cannot be avoided. There is a clear need for interventions to decrease maternal stress among MLWHs. An underutilized approach for doing so is to improve parenting skills among MLWHs.

2 Theoretical Frameworks

The MOMS Study was guided by tenets of two theoretical frameworks: Family Systems Theory and Social Cognitive Theory. First, we used Family Systems Theory to increase our understanding of the complex familial issues that challenged optimal family functioning in our population. Then, we used Social Cognitive Theory to develop the program components.

Most family theories (including Family Systems Theory and Family Development Theory) are grounded in the fundamental notion of dynamic interaction, which states that the individual and his/her environment interact in ways that change both. Development is not seen as linear but spiral, where this constant interaction and reciprocal influence leads to future interactions that have been influenced by the perception of past interactions. Bowen's (1978) Family Systems Theory (FST) is a comprehensive model of human behavior that represents a family's emotional and relational life. FST posits several constructs that shape family functioning that are particularly relevant to the life circumstances of MLWHs. First, all families can be characterized on a continuum of *differentiation* that reflects each family member's tolerance for individuality and intimacy. A well-differentiated individual demonstrates intact personal boundaries and effective problem-solving skills, while an undifferentiated person may largely base his or her decisions on the attitudes and opinions of significant others.

FST further asserts that the nuclear family is the *emotional system*, which functions as one emotional unit rather than many individuals with their own emotions. Because the actions of one affect everyone else, anxiety is infectious, easily passed from one person to another in the group. The concept of *emotional cutoff* reflects how, in the presence of excessive emotional intensity, a family member separates from the rest of the family or vice versa. This occurs when individuals behave in such a way that they are cut off emotionally from the rest of the family. HIV, homosexuality, disapproval of partner choice, and addiction are common situations leading to emotional cutoff. The *multigenerational transmission process* reflects how family functioning is repeated over several generations. FST proposes that the transmission of pathology transcends generations and affects the patterns of familial behavior, such that in dysfunctional families, each generation creates members with increasingly poorer differentiation, leaving them highly vulnerable to anxiety and fusion (Goldenberg and Goldenberg 1991; Coco and Courtney 1998).

With this insight, we used Social Cognitive Theory to guide the development of specific intervention components most likely to enhance maternal self-efficacy and build key parenting skills. According to Bandura's (1986) Social Cognitive Theory (SCT), human behavior is best explained by triadic reciprocal determinism in which the three primary behavioral determinants (behavior, cognitive and other personal factors, and environmental influences) interact to influence each other bidirectionally. While SCT does not assume that all sources have equal influence or act simultaneously to shape behavior, it does argue that these factors are not independent of one another nor are they static. Rather, they are reciprocal and dynamic. Another central construct of SCT is observational or social learning, which states that people learn by watching the behavior (and subsequent consequences) of others. These SCT constructs were translated into specific intervention strategies in the MOMS parenting intervention (described in the intervention section below).

3   The MOMS (Making Our Mothers Stronger) Project

MOMS was developed to address the concerns shared by mothers living with HIV during their clinic visits, who expressed a sense of being overwhelmed by the competing demands of being a parent and living with a serious health condition. Unlike most secondary prevention trials that aim to reduce HIV transmission and reinfection via sexual risk reduction strategies, MOMS aimed to enhance quality of life issues by focusing on the specific needs of mothers and children affected by the HIV epidemic. While MOMS was designed for women across the sociodemographic spectrum, our population closely reflects that of the larger population of persons living with HIV in the USA: predominantly those of color (88% African American) and of low socio-economic status (SES). As such, our intervention aims to meet the stress reduction needs of mothers living with HIV and the stresses of stigma, multiple responsibilities, very limited resources, and, frequently, discrimination. The Institutional Review Board at the University of Alabama at Birmingham, USA, approved the study.

The target population for the MOMS Project included women who were over 18 years of age, HIV-positive, and a primary caregiver of a child between 4 and 12 years of age. Knowing we would need broad support in accessing and engaging this very hard-to-reach population, we placed high priority on developing our recruitment strategies. We collaborated with all local HIV organizations as our community partners, which included three HIV/AIDS community agencies, three health care clinics specializing in HIV care, and a statewide HIV coalition. We invited their involvement from the beginning and sought their expertise and input on program promotion, participant recruitment, and intervention content. In addition, we created a Community Leadership Advisory Board, composed of community health advocates and key staff from our partner agencies. This Board provided ongoing guidance to the MOMS study team throughout the project period. From the front lines of patient care and case management, these individuals were an invaluable asset, making suggestions that often turned out to be crucial. Their input ensured that our intervention was responsive to the social and cultural characteristics of the participants, enabling us to more effectively engage mothers living with HIV into care.

Focus groups were conducted with women from the target population and the members of the advisory committee. In addition, semi-structured interviews were conducted with HIV service providers. Data obtained from this formative research helped to determine the perceived needs of HIV-positive mothers, desired intervention content, intervention process, and structure. The project advisors reviewed all MOMS session materials and even participated in mock intervention sessions, providing a friendly audience as well as invaluable feedback as our health educators were practicing intervention delivery.

The MOMS Project was a pretest-posttest, randomized-controlled behavioral trial that aimed to improve functioning of families affected by HIV by reducing childbearing stressors among HIV-positive mothers. Participants ($N = 106$) were randomly assigned to one of two intervention conditions: a Social Cognitive Theory (SCT)-based intervention focused on reducing parenting stress ("Parenting Skills for MOMS") or an attention-control intervention focused on reducing health-related stress ("Healthy MOMS"). The primary outcome of the trial was positive parenting skills; secondary outcomes included maternal stress, parenting self-efficacy, depression, and physical and mental health status.

Because of the dearth of existing resources for MLWHs, it was important that both interventions provided meaningful information and assistance to better cope and function with their HIV. So, while the study used an attention-control design, both interventions were significantly above and beyond "usual care" for MLWHs. Perhaps most important, both groups received the social support aspect inherent in small group-based intervention programs. However, the attention-control condition did not receive any parenting-specific information or skills training to enhance their parenting skills, which was the primary outcome of the study.

Through weekly 2½-h sessions over a 6-week period, participants came together for small group sessions of five to eight women and one health educator. Each cohort of women was stable and did not allow for new participants joining the group midway through the sequence of sessions. This design enhanced group cohesion, trust, and confidentiality and provided a safe environment for the expression of thoughts and feelings. During the first intervention session, ground rules were presented and discussed; these include items such as "Whatever we hear in this room stays in this room," "Listen, be nonjudgmental, and keep an open mind on issues" and were designed to maximize confidentiality and respect for individuals within the group. All participants were able to appreciate the shared experience of dealing with HIV while also functioning as a parent. Incentives such as timers, toys, games, candles, inspirational books, framed poems, recipes, and exercise bands were provided at each session to both intervention groups to encourage participants to continue at home what they learned in their sessions. Table 18.1 provides an overview and objectives of each group session for each intervention condition.

3.1 MOMS Parenting Skills Intervention

The parenting intervention included some general topics related to parenting and also included some components to address the specific needs of MLWHs and their children. Social Cognitive Theory guided the development of individual program components. The intervention focused on building four key skills: (1) *communicating clearly and effectively* with their children, (2) using *positive and negative consequences* with their children to effectively change child's behavior, (3) enjoying their children more by finding ways to *build quality time together* into their normal routine, and (4) *taking care of themselves* so they can best care for their children.

The parenting intervention aimed to improve communication and monitoring skills of MLWHs. Effective communication involves listening to children and giving them clear instructions of what is expected from them. Further, moms were taught effective discipline strategies to teach their children desirable behavior, while changing the unwanted behavior. Parents are responsible for setting family rules and implementing consistent disciplinary strategies to make sure that those rules are followed. The participating moms were taught how they can establish some ground rules in their home and can use positive and negative consequences to reinforce the desired behavior in their children. The self-control activity was used to teach moms how they can handle frustrating or challenging situations. Further, moms were encouraged to

Table 18.1 MOMS intervention overview

MOMS parenting skills intervention	Healthy MOMS intervention
Session 1: Communicating expectations	*Session 1*: Effective communication
Learning objectives:	*Learning objectives*:
Identify age-appropriate expectations for children	Identify barriers to communicating needs and concerns to health care providers
Demonstrate appropriate techniques for active listening and reflective statements	Identify strategies to most effectively communicate her needs and concerns and have her questions answered
Describe child behavior using clear and descriptive words	Identify points to an effective telephone call with a health care provider
Exhibit ability to draft family purpose statement	
Theme/inspiration: Differences in teaching vs. punishment; set realistic and appropriate expectations for children	*Theme/inspiration*: "Most important is hearing what isn't being said"
Session 2: Focus on discipline	*Session 2*: Adherence
Learning objectives:	*Learning objectives*:
Demonstrate appropriate strategies to communicate effectively with their children	Identify personal barriers to following health care provider's advice
Demonstrate appropriate use of positive and negative consequences	Identify strategies for improving adherence to health care provider's advice
Develop a plan for establishing ground rules	Identify personal barriers to following prescription protocol
Demonstrate ability to be consistent in applying strategies	Identify strategies for improving prescription adherence
	Identify the importance of keeping her providers advised about her adherence
Theme/inspiration: Children only know after we teach them, and "teaching" requires more than just "telling"	*Theme/inspiration*: "Incurable simply means you have to go inside to find the cure"
Session 3: Building and maintaining social support/contemplating disclosure	*Session 3*: Nutrition
Learning objectives:	*Learning objectives*:
Present and receive feedback on communication basics	Identify special nutritional needs of individuals living with HIV.
Distinguish between types of support	Identify several high calorie and protein food options to incorporate into their usual meals.
Identify and maintain social support network	Discuss the healthy food pyramid
Increase ability to seek and request help	Identify several barriers and strategies to overcome barriers to good nutrition.
Identify the pros and cons of disclosure	Identify safe and healthy food storage and preparation techniques
Increase awareness of feelings and beliefs about disclosure	
Evaluate the consequences of disclosing to particular people	

(continued)

Table 18.1 (continued)

MOMS parenting skills intervention	Healthy MOMS intervention
Theme/inspiration: "Good parenting takes time"	*Theme/inspiration*: "Love is a fruit in season at all times and within reach of every hand"
Session 4: Taking care of yourself	*Session 4*: Physical activity
Learning objectives:	*Learning objectives*:
Identify stressors and use strategies to make a coping plan	Identify benefits of regular physical activity
Demonstrate ability to let go of grudges	Increase understanding of the barriers they perceive that keep them from regular activity
Practice relaxation technique	Learn strategies for overcoming these identified barriers
Identify good things about themselves and increase knowledge of self-care	Increase knowledge about methods of safe exercise
Practice positive mom-child connections	
Increase use of stress-reducing strategies	
Theme/inspiration: "Conflicts are inevitable. Anger, grudges, hurt, and blame are not"	*Theme/inspiration*: "There is no better exercise for the heart than reaching down and lifting someone up"
Session 5: Focus on me/my children	*Session 5*: Sexual health risk reduction
Learning objectives:	*Learning objectives*:
Demonstrate appropriate techniques for parenting in high-stress situations	Identify the benefits to their own and other's health by reducing risky sexual activity
Demonstrate their ability to describe and understand emotions	Show increased knowledge about STDs and HIV reinfection; dispel common myths about barrier methods of protection
Encourage open communication about death with children	Demonstrate skills necessary to reduce risky behaviors (i.e., proper condom and barrier use skills)
Evaluate knowledge of future planning	Identify high, low, and no risk sexual activities and benefits of barrier protection
Demonstrate ability to set goals for children	Develop more positive attitudes toward using protection consistently
Theme/inspiration: "Staying calm is the key to curbing your child's poor behavior"	*Theme/inspiration*: "The secret of good health for both mind and body is not to mourn for the past, nor to worry about the future, but to live the present moment wisely and earnestly"
Session 6: How far we've come and graduation	*Session 6*: Stress reduction
Learning objectives:	*Learning objectives*:
Compare past and current views of "discipline"	Increase knowledge of ways to positively react to stress
Demonstrate knowledge of disciplinary strategies and terminology	Review and recognize what you have learned since the first MOMS session
Identify gifts and strengths of other moms in the group	Celebrate your accomplishments and those of your group members
Participate in a graduation ceremony to show successful completion of the program	

(continued)

Table 18.1 (continued)

MOMS parenting skills intervention	Healthy MOMS intervention
Theme/inspiration: "How far we've come."	*Theme/inspiration*: "There comes a time when you learn to step right into and through your fears because you know that whatever happens, you can handle it and to give in to fear is to give away the right to live life on your terms."

teach their children self-control. By learning and exercising self-control, children can make appropriate decisions and choose behaviors that are more likely to have positive outcomes. These parenting skills can help MLWHs manage children's misbehavior in high-risk situations such as school and community settings.

MLWHs face many physical, psychological, financial, and social issues that are difficult to manage on their own. The parenting intervention encouraged moms to identify and build their social support networks. The program emphasized that moms can improve their quality of life by accessing social support and most importantly, being comfortable asking for help for themselves and their children.

The parenting intervention also focused on strategies to reduce stress faced by MLWHs. The first step to alleviate stress is to recognize stressors and the symptoms of stress. In addition to the health condition, things like past regrets, painful memories, and feeling of guilt can lead to stress. Therefore, the intervention emphasized the need to resolve grudges and conflicts. Other stress-reducing activities included relaxation and deep breathing exercises. Moms were also encouraged to take care of themselves so that they can take care of their children. While coping with HIV and raising children, it is important that MLWHs are able to manage their own emotions.

Recognizing the difficulty many MLWHs have in deciding whether or not to disclose their status to their children (Tompkins 2007: see also Chap. 8 in this volume), this was a priority focus of the parenting intervention. There are pros and cons of HIV self-disclosure, in that it both causes and alleviates tension (Smith et al. 2008) and that it can lead to increased receipt of social support from some individuals and stigma, shame, and/or rejection by others. Because there is no clear answer on whether it is beneficial to disclose or not, our intervention discussed the factors that contribute to better decision-making regarding disclosure. Other topics specific to the need of MLWHs included talking with children about death and planning for the future, planning for what will happen and who will take care of their children if something happens to them.

With SCT as its foundation, the MOMS Parenting Intervention incorporated goal setting, role modeling, skills practise with guided feedback, self-monitoring via homework assignments, and reinforcement. Educational activities, problem solving, group discussion, and social support were employed to increase participants' ability to cope with various issues related to living with HIV.

3.2 Healthy MOMS Intervention

The attention-control condition provided up-to-date information and education related to living optimally with HIV. Gleaned from formative focus groups conducted to obtain input on the needs of our intended audience, the Healthy MOMS intervention included the topics of medication adherence, nutrition, physical activity, and STDs and HIV and was directly responsive to expressed desires for enhanced knowledge in each of these areas. Additionally, information about effective communication techniques, risk reduction strategies, and strategies for coping with stress are components of the intervention that were indicated as important by women in the focus groups. Finally, there are a number of aspects of the intervention group structure and process that were designed to meet the needs expressed by women and service providers. Sessions were formatted to address each participant as a whole person rather than solely focusing on the topic of HIV; for example, each session involves a "cut and paste" activity, which entails self-reflection about various aspects of the participants' lives.

The content of the health-focused intervention provided HIV-infected mothers with the following information: (1) improving their overall health by maintaining a healthy diet and being physically active, (2) adhering to medication regimens and keeping clinic appointments, (3) being knowledgeable about their condition so that they can better communicate with health care providers, (4) and maintaining an awareness of their sexual and physical anatomy. Broad ranges of strategies were used including educational activities, problem solving, group discussion, self-reflection, and social support building.

4 Preliminary Quantitative and Qualitative Findings

4.1 Preliminary Quantitative Findings for Parenting Stress Reduction

While the final dataset is still being prepared for analysis of primary intervention outcomes, a preliminary analysis was conducted to examine intervention effects on maternal stress as measured by the Parental Stress Index–Short Form (PSI/SF). The PSI/SF is a 36-item scale with three subscales: parental distress, parent–child dysfunctional interaction, and difficult child (each with a range of scores from 12 to 60). The Total Stress Index (PSI) is calculated by summing subscale scores (range of scores, 36–180). The PSI/SF has a reliability coefficient of 0.91 (Abidin 1995). The normal range of PSI scores (e.g., 15th–80th percentile) ranges from 27 to 144; scores of 162 and over ($\geq$90th percentile) are considered clinically relevant levels of stress (Abidin 1995). Analyses indicate that (1) both intervention conditions experienced a statistically significant decline in parental stress levels at the post-intervention follow-up visit, compared to baseline scores (82.9 ± 18.5 vs.

79.2 ± 19.4; p-value ≤ 0.0001) and (2) while MLWHs in the parenting-focused intervention achieved higher decreases in PSI-SF scores than those who participated in the health-focused intervention, these differences were not statistically significant.

These findings suggest that the group support component may be more beneficial in reducing parental stress levels than the educational elements (parenting skills vs. general health). Group support interventions have been shown to enhance social support, improve overall coping capabilities, and reduce the burden of stress among HIV-infected individuals. Further, a supportive environment in which HIV-infected mothers can learn to cope with life stressors can promote healthier parenting behaviors (Hansell et al. 1998), which may account for the decrease in parenting stress that was seen in both groups. This is consistent with previous studies that suggest that a supportive environment can be beneficial in relieving the burden of HIV-related stressors (Friedland et al. 1996), such as the burden of caregiver stress (Silver et al. 2003).

4.2   Post-intervention Qualitative Focus Group Findings

Qualitative methods were used to compliment quantitative analyses in describing overall program effects and identifying the most useful elements of each behavioral intervention for mothers living with HIV. We conducted post-intervention focus groups ($N=4$) to elicit participants' ($N=16$) perceived responses to MOMS participation. Two focus groups were conducted with participants from each intervention condition. Constant comparison analyses of transcripts by three independent coders led to the development of a codebook outlining primary and supporting themes.

Participants from both groups expressed significant emotional benefits from the group support and connection (meeting new people, having others identify with their experiences). Both groups expressed that the MOMS sessions provided a sense of community, which was highly valued in this previously isolated population. Participants stated how MOMS gave them a chance to really relax and just "be" in a room where everyone knew the familiar stressors that they were dealing with. The group sessions also gave them a place where they could talk openly about the intense feelings they often have but seldom share because few of them knew other HIV-positive mothers before the MOMS program. They also described how the MOMS staff went out of their way to make them feel comfortable and how the recruiter's gentle persistence in a way that showed true concern for their well-being was what led them to enroll in MOMS, despite their initial hesitation and fears.

While the above themes were echoed in every focus group across intervention conditions, there were a few notable differences between intervention conditions. Benefits identified only by the parenting intervention participants included acquired parenting skills (i.e., family management, less harsh discipline, consistent use of rewards and consequences) and increased acceptance of their child (and feeling "at peace" with their child). Benefits expressed only by the health-focused intervention participants included better medication adherence and increased reliance on prayer as a coping tool. While intervention content varied greatly, participants in both conditions valued the group support, experience of sharing, trusting group members, and being a resource for others. Using a qualitative, phenomenological approach to gain insight on participant experiences in this way can inform future efforts to engage similarly vulnerable, socially isolated populations currently underserved for HIV and other services.

Results of the preliminary quantitative analyses and the qualitative focus group discussions together suggest that relief of social isolation and validation of self-worth may have a more therapeutic effect than anything else covered in the MOMS intervention sessions, including stress management exercises, medication adherence education, parenting skills training, and communication building activities. And not only do they benefit from this, their children do as well. Future interventions to support MLWHs should focus on reducing stress, increasing coping skills, and fostering supportive networks. While the educational and problem-solving activities are an important part of the intervention, the peer-based support system provides an equally vital component: a sense of community for this previously isolated population.

5   Conclusion

While the science related to HIV continues to make tremendous gains, HIV unfortunately continues to spread, especially among those most vulnerable, as the result of insufficient physical resources or political will to expand education, to increase awareness, and to provide testing and counseling services (Plowden et al. 2005).

It is imperative that African American mothers living with or at risk for HIV in the southern USA be given priority in future research, policy, and practise. Recruitment and intervention strategies must be identified that take into account the unique stressors and strengths of this population and the communities in which they live. Because MLWHs are more likely to experience multiple stressors that negatively affect parenting skills, increased efforts are needed to decrease parenting-related stress among MLWHs.

Preliminary analyses indicate that both MOMS intervention conditions ("Parenting Skills for MOMS" and "Healthy MOMS") decreased parental stress levels significantly over baseline levels. Further work is needed in both the research and practise arenas to reduce childrearing stressors among MLWHs, improve their social support networks, and ultimately improve functioning of families affected by HIV.

References

Abidin RR (1995) Parenting stress index, 3rd edn: professional manual. Psychological Assessment Resources, Inc., Odessa

Adimora AA, Schoenbach VJ (2002) Contextual factors and the Black-White disparity in heterosexual HIV transmission. Epidemiology 13(6):707–712

amfAR (2008) Women and HIV/AIDS. amfAR AIDS Research, Fact sheet No. 2

Andrews S, Williams AB, Neil K (1993) The mother-child relationship in the HIV-1 positive family. Image J Nurs Sch 25(3):193–198

Bandura A (1986) Social foundations of thought and action: a social cognitive theory. Prentice-Hall, Inc., Englewood Cliffs

Bowen M (1978) Family therapy in clinical practice. Jason Aronson, New York

Boyce WT (2009) The family is (still) the patient. Arch Pediatr Adolesc Med 163(8):768–770

Center for Disease Control and Prevention (CDC) (2010a) Diagnoses of HIV infection and AIDS in the United States and dependent areas, 2008: HIV surveillance report, vol 20. US Department of Health and Human Services, Atlanta. http://www.cdc.gov/hiv/surveillance/resources/reports/2008report/index.htm. Accessed 19 Oct 2011

Center for Disease Control and Prevention (CDC) (2010b) HIV among African Americans. National Center for HIV/AIDS, Hepatitis, STD, and TB Prevention. Division of HIV/AIDS Prevention, Atlanta. http://www.cdc.gov/hiv/topics/aa/pdf/aa.pdf. Accessed 19 Oct 2011

Center for Disease Control and Prevention (CDC) (2011) Disparities in diagnoses of HIV infection between Blacks/African Americans and other racial/ethnic populations – 37 States, 2005–2008. Morb Mortal Wkly Rep 60(04):93–98

Ciambrone D (2002) Informal networks among women with HIV/AIDS: present support and future prospects. Qual Health Res 12(7):876–896

Ciesla JA, Roberts JE (2001) Meta-analysis of the relationship between HIV infection and risk for depressive disorders. Am J Psychiatry 158(5):725–730

Clark HJ, Lindner G, Armistead L, Austin BJ (2003) Stigma, disclosure, and psychological functioning among HIV-infected and non-infected African-American women. Women Health 38(4):57–71

Coco EL, Courtney LJ (1998) A family systems approach for preventing adolescent runaway behavior. Adolescence 33(130):485–496

Corrigan PW, River LP, Lundin R, Wasowski K, Campion J, Mathisen J et al (2000) Stigmatizing attributions about mental illness. J Community Psychol 28(1):91–102

Crawford AM (1996) Stigma associated with AIDS: a meta-analysis. J Appl Soc Psychol 26(5):398–416

Emlet CA (2007) Experiences of stigma in older adults living with HIV/AIDS: a mixed-methods analysis. AIDS Patient Care STDS 21(10):740–752

Friedland J, Renwick R, McColl M (1996) Coping and social support as determinants of quality of life in HIV/AIDS. AIDS Care 8(1):15–31

Fullilove MT, Fullilove RE III (1999) Stigma as an obstacle to AIDS action. Am Behav Sci 42(1):117–129

Glover DA, Garcia-Aracena EF, Lester P, Rice E, Rothram-Borus MJ (2010) Stress biomarkers as outcomes for HIV+ prevention: participation, feasibility and findings among HIV+ Latina and African American mothers. AIDS Behav 14(2):339–350

Goldenberg I, Goldenberg H (1991) Family therapy: an overview. Brooks/Cole, Pacific Grove

Haile R, Padilla MB, Parker EA (2011) 'Stuck in the quagmire of an HIV ghetto': the meaning of stigma in the lives of older black gay and bisexual men living with HIV in New York City. Cult Health Sex 13(4):429–442

Hall HI, An Q, Hutchinson AB, Sansom S (2008) Estimating the lifetime risk of a diagnosis of the HIV infection in 33 states, 2004–2005. J Acquir Immune Defic Syndr 49(3):294–297

Hansell P, Hughes C, Caliandro G, Russo P, Budin W, Hartman B et al (1998) The effect of a social support boosting intervention on stress, coping, and social support in caregivers of children with HIV/AIDS. Nurs Res 47(2):79–86

Herek GM, Capitanio JP (1994) Conspiracies, contagion, and compassion: trust and public reactions to AIDS. AIDS Educ Prev 6:365–375

Herek GM, Capitanio JP, Widaman KF (2002) HIV-related stigma and knowledge in the U.S.: prevalence and trends, 1991–1999. Am J Public Health 92:371–377

Hudson AL, Lee KA, Miramontes H, Portillo CJ (2001) Social interactions, perceived support, and level of distress in HIV-positive women. J Assoc Nurses AIDS Care 12(4):68–76

Hutchinson AB, Corbie-Smith G, Thomas SB, Mohanan S, del Rio C (2004) Understanding the patient's perspective on rapid and routine HIV testing in an inner-city urgent care center. AIDS Educ Prev 16(2):101–114

Imber-Black E (1998) The secret life of families: truth- telling, privacy and reconciliation in a tell-all society. Bantam, New York

Kempf MC, McLeod J, Boehme AK, Walcott MW, Wright L, Seal P et al (2010) A qualitative study of the barriers and facilitators to retention-in-care among HIV-positive women in the rural southeastern United States: implications for targeted interventions. AIDS Patient Care STDS 24(8):515–520

Kojic EM, Cu-Uvin S (2007) Special care issues of women living with HIV-AIDS. Infect Dis Clin N Am 21(1):133–148

Konkle-Parker DJ, Erlen JA, Dubbert PM (2008) Barriers and facilitators to medication adherence in a southern minority population with HIV disease. J Assoc Nurses AIDS Care 19(2):98–104

Kopnisky KL, Stoff DM, Rausch DM (2004) Workshop report: the effects of psychological variables on the progression of HIV-1 disease. Brain Behav Immun 18(3):246–261

Lee M, Rotheram-Borus M (2001) Challenges associated with increased survival among parents living with HIV. Am J Public Health 91(8):1303–1309

Liamputtong P (ed) (2013) Stigma, discrimination and living with HIV/AIDS: a cross-cultural perspective. Springer, Dordrecht

McCubbin HL, McCubbin MA, Thompson AL, Han S, Allen CT (1997) Families under stress: what makes them resilient? JFam Consum Sci 89(3):2–12

McKinney MM (2002) Variations in rural AIDS epidemiology and service delivery models in the United States. J Rural Health 18:455–466

Mellins CA, Havens JF, McCaskill EO, Leu CS, Brudney K, Chesney MA (2002) Mental health, substance use and disclosure are significantly associated with the medical treatment adherence of HIV-infected mothers. Psychol Health Med 7(4):451–460

Moneyham L, Sowell R, Seals B, Demi A (2000) Depressive symptoms among African American women with HIV disease. Sch Inquir Nurs Pract 14(1):9–39

Murphy D, Austin E, Greenwell L (2006) Correlates of HIV-related stigma among HIV-positive mothers and their uninfected adolescent children. Women Health 44(3):19–42

Murphy DA, Marelich WD, Armistead L, Herbeck DM, Payne DL (2010) Anxiety/stress among mothers living with HIV: effects on parenting skills and child outcomes. AIDS Care 22(12):1449–1458

Murphy DA, Armistead L, Marelich WD, Payne DL, Herbeck DM (2011) Pilot trial of a disclosure intervention for HIV+ mothers: the TRACK program. J Consult Clin Psychol 79(2):203–214

Muturi N, An S (2010) HIV/AIDS stigma and religiosity among African American women. J Health Commun 15(4):388–401

Nöstlinger C, Bartoli G, Gordillo V, Roberfroid D, Colebunders R (2006) Children and adolescents living with HIV positive parents: emotional and behavioral problems. Vulnerable Child Youth Stud 1(1):29–43

Payne NS, Beckwith CG, Davis M, Flanigan T, Simmons EM, Crockett K et al (2006) Acceptance of HIV testing among African-American college students at a historically black university in the south. J Natl Med Assoc 98(12):1912–1916

Pence B, Reif S, Whetten K, Leserman J, Stangl D, Swartz M, Thielman N, Mugavero M (2007) Minorities, the poor, and survivors of abuse: HIV-infected patients in the US Deep South. South Med J 100(11):1114–1122

Pennebaker JW, Hughes CF, O'Heeron RC (1987) The psychophysiology of confession: linking inhibitory and psychosomatic processes. J Pers Soc Psychol 52:781–793

Pennebaker JW, Colder M, Sharp LK (1990) Accelerating the coping process. J Pers Soc Psychol 58:528–537

Peterman T, Lindsey C, Selik R (2005) This place is killing me: a comparison of counties where the incidence rates of AIDS increased the most and the least. J Infect Dis 191:S123–S126

Phillips KD, Moneyham L, Thomas SP, Gunther M, Vyavaharkar M (2011) Social context of rural women with HIV/AIDS. Issues Ment Health Nurs 32(6):374–381

Pilowsky D, Zybert P, Hsieh P, Vlahov D, Susser E (2003) Children of HIV-positive drug-using parent. J Am Acad Child Adolesc Psychiatry 42(8):950

Plowden KO, Fletcher A, Miller JL (2005) Factors influencing HIV-risk behaviors among HIV-positive urban African Americans. J Assoc Nurses AIDS Care 16(1):21–28

Price V, Hsu M (1992) Public opinion about AIDS policies: the role of misinformation and attitudes toward homosexuals. Public Opin Q 56:29–52

Reid MJ, Webster-Stratton C, Beauchaine TP (2001) Parent training in head start: a comparison of program response among African American, Asian American, Caucasian, and Hispanic mothers. Prev Sci 2(4):209–227

Reif S, Geonnotti KL, Whetten K (2006) HIV infection and AIDS in the Deep South. Am J Public Health 96(6):970–973

Sayles JN, Ryan GW, Silver JS, Sarkisian CA, Cunningham WE (2007) Experiences of social stigma and implications for healthcare among a diverse population of HIV positive adults. J Urban Health 84(6):814–828

Sengupta S, Strauss RP, Miles MS, Roman-Isler M, Banks B, Corbie-Smith G (2010) A conceptual model exploring the relationship between HIV stigma and implementing HIV clinical trials in rural communities of North Carolina. N C Med J 71(2):113–122

Serovich JM (2001) A test of two HIV disclosure theories. AIDS Educ Prev 13(4):355–364

Silver EJ, Bauman L, Camacho S, Hudis J (2003) Factors associated with psychological distress in urban mothers with late-stage HIV/AIDS. AIDS Behav 7(4):421–431

Smith R, Rossetto K, Peterson BL (2008) A meta-analysis of disclosure of one's HIV-positive status, stigma and social support. AIDS Care 20(10):1266–1275

Stein M, Crystal S, Cunningham W, Ananthanarayanan A, Anderson R, Turner B et al (2000) Delays in seeking HIV care due to competing caregiver responsibilities. Am J Public Health 90(7):1138–1140

Stormshak EA, Kaminski RA, Goodman MR (2002) Enhancing the parenting skills of head start families during the transition to kindergarten. Prev Sci 3(3):223–234

Tompkins T (2007) Disclosure of maternal HIV status to children: to tell or not to tell…that is the question. J Child Fam Stud 16(6):773–788

Tompkins TL, Wyatt G (2008) Child psychosocial adjustment and parenting in families affected by maternal HIV/AIDS. J Child Fam Stud 17:823–838

Van Loon RA (2000) Redefining motherhood: adaptation to role change for women with AIDS. Fam Soc 81(2):152–161

Vyavaharkar M, Moneyham L, Corwin S, Saunders R, Annang L, Tavakoli A (2010) Relationships between stigma, social support, and depression in HIV-infected African American women living in the rural Southeastern United States. J Assoc Nurses AIDS Care 21(2):144–152

Wallace SA, McLellan-Lemal E, Harris MJ, Townsend TG, Miller KS (2011) Why take an HIV test? Concerns, benefits, and strategies to promote HIV testing among low-income heterosexual African American young adults. Health Educ Behav 38(5):462–470

Webster-Stratton C, Hammond M (1990) Predictors of treatment outcome in parent training for families with conduct problem children. Behav Ther 21:319–337

Wiener LS, Battles HB, Heilman NE (1998) Factors associated with parents' decision to disclose their HIV diagnosis to their children. Child Welfare 77:115–135

Wood S, Tobias C, McCree J (2004) Medication adherence for HIV positive women caring for children: in their own words. AIDS Care 16(7):909–913

Chapter 19
Coping with Patriarchy and HIV/AIDS: Female Sexism in Infant Feeding Counseling in Southern Africa

Ineke Buskens and Alan Jaffe[†]

1 Introduction

HIV-positive mothers in resource-poor settings in developing countries are faced with an appalling choice, between considerable risk of postnatal mother-to-child transmission (MTCT) of HIV through breastfeeding and considerable risk from infectious disease and malnutrition to these infants from not breastfeeding (WHO 2000). Policy makers have been given hope by studies that indicate that infants who are exclusively breastfed have a risk of being HIV-infected that is manyfold lower than those who are partially breastfed or receive mixed feeding (Coovadia et al. 2007). The availability of antiretroviral treatment (ART), also in highly active (HAART) combinations, holds potential both as treatment and as prophylaxis by lowering viral loads in breast milk (Arendt et al. 2007; Kilewo et al. 2007). Together, these strategies promise to revive the dream of an AIDS-free generation in southern Africa. See also Chaps. 9, 10, and 16 in this volume.

Yet, caution has to be expressed in making HAART the panacea of preventing MTCT (PMTCT); the dispensing of the drugs takes place within the PMTCT counselor-client relationship, and the challenges of adherence and the risks of toxicity and resistance make the effectiveness of HAART dependent on the quality of the counseling encounter. Research has indicated that these encounters have significant weaknesses (Chopra et al. 2005), disappointing impact (Rollins et al. 2006), and are fraught with problems (Buskens and Jaffe 2008).

[†]Dr Alan Jaffe passed away in 2009.

I. Buskens (✉)
Research for the Future, P.O. Box 170, Elgin 7180, South Africa
e-mail: ineke@researchforthefuture.com

P. Liamputtong (ed.), *Women, Motherhood and Living with HIV/AIDS:*
A Cross-Cultural Perspective, DOI 10.1007/978-94-007-5887-2_19,
© Springer Science+Business Media Dordrecht 2013

PMTCT counseling is drawn into a medico-moral discourse that emphasizes the values of chastity and fidelity, predominantly for women; patriarchy exalts motherhood and male sexuality, while regarding female sexuality with contempt (Seidel 1993). Because of the association of HIV/AIDS as a sexual and immoral disease, HIV-positive pregnant women carry a threefold burden of stigma: as women, as HIV-positive women, and as HIV-positive women who are presumed to have allowed themselves to fall pregnant (Panos Report 2001). This triple stigma casts HIV-positive women and mothers as sexually immoral, even when they would be married, have been faithful to their (often polygamous) partner and, most probably, would have been exposed to the disease through their partner (see also Chap. 15 in this volume). At the same time, the public health agenda has framed antenatal care as an opportune moment for monitoring and intervening to control the HIV epidemic. This implies that the persons who would be least positioned to bring the message of HIV infection into their families will be these women and that at a time when they are least equipped psychologically to face such a challenge because of pregnancy and breastfeeding. Furthermore, what is required for an HIV-positive pregnant woman or feeding mother to prevent vertical transmission – disclosure, negotiating safe sex with male partners, and engaging infant feeding that is exclusive of water, medicine, and solids – are profound behavior changes for them, their partners, and their families. This set of behavior changes is a challenge to the identity of the "decent" woman who respects her partner, family, and community, as it requires that she challenge traditional systems of belief, influence, and authority (Buskens et al. 2007a).

This chapter examines to what extent the infant feeding (IF) counselor-client interaction is capable of meeting current and future health expectations and requirements, including those of ART and HAART, by focusing on the nature of the interpersonal dynamics between the IF counselors and their clients during the counseling encounter.

2 The Study

The research on which this chapter is based consisted of ethnographic fieldwork done over a period of 7 months in 2003 across 11 sites in 3 southern African countries: Namibia, Swaziland, and South Africa. Sites were selected to include a range of settings (urban, peri-urban, and rural; formal, traditional, and informal settlements) to facilitate the development of a cross-sectional analysis of infant feeding practises in the region (Bechhofer and Paterson 2000). Researchers were female indigenous language speakers trained in the use of participant observation, observations, formal and informal interviews, and focus groups. Primary research respondents were pregnant women and mothers with infants of up to a year old (jointly termed "mothers" in this chapter). A total of 11 pregnant women, 167 mothers of infants, 32 relatives (fathers, grandmothers, and caregivers), 22 health workers (nurses, counselors, PMTCT co-coordinators, and a doctor), and 7 traditional healers were formally interviewed. The interviews were transcribed and translated. The data comprised field notes, reflective diaries, informal interview notes, and formal interview transcriptions. Data analysis was done in 2004 using internal and external analysts. First, the researchers analyzed their own data using the initial steps of a conceptual framework analysis designed for health policy research (Ritchie and Spencer 1994). Then, the principal researchers and an external analyst analyzed the total data set independent of each other. Finally, the principal investigator applied "analytic retroduction," a double-fitting of analysis and data collection (Ragin 1994). This is a refinement of a general "inductive" approach widely used to allow themes to emerge from qualitative data (Thomas 2006).

3   Mothers and Female Health Workers: A Troubled Relationship

An evaluation of HIV/AIDS counseling in South Africa found that counselors were disadvantaged as role models because just like their clients, they would tend to be in relationships that would inhibit safe sex practices. This would create incongruence with the health messages they would be giving (Richter et al. 1999).

A semiotic analysis was conducted on ethnographic interviews with obstetric nurses involved directly or indirectly with infant feeding and counseling in South Africa. This analysis found that obstetric nurses judge, "otherize," and marginalize young female clients as if their welfare was not a legitimate concern for these nurses. Health care workers were found to judge – sometimes even harshly – vulnerable and unmarried mothers, regardless of their HIV status. Seidel (1993) notes how nurses' perceptions of these women as shaped by a "medico-moral discourse" which gives positive value to "compliance" rather than to individual rights. This would explain why some nurses would not see their role as supporting vulnerable patients but as needing to tell them how to behave (Seidel 2000).

Our findings on the counseling encounter were previously reported in an article from this same study (Buskens and Jaffe 2008). In summary, most infant feeding encounters were found to be discordant, with both parties talking past one another; two opposing subtexts inform counselors' and mothers' perspectives, attitudes, and behaviors. Mothers were seeking counsel from the "consultation," yet counselors confronted clients with their risks, so as to persuade them to "correct" their behavior. Mothers reported feelings of being judged, stigmatized, and shamed; counselors confirmed that they revert at times to "confronting, judging, and shaming mothers." To avoid these feelings, mothers admit to telling nurses what they think the nurses want to hear. Counseling nurses complained of feelings of frustration and anger that women clients would neither tell them the truth about their infant feeding habits nor heed their best advice. Many counselors were noted to suffer from stress, depression, and burnout. Counselors were seldom able to create an environment where choice became an option for the mothers.

While the IF counseling literature mentioned thus far makes note of the troubled nature of the IF counseling encounter and its inability to deliver what is expected, the authors found a dearth of in-depth analysis. It was therefore deemed necessary to spread the net wider; hence, we include here research into other health and caring relationships in southern Africa that made mention of similar health worker attitudes.

A study on TB in South Africa found that nurses' recognition of excessive identification with their patients tends to trigger strategies of distancing and judgment, causing them to hide behind a mask of defensive coping mechanisms when nurses identified "too close for comfort" with patients sharing the same ethnicity (Van der Walt 2002). The authors explain that nurses' anxiety has its roots in incongruous roles: epidemic infection control (including quarantine) versus caring for patients (and their rights, e.g., to access and free movement). Where nurses share ethnicity, there may be further fears of psychological contamination, as if their shared history might rub off and negate nurses' social gains: "the professional role may represent a way for nurses to advance socio-economically... the implicit threat (is) of never being able to get away" (Van der Walt and Swartz 2002: 1007; Van der Walt 2002). Nurses tend to take refuge against this "emotional invasion" of ethnic contamination by hiding behind a "mask" of roles and routines: the uniform, epaulettes, and stethoscope help to shield her behind a professional status; tasks shield her from the total reality. According to Van der Walt and Swartz (2002: 1006), "it is safer for the nurse to acknowledge the control of the disease and the bacteria than to open themselves up to the illness experience and the human needs of the person." The authors quote extensively from their earlier article (Van der Walt and Swartz 1999) on the work of the psychoanalyst Menzies-Lyth and how psychological defense mechanisms are integrated into institutional and organizational culture and how these manifest as rigid routines and procedures to protect nurses against "emotional contagion" (Menzies-Lyth 1960).

An earlier South African study had reported extraordinarily incongruous carer behavior in obstetric services, taking the form of clinical neglect, verbal abuse, and physical abuse; this was interpreted as a need from the nurses to assert control over an often unpredictable environment and challenges to their status, power, and authority. Nurses deployed coercion and violence as a means of creating "social distance" in a struggle to assert fantasies of professional and moral superiority and their middle-class aspirations and identity (Jewkes et al. 1998).

Anecdotal evidence from across southern Africa has confirmed incidences of abuse and troubled nurse-patient relationships. Reports that emanated from maternity wards in Swaziland revealed that pregnant women preferred to be delivered by male midwives because they found the males to be more gentle and compassionate with them.[1]

In our study, mothers have been reporting on clinical encounters with midwives and nurses in obstetric wards and clinics – maternity, antenatal, and postnatal. Obstetric services provide the physical setting and the professional context for infant feeding counseling encounters. Furthermore, clinical practise is part of the

---

[1] These reports were verified by a Swazi Department of Health official (Nhlabatsi 2004; personal correspondence).

psychological context for infant feeding counselors who are nurses (or in the case of South Africa, lay counselors who were previously nurses).

3.1 *"They Run Away"*

We found that most counseling sessions were combined with maternal VCT, with clients being expected to make an infant feeding decision while they are still reeling, in emotional turmoil from the news of their HIV status. Counselors confirmed an exclusive focus on the health of the infant as the purpose of PMTCT:

> They only speak about what you must do with the baby, and nothing is being said about you and how to cope with the news they just told you. I mean counseling you to understand about your status is the most important, but they run away from that. (34-year-old HIV-positive mother, Soweto)

3.2 *"They Will Shout at You"*

Although mothers agree that nurses are not all the same, many HIV-positive mothers report experiences of verbal abuse and belittling, in this case, with information that implicitly exposes their HIV status:

> You know if you go to the clinic with a bottle, they will shout at you and say that you are lazy to breastfeed. What I don't like about them saying that is they talk very loud so that everybody could hear. What for, we are all human, and we also need to be treated like everybody else, and they must remember that we are not children. (HIV-positive focus group participant, Soweto)

3.3 *"Yah, You Know Your Disease"*

Mothers reported numerous frank breaches of confidentiality within public contexts, often in ways that were unequivocally unkind and stigmatizing, if not cruel or brutal. In this quote, the nurse reveals also the baby's HIV status, as well as the mothers CD 4 result, signifying late-stage disease: AIDS. This mother seems to cooperate reluctantly in this disclosure but explains her apparent collusion as mediated by her fear and dependence on the nurse for information:

> The sister is just asking things on HIV in front of other people. When I went back for the baby's results, the registered nurse asked me "You ought to know what your problem is." (I answered) "Yes," and the registered nurse asked me again "what type of disease." I first kept quiet and later responded "AIDS." There were many people. An older woman sat next to me when the nurse asked me all these questions. There is no privacy there, unlike the ANC (antenatal clinic). After asking these questions, the nurse told me, "yah you know your disease, the baby has it also, but it is not (the) worst." She said something about 58. But I did not want to ask, as I feared that this sister will maybe not expla in nicely or she will just talk everything in front of the people. (26-year-old HIV-positive shack dweller and mother of two, Windhoek)

3.4 "That Is What Scares Us"

Other quotes give an indication of the depths of fear that some mothers have of the abuse of power differentials by some carers:

> It makes us feel bad, but we have decided to allow it in our hearts that even if a nurse does what (–ever), you just tell yourself that is how they are, simply that is how they are. Because if you could begin to question them, there is a danger that you will never get well – remember they have all the injections so that is what scares us. (Researcher laughs at this; the mother expands.) At times, you see them manhandling your child but what do you say – nothing because they can kill your child with their injections and what would you say. Nurses are capable of anything. So you must just keep quiet. (45-year-old HIV-positive rural mother and grandmother and traditional and religious healer, Kwazulu Natal)

3.5 "Then You Really Suffer"

Some mothers display good insight into nurse's burnout and defensive coping mechanisms, in this case displacement:

> Nurses, they differ. Some maybe come to work with their frustrations; others maybe have marital problems or something, and they offload all their frustrations on you. Some are good because you can never tell whether they are happy or angry. One must just accept all this because you need help…Sometimes, I think the nurses are also tired. Maybe the number of patients has increased so much that they are tired of helping people. And if you find them after having quarreled with their husbands, then you really suffer. You will wonder if you are now the husband because they will take out their frustrations on you. (30-year-old mother of three girls, Windhoek)

4 Discussion

It warrants repeating that we did not find these forms of overt maltreatment or abuse in the counselor-client encounters; what we did find was mothers' accounts of stigma and counselors' confirmation that they revert at times to "confronting, judging, and shaming mothers." However, we found the most significant dynamic, common to both these sets of encounters, nurse-patient and counselor-client, to be judgment. Judgment is diametrically opposed to the stance that counselors have been trained to adopt within the IF counseling relationship, namely, client-centered unconditional positive regard. This raises the question: What would be the rationality of judgment from the side of the counselor in this interaction and relationship?

4.1 Too Close for Comfort?

Ethnicity is very often shared in the PMTCT relationship. Could the judgments that we noticed in PMTCT encounters be explained in the same vein as did Van der Walt

(2002) and Van der Walt and Swartz (2002), a distancing dynamic between counselor and client and one that is triggered when their shared ethnicity provides the "mirror" in which counselors see the reflection of their own personal predicaments or risks?

Adopting and extending their psychoanalytic interpretation, when a particular patient feels "too similar" or their suffering feels "too close," counselors may well evade such potentially overwhelming feelings in several ways. Such evasion would happen through projection (the attribution of one's own unaccepted and repressed attitudes or emotions to others), through displacement, or through transferring repressed emotions and reactions onto an available substitute. The rationality of coping mechanisms (Freud 1937), including the distancing as a "denial of shared vulnerability," can thus be seen as defensive attempts at boundary management, with judgment as a form of projection, and blaming the client as a form of displacement.

Yet, in the case of the PMTCT counseling relationship, another factor besides shared ethnicity could play a role and that would be shared gender; all PMTCT clients are female, as are almost all counselors.

As noted in the literature section, reports from maternity wards in Swaziland revealed that pregnant women preferred to be delivered by male midwives because they found the males to be more compassionate with them. Ethnicity is an unlikely cause in the Swaziland settings, as both male and female midwives would share ethnicity with their patients. Could it be that in the PMTCT relationship, gender plays a similar role in the "too close for comfort" dynamic as ethnicity does in the TB relationships that Van der Walt (2002) and Van der Walt and Swartz (2002) studied? This finding is at odds with gendered roles but has been corroborated by the study conducted by Jewkes et al. (1998): although these authors do not discuss this specific finding, the article notes that mothers found particularly the male midwives being "nice" to them.

To rephrase this question, Is it exclusively in the female dyad where the reported and observed abuse of clients by health workers takes place? Reviewing the three sets of South African articles that discuss these dynamics Van der Walt (2002), Van der Walt and Swartz (2002), Jewkes et al. (1998), and Seidel (1993, 2000), it can be noted that nurses' judgment, moral confrontation, and shaming toward their clients seem to indeed be confined to female dyads. In addition, the verbal and physical abuse of obstetric patients by midwives noted by Jewkes and colleagues have, to our knowledge never before or since, been reported in other health care settings, settings not confined to female dyads.

4.2   The Dynamics of Benevolent Female Sexism

According to a seminal volume entitled "woman's inhumanity to woman," in a context of profound sexism and patriarchy, women tend to collude with internalized patriarchal values, manifesting mostly as female "benevolent sexism," and less commonly among women, as overt hostility toward other women (Chesler 2001).

Female benevolent sexism serves to maintain the status quo by, on the one hand, idealizing the "good" woman that adheres to traditional values, while condemning or even demonizing any woman who "breaks the mold" (Glick et al. 2000). This hostility toward other women expresses itself predominantly indirectly in the form of shunning, gossiping, shaming, judging, and stigmatizing (Chesler 2001). The realization that one, as a woman, could be in the same situation as another woman who is suffering (from rape or discrimination for instance) could be too painful for one's sense of self and sense of vulnerability, as a woman, to entertain. For example, women jurors are said to use judgment and blame to avoid identifying with the woman survivor in an attempt to keep themselves out the "possible victim category" in their own minds (Chesler 2001). Such a "defensive distancing" dynamic translated to the counselors' perspective in an IF encounter could lead a counselor to entertain the following train of thought: "It could not happen to me because, although I find myself in a similar situation, I myself am a very different woman than this woman, so she (the mother) must be to blame individually and personally for what has happened to her."

Defensive psychodynamics are socialized as ubiquitous social norms, so only the behaviors and their impact may be apparent while the thinking underlying the behavior may remain subconscious. A study among college students found that women who self-identify as feminists or score as feminist on psychometric measures were, disappointingly, not anymore aware of their hostility to other women than nonfeminist students were (Cowan 2000, 2001). This illustrates the degree to which benevolent female sexism is subconscious.

A comparative study over five continents found a direct relation between a country's sexism rate and its degree of benevolent female sexism; it also found that southern African countries were among the most sexist (Glick and Fiske 1997).

Given these findings, one can expect that the PMTCT counseling female dyad in southern Africa would be prone to evoke subconscious internalized sexism in both counselor and client, especially, as both these women and their encounter are embedded in the triple burden of stigma that is laid upon HIV-positive pregnant women and mothers.

4.3 Benevolent Female Sexism in Infant Feeding Counseling in Southern Africa

A hypothesis emerged from this analysis: infant feeding counselors that have internalized sexism subconsciously deploy judgment, moral confrontation, and shaming to create emotional distance when, as women, they see their own subconscious vulnerabilities reflected in the predicaments, risks, or dilemmas of the mothers they are counseling, especially when these reflections are "too close" to their own unhealed past hurts or current personal predicaments as women in profoundly patriarchal societies in a time of AIDS.

4.4 The Mental Risks to Counselors of Defensive Judgment and Distancing

Defense mechanisms are considered functionally adaptive as tactics to evade overwhelming emotions for a few days (Suls and Fletcher 1985). Defensive judgment as a manifestation of this "denial of shared vulnerability" is an effective coping strategy because it makes the fear that is nowhere acknowledged invisible. As psychological defenses are mostly subconscious, counselors may be unaware of these dynamics and be aware only of their manifestation as ineffective and dissatisfying encounters, with reluctant, resistant, or resentful clients.

However, as Van der Walt (2002) and Van der Walt and Swartz (2002) argue, distancing, deployed as a social defense, leaves carers with a burden by preventing them from sharing their load of responsibility, their stress, or their emotional pain through more reciprocal collaboration with their patients: "distancing as a social defense could in itself cause "secondary stress" because it leads to evasion which inhibits the development of more effective mastery of anxiety." International mental health literature shows that counselors' fears of being vulnerable to what Van der Walt and Swartz term "psychological contamination" and "secondary stress" are in fact justified. Especially, when a female counselor has a history of personal trauma (Kassam-Adams 1995), then exposure to a clients' predicament or trauma can trigger a syndrome of "vicarious traumatization" (VT), previously described as "secondary traumatic stress." This syndrome is formally recognized as a form of post-traumatic stress disorder (Dunkley and Whelan 2006). Put plainly, "compassion fatigue" and cognitive rigidity can leave one mentally vulnerable; in the long term, defensive attempts to regain control can aggravate the same stress, which, in the short term, they try to alleviate.

5 Conclusion

Managers, health researchers, and policy makers are aware of the evidence of lack of compassion by carers and even abuse by nurses, but this is often blamed on junior individuals, framed as aberrant behavior, or excused by the fact that health workers are overworked and underpaid. While these factors may contribute, perhaps as precipitants, they cannot explain the range or depth of hazardous malpractise found in this and other studies.

Applying Van der Walt and Swartz's (2002) analysis to our finding of judgmental distancing provides the insight of counselors coping defensively with the threat of being overwhelmed emotionally.

Chesler's (2001) analysis of woman's inhumanity to woman presents the insight that infant feeding counselors who have internalized aspects of female benevolent sexism would be almost "set up" to judge, shame, and blame their clients. They themselves will most probably not have made the change in attitudes and behavior that they implicitly require of their clients. They will therefore not be able or willing to envision the changes that their clients need to make in order to adhere to their infant feeding advice. To the extent that these counselors subconsciously identify with the image of "the good" traditional woman, they will not be able to see the dangers inherent in the traditional sexist gender stereotypes that they entertain (Buskens et al. 2006).

The interpretation of judgment as defensive coping with subconscious displacement of disowned feelings onto the patient helps explain our findings of blame and verbal abuse in the form of shouting, belittling, and breaching of confidentiality in nurse-patient encounters. Subconscious denial by counselors of their own and of clients' feelings and states of being must subvert the purpose of counseling, especially when they cause counselors to deploy subconscious but demotivating manipulations such as moral confrontation and shame. These dysfunctional carer behaviors can cause secondary stress and even VT by aggravating the very anxiety they attempt to evade. The emotional blunting that can be expected from undiagnosed VT can be expected to entrench repressive and self-deceptive coping styles, both within the personality (Werhan and Cox 1999) and within institutional health culture (Menzies-Lyth 1991). If judgment is reflected back onto the self, it can also be expected to result in recriminating guilt and shame. These cumulative psychosocial effects would help to explain our findings of counselors reporting stress, depression, and burnout (Buskens et al. 2007b).

It is important that counselors feel safe and respected in their work environment (Roosenbloom et al. 1995). If counselors who need support to help face their fears, or manage their behavior, are unlikely to find it within their working environment as the dynamics of defensive distancing are not well appreciated, and the risks of VT are not yet acknowledged as being real by the health services in southern Africa, their sense of alienation and hence their stress will be agumented (Dutton and Rubinstein 1995). The concept of female sexism, especially, is unspeakable, not only among those traditionalists who have no words for it but also for feminists who adhere firmly to an assumption of a universal sisterhood (Siegal and Baumgardner 2007), termed "umbokodo" in southern Africa, because the concept of woman's inhumanity to woman could be construed as treachery, a betrayal of the sisterhood. In her introduction, Chesler (2001) illustrates how, to a feminist who adheres to an assumption that blames the male gender, the thought of an "enemy within" is too abhorrent to contemplate. Chesler recommends a discipline of sisterhood that requires self-awareness together with self-care of loving rather than judging oneself. This is a daily self-discipline of reflection with self-compassion, acknowledging one's own prejudice as inevitable as one cannot change what one is not yet aware of or not ready and willing to acknowledge and face. This practise also requires an independent mind and a strong spirit to be very clear of one's own psychological boundaries and to guard them well. "Only then will she have the capacity to respect and not violate another woman's boundaries" (Chesler 2001: 475).

6   Returning to Our Introduction: The Promise of HAART

There may be a hope that ART might somehow obviate the need for counselors to manage their relationships with mothers. Our findings suggest that it could as easily reinforce distancing dynamics by providing a new opportunity for carers to sublimate, in treatment details, their fear that despite ART death remains too real a possibility to the mother and HIV infection a repressed possibility or a threat to the counselor. It is our contention that for PMTCT to become a success, the relationship between counselor and client needs to be understood and even more importantly, what this relationship has to face up to. Dysfunctional IF counseling is a manifestation of what has not been resolved in the society at large in terms of general sexism and female sexism in particular. Expecting the female dyad of counselor and mother to deal with the inherent gender relation tensions at a moment of great emotional vulnerability and stress is not rational or realistic. Most importantly, however, it is not humane.

7   Recommendations

The advent of HAART revives the dream of an AIDS-free generation in southern Africa; PMTCT with exclusive infant feeding provides a unique opportunity to spearhead this dream. However, to realize these opportunities, infant feeding counselors need far more support. For such support to take form, it is important that health researchers, policy makers, and managers cease to deny the sexist realities in which mothers live and in which counselors work, that they acknowledge the moral and defensive rationalities that underpin women's behaviors in these settings, and not underestimate the risks to which both sets of women are exposed to because of the dysfunctional counseling that results from these dynamics. It is time to name internalized female sexism for what it is and understand it from within the prevalent patriarchal settings.

We, therefore, recommend that the training of health care workers and their managers be enriched with a focus on an inclusive form of gender awareness that not only focuses on the ways how general sexism gets internalized in the female self but also how it expresses itself in relation to other women (especially clients) and how it can be overcome.

Change does not come easily. However, as counselors implicitly expect their clients to change – to adhere to infant feeding advice means profound change for traditional African women – asking the health services to commit to change in this context seems fair enough. One of the underlying assumptions of counseling is that there is nothing that is not speakable; the instant we are able to name the monster, we take back a power we have at some point given away. And as awareness and compassion should not be foreign to health care as a discipline, it should be entirely possible and feasible to integrate inclusive gender awareness in existing counseling training. It will not only make life better for mothers during the probably most challenging moments of their lives, it will enrich and empower the female counselors also.

Acknowledgements We acknowledge the funder Secure the Future, an initiative of Bristol Myers Squibb, for their contribution and trust. We appreciate all our researchers for their commitment, courage, and tenacity: Raylene Titus, Ieshrit Sayeed, Nobantu Gantana, Josephine Malala, Zodwa Radebe, Joolekeni Komati, Kaarina Amutenya, Kathe Hofnie, Olivia Ndjadila, Gregentia Shapumba, Kholeka Mooi, Ndumi Sikotoyi, Sindisiwe Sikotoyi, Zaheeda Kadir, Happiness Mkhatshwa, and Nomsa Magagula. We thank their mentors for their field research support: Ezelle Theunissen, Nokuthula Skhosana, Scholastika Iipinge, Ndapeua Shifiona, Teresa Connor, Anna Voce, and Gladys Matsebula. We thank our core team for guiding the process: Judy Dick, Jenni Gordon, and Pia Bombardella for guiding the process and Katy Menell for comments on this article. We appreciate the support of the Swaziland, Namibian, and South African Ministries and Directorates of Health and Social Services/Welfare, their hospitals, as well as the Universities of Stellenbosch, Namibia, and Swaziland. Our deepest gratitude is reserved for the courageous women respondents, especially those living openly with HIV.

References

Arendt V, Ndimubanzi P, Vyankandondera J, Ndayisaba G, Muganda J, Courteille O et al (2007) AMATA study: effectiveness of antiretroviral therapy in breastfeeding mothers to prevent post-natal vertical transmission in Rwanda. In: Proceedings of the fourth international AIDS Society conference, Sydney, Australia, 22–25 July 2007. http://www.ias2007.org/pag/Abstracts. aspx?SID=52&AID=5043. Accessed 23 Oct 2011

Bechhofer F, Paterson L (2000) Principles of research design in the social sciences. Routledge, London

Buskens I, Jaffe A (2008) Demotivating infant feeding counselling encounters in southern Africa: do counsellors need more or different training? AIDS Care 20(3):337–345

Buskens I, Menell K, Jaffe A, Mkhatshwa H, Shifiona N, Sayeed I, et al (2006) Woman's inhumanity to woman in infant feeding counselling in southern Africa. Paper presented at the XVI international AIDS conference, Toronto, Canada, 13–18 Aug 2006 [Poster abstract no.: TUPE0605]

Buskens I, Jaffe A, Mkhatshwa H (2007a) Infant feeding practices: realities and mind sets of mothers in southern Africa. AIDS Care 19(9):1101–1109

Buskens I, Jaffe A, Menell K (2007b) Stigma, secondary stress and sexism in infant feeding counselling in southern Africa: jeopardizing mental health. Poster presented at the 3rd South African Aids conference, Durban, South Africa, 6–8 June 2007 [Poster abstract 242]

Chesler P (2001) Woman's inhumanity to woman. Thunder's Mouth Press/Nation Books, New York

Chopra M, Doherty T, Jackson D, Ashworth A (2005) Preventing HIV transmission to children: quality of counselling of mothers in South Africa. Acta Paediatr 94:357–363

Coovadia HM, Rollins NC, Bland RM, Little K, Coutsoudis A, Bennish ML, Newell M-L (2007) Mother-to-child transmission of HIV-1 infection during exclusive breastfeeding in the first 6 months of life: an intervention cohort study. Lancet 369:1107–1116

Cowan G (2000) Women's hostility to women and rape and sexual harassment myths. Violence Against Women 6:236–246

Cowan G (2001) Personal correspondence on her study. Quoted in Chesler, P. Woman's inhumanity to woman. Thunder's Mouth Press/Nation Books, New York p.150

Dunkley J, Whelan TA (2006) Vicarious traumatisation: current status and future directions. Br J Guid Couns 34(1):107–116

Dutton MR, Rubinstein FL (1995) Working with people with PTSD: research implications. In: Figley CR (ed) Compassion fatigue: coping with secondary traumatic stress disorder in those who treat the traumatized. Brunner/Mazel, New York, pp 82–100

Freud A (1937) The ego and the mechanisms of defense. Hogarth Press and Institute of Psycho-Analysis, London

Glick P, Fiske ST (1997) Hostile and benevolent sexism: measuring ambivalent sexist attitudes to women. Psychol Women Q 21:119–135

Glick P, Fiske ST, Mladinic A, Saiz JL, Abrams D, Masser B et al (2000) Beyond prejudice as simple antipathy: hostile and benevolent sexism across cultures. J Pers Soc Psychol 70(5):763–775

Jewkes R, Abrahams A, Mvo Z (1998) Why do nurses abuse patients? Reflections from South African obstetric services. Soc Sci Med 47:1781–1795

Kassam-Adams N (1995) The risk of treating sexual trauma: stress and secondary trauma in psychotherapists. In: Stamm BH (ed) Secondary traumatic stress: self-care issues for clinicians, researchers and educators. Sidiran Press, Baltimore, pp 37–48

Kilewo C, Karlsson K, Ngarina, Massawe A, Lyamuya E, Swai A, Mhalu F, Biberfeld G (2007) Prevention of mother to child transmission of HIV-1 through breastfeeding by treating mothers prophylactically with triple antiretroviral therapy in Dar es Salaam, Tanzania – the MITRA plus study. Paper presented at the 4th international AIDS Society conference, Sydney, 2007. Oral abstract TUAX101

Menzies-Lyth IEP (1960) A case in the functioning of social systems as a defence against anxiety: a report on a study of the nursing service of a general hospital. Human Relat 13:95–121; reprinted in Menzies-Lyth IEP (ed) (1988) Containing anxiety in institutions: selected essays, vol 1. Free Association Books, London, pp 43–85

Menzies-Lyth IEP (1991) Changing organisations and individuals: psychoanalytic insights for improving organisational health. In: Kets de Vries MFR (ed) Organisations on the couch: clinical perspectives on organisational behaviour and change. Jossey-Bass, San Francisco, pp 361–364

Panos Report (2001) Stigma, HIV/AIDS and prevention of mother to child transmission: a pilot study in Zambia, India, Ukraine and Burkina Faso. The PANOS Institute, UNICEF, London

Ragin CC (1994) Constructing social research. Pine Forge Press, Thousand Oaks

Richter L, Durrheim K, Griesel R, Solomon V, Van Rooyen H (1999) Evaluation of HIV/AIDS counselling in South Africa: report to the Department of Health, Pretoria. School of Psychology, University of Natal publications, Pietermaritzburg

Ritchie J, Spencer L (1994) Qualitative data analysis for applied policy research. In: Bryman A, Burgess RG (eds) Analysing qualitative data. Routledge, New York, pp 173–194

Rollins N, Mzolo S, Little K, Horwood C, Newell ML (2006) HIV prevalence rates amongst 6 week old infants in South Africa: the case for universal screening at immunization clinics. Paper presented at the XVI international AIDS conference, 2006, Toronto (Oral abstract THAC0104)

Roosenbloom DJ, Pratt AC, Pearlmann LA (1995) Helpers responses to trauma work: understanding and intervening in an organisation. In: Stamm BH (ed) Secondary traumatic stress: self care issues for clinicians, researchers and educators. Sidran Press, Baltimore, pp 65–79

Seidel G (1993) The competing discourses of AIDS in Africa. Soc Sci Med 26(3):175–194

Seidel G (2000) Reconceptualising the issues surrounding HIV and breastfeeding advice: competing rights and representations of 'motherhood'. Findings from sociological research in KwaZulu-Natal, South Africa. In: Baylies C, Bujra J (eds) Review of African political economy, No 86, special issue on AIDS. Routledge/Taylor & Francis, London, pp 501–518

Siegal D, Baumgardner J (2007) Sisterhood interrupted: from radical women to grrls gone wild. Palgrave Macmillan, New York

Suls J, Fletcher B (1985) The relative efficacy of avoidant and nonavoidant coping strategies: a meta-analysis. Health Psychol 4(3):249–288

Thomas DR (2006) A general inductive approach for analyzing qualitative evaluation data. Am J Eval 27(2):237–246

Van der Walt H (2002) Too close for comfort: emotional ties between nurses and patients in Swartz. In: Gibson K, Gelman T (eds) Reflective practice – psychodynamic ideas in the community. HSRC Press, Pretoria, pp 73–83

Van Der Walt H, Swartz L (1999) Isabel Menzies Lyth revisited. Institutional defences in public health nursing in South Africa during the 1990's. Psychodyn Couns 5:483–495

Van Der Walt H, Swartz L (2002) Task oriented nursing in South Africa: where does it come from and what keeps it going? Soc Sci Med 54(7):1001–1009

Werhan CD, Cox BJ (1999) Levels of anxiety sensitivity in relation to repressive and self-deceptive coping styles. J Anxiety Disord 13(6):601–609

WHO Collaborative Study Team on the Role of Breastfeeding on the Prevention of Infant Mortality (2000) Effect of breastfeeding on infant and child mortality due to infectious diseases in less developed countries: a pooled analysis. Lancet 355:451–455

CPSIA information can be obtained at www.ICGtesting.com
Printed in the USA
LVOW07*1108210713

343877LV00010BA/351/P

9 789400 758865